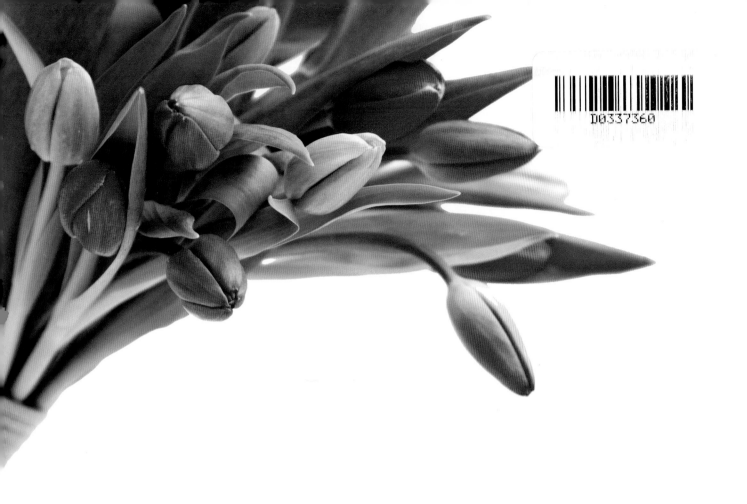

Breast cancer has invaded my body,
but it need not invade my spirit.

There may be scars on my chest,
but there need not be scars on my heart.

– Judy Kneece

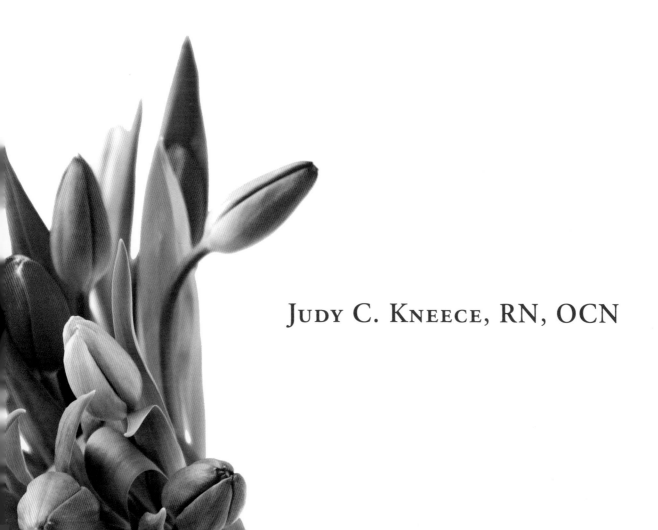

Breast Cancer

Treatment Handbook

Understanding the Disease, Treatments, Emotions and Recovery from Breast Cancer

Judy C. Kneece, RN, OCN

ISBN: 978-1-886665-33-0

Library of Congress Control Number: 2017934797

Printed in the United States of America

Published by EduCareInc.com

Illustrations: Renee Cannon, Debra Strange

To Order:
EduCare
8420 Dorchester Road, Suite 203
North Charleston, SC 29420
1-800-849-9271 or Fax: 843-760-6988
www.educareinc.com

Publisher's Cataloging-In-Publication Data
(Prepared by The Donohue Group, Inc.)

Names: Kneece, Judy C. | Cannon, Renee, illustrator. | Strange, Debra, illustrator.

Title: Breast cancer treatment handbook : understanding the disease, treatments, emotions and recovery from breast cancer / Judy C. Kneece, RN, OCN ; illustrations: Renee Cannon, Debra Strange.

Other Titles: Your breast cancer treatment handbook. 2017 | Your breast cancer recovery guide

Description: 9th edition. | North Charleston, SC : EduCareInc.com, 2017. | "The Comprehensive Patient Navigation Guide"--Cover. | Originally published as: Your breast cancer treatment handbook : a patient's guide to understanding the disease, treatment options, and the physical and emotional recovery from breast cancer. | Includes bibliographical references and index.

Identifiers: LCCN 2017934797 | ISBN 978-1-886665-33-0

Subjects: LCSH: Breast--Cancer--Patients. | Cancer--Treatment.

Classification: LCC RC280.B8 K54 2017 | DDC 616.99/449/06--dc23

Dedication

This book is dedicated to all of the brave women who have faced the pain of diagnosis and the challenge of physical and emotional recovery from breast cancer.

A special tribute is extended to the hundreds of women and families who shared openly and honestly as I served as their Breast Health Navigator. Their openness about their fears, questions, challenges and hopes during their breast cancer journey made this book possible. From the privilege of being there with them, I learned the basic educational and recovery needs of women diagnosed with breast cancer. They shared their struggles and how they learned to cope so that other patients could benefit from their journey.

I am especially grateful to my first mentor in breast disease, Henry Patrick Leis, Jr, MD, FACS, who spent over 50 years promoting increased humanity in patient breast care delivery. Dr. Leis was a pioneer as he became one of America's first dedicated breast surgeons in the early 1940s. He served as a clinical professor at New York Medical Center where he founded the Institute of Breast Disease; co-authored 17 textbooks; authored over 300 clinical articles; held membership in over 50 international organizations; received over 25 honorary degrees; and served as President of the International College of Surgeons. In his final years, Dr. Leis graciously spent much time with me, a nurse, sharing one-on-one clinical information and how breast care delivery could be improved. At his death in 2003, hopefully, I picked up his torch of caring and continue his efforts to improve the breast cancer experience for every woman.

A special dedication to Cindy Dreher, MPHA, MAT, former Director of Women's Services at Baptist Medical Center in Columbia, SC. Cindy gave me the opportunity to develop and implement the concept of breast health navigation in a hospital setting. Because of her support, constant encouragement and unique insight into the psychosocial needs of women, I was able to develop a program of education and support for breast cancer patients.

My gratefulness to Kevin Hughes, MD, FACS, Massachusetts General Breast Center and assistant professor at Harvard Medical School for his unwavering support for my work for over 25 years. I would also like to thank Maurice Nahabedian, MD, FACS, professor at Georgetown University, and Ned Dalton, MD, FACS, Director of Elliot Hospital Breast Center, for their continued clinical support and input.

My gratefulness is extended to my support staff. No words would ever suffice to express my appreciation to Mindy Wilson for her oversight in all areas of production—planning, editing, layout, design and project management. Mindy's dedication is unequaled. A thank you also to Constance Hickman for her support in all aspects of this project. Their dedication to serve breast cancer patients unselfishly brought this project to fruition.

Someone once asked, *"Have you had breast cancer?"* My reply was, *"No, my body has not, but my heart has been diagnosed hundreds of times as I shared the pain my patients were feeling as they walked through their unexpected journey with cancer."* It is to those of you who now face the same experience that I make this final dedication. You are the reason for this book!

Acknowledgements

A special word of appreciation to the following people for their contributions to this work:

Peg Baim, MS, NP
Associate in Medicine, Harvard Medical
School; Clinical Director, Center for Training,
Benson Henry Institute of Mind/Body
Medicine at Massachusetts General Hospital

Anna Cluxton, MBA
Survivor; President, Young Survival
Coalition, Columbus, Ohio

Edward P. Dalton, MD, FACS
Elliot Hospital Breast Center, Manchester,
New Hampshire; Past President, National
Consortium of Breast Centers

Carla J. Daniels, MSN, AOCNP
Springfield Clinic, Oncology Department,
Springfield, Illinois

Robert Karl Hetz, MD
Family Practice, Charleston, South Carolina

Kevin Hughes, MD, FACS
Surgical Director, Avon Foundation
Comprehensive Breast Evaluation Center,
Massachusetts General; Co-Director, Breast
and Ovarian Cancer Genetics and Risk
Assessment Program; Assistant Professor of
Surgery, Harvard Medical School

Lisa Martinez, RN, BSNM, JD
Survivor, Founder and Executive Director
of The Women's Sexual Health Foundation,
Cleveland, Ohio

Maurice Nahabedian, MD, FACS
Professor of Plastic Surgery,
Georgetown University, Washington, DC

Ervin Shaw, MD
Chief of Pathology, Lexington Medical Center,
West Columbia, South Carolina

**Harriett Barrineau, Earnestine Brown,
Anna Cluxton and Lisa DelGuidice**
The Voices of Experience, Breast Cancer
Survivors

Mindy Wilson
Graphic Design, Layout and Production

Renee Cannon and Debra Strange
Medical Illustrations

Jerri White and Saralyn White
Copyediting

About the Author

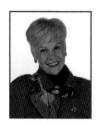

Judy C. Kneece, RN, OCN, is a certified oncology nurse with a specialty in breast cancer. She began her career as a Breast Health Navigator in a hospital where she developed her concept of nursing patient navigation in 1991. She started EduCare Inc. in 1994 to train other nurses in patient navigation.

During the past twenty-four years, EduCare has been a leader in developing educational materials and in training nurses to support breast cancer patients. Judy has trained over 2,300 registered nurses to fill the Breast Health Navigator role in hospitals, breast centers and physicians' offices. In 1998, she began holding Comprehensive Strategic Planning trainings for breast centers and hospital administrators. Over 500 hospitals and breast centers have used her principles to implement breast care programs that include patient pre-treatment interdisciplinary care conferences and a patient Nurse Navigator.

The first edition of the *Breast Cancer Treatment Handbook* was published in 1995. It has been in continuous publication and is now in its fully revised ninth edition. A companion book for the support person, the *Breast Cancer Support Partner Handbook* was also published in 1995 and is in its ninth edition. The *Breast Cancer Survivorship Handbook*, released in 2013, is designed as a patient's guide for life after cancer. Judy has authored four other books, including the *Breast Health Navigator Manual* and *Sexuality After Cancer Treatment* (May, 2017). She also created the *COPE Library: Breast Health Edition*, a collection of over 450 topics designed to help nurses and doctors support and educate their patients.

Her background working in a hospital as a Breast Health Navigator gave her new insights into the needs of women and their families going through breast cancer. Judy has also conducted extensive research on the experiences of breast cancer patients by holding national focus groups on breast cancer, recurrent breast cancer and sexuality issues after chemotherapy treatments. Her research serves as a basis for understanding the needs of patients and their families.

When being interviewed in *Cope* magazine in 1994, Tricia Brown, *Cope's* editor, asked Judy about her motivation to start breast health navigation for patients. Judy replied, *"Empowering patients with an understanding of their disease, treatment options and providing tools for recovery management are essential for complete recovery. Breast cancer is more than scars on the breast; it can also scar the heart. We must address the psychological and social issues breast cancer brings if a woman is to successfully manage her disease. Getting well is more than surgery and treatments; it is a woman understanding the vital role she can play in managing her own recovery."*

In 2015, the National Consortium of Breast Centers (NCBC) awarded Judy the Inspiration Award for her work in breast cancer, citing: *"For unrelenting devotion to the journey of women with breast cancer, for developing the field of patient navigation from diagnosis to survivorship, and for providing education to breast care professionals and for all those in need, the National Consortium of Breast Centers expresses its deepest gratitude for your service to our patients."*

You Are Not Alone...

Unwanted as the diagnosis must be, you have joined a host of other women who have experienced the overwhelming anxiety of hearing the words, *"You have breast cancer,"* and are now living examples of survivorship. Among those survivors are:

Christina Applegate	Peggy Fleming	Cynthia Nixon
Kathy Bates	Jane Fonda	Kim Novak
Judy Blume	Dorothy Hamill	Sharon Osbourne
Diahann Carroll	Laura Ingraham	Giuliana Rancic
Sheryl Crow	Kate Jackson	Cokie Roberts
Shannen Doherty	Ann Jillian	Robin Roberts
Jill Eikenberry	Hoda Kotb	Carly Simon
Linda Ellerbee	Joan Lunden	Jaclyn Smith
Melissa Etheridge	Kylie Minogue	Suzanne Somers
Edie Falco	Martina Navratilova	Gloria Steinem
Carly Fiorina	Olivia Newton-John	Wanda Sykes

As you can see from this list, although breast cancer is an unwelcome experience, it is one that can add depth and influence to your life. These well-known women are now advocates in education and support for other women living with cancer. As you begin your journey to understand and recover from breast cancer, be assured that you, too, can master the experience. You can learn, as they learned, how to take the crisis of breast cancer and transform it into an opportunity for personal growth. You can become a triumphant survivor.

Seeds of faith are always within us; sometimes it takes a crisis to nourish and encourage their growth.

— Susan Taylor

Dear Survivor

I almost began this letter "Dear Patient," but then I changed my mind. I do not want you to see yourself or think of yourself as only a patient. You will be a patient for a short time. You will be a survivor for the rest of your life. I want you to know that you are, from the innermost parts of your being, a breast cancer survivor.

"You have breast cancer" are four words that have changed your life. A cancer diagnosis is most often an unexpected journey—a journey that you did not choose. Cancer has not only invaded your body, but it has also invaded your life. It has interrupted all of your plans and probably left you feeling unprepared to face this new challenge. If you feel this way, you are sharing the feelings of thousands of other women after their diagnoses. Diane Rice, one of my patients, said shortly after her diagnosis, *"The first 24 hours were dreadful for me because I didn't have any answers and didn't know who would help me find them. For me, losing control over what was happening in my life was the most difficult part."*

Like Diane, most women find that not knowing what to do and what is ahead—the loss of personal control over their bodies and their lives—is the hardest part to deal with. Most likely, this may be your feeling. How do you regain your control? This is my job. From my personal experience, first as a Breast Health Navigator working directly with patients and then in twenty-four years of training other Breast Health Navigators to educate and support patients, I write this book as your guide. In the following chapters of this book, we will go step-by-step through breast cancer treatment and recovery, but this book is about more than just breast cancer treatment. It is also about you regaining your control and planning to emerge stronger emotionally and physically.

The goal is to convert your emotional distress and helplessness into a plan for action. The challenge is to take this time to make positive changes and emerge with a new and improved life. At this time in your diagnosis, this statement may seem trite. The truth is that no one likes the process, but people most often emerge stronger from their personal struggles with cancer. Now is the time to re-examine your life and plan how you want to redefine your life's goals.

Cancer is certainly not a good thing, but good things can come from the cancer experience. Let's get started on our journey to making cancer a positive change. By learning about your disease, you are beginning your journey to survivorship like millions of other women.

It is my privilege to share this journey with you,

Judy

The Voices of Experience

As I worked with newly diagnosed breast cancer patients, I quickly learned the value of their early interaction with other women who had experienced breast cancer. They needed to talk to a peer who had survived all of the decisions that they were going to have to make over the next weeks and months. While writing this guide for you, I immediately decided to include other women's experiences with breast cancer so that you, too, could benefit from what they have learned. To serve as your peers throughout this book, four women from very different situations share their experiences, fears and thoughts on their journeys with breast cancer. Let me introduce you to Earnestine Brown, Anna Cluxton, Lisa DelGuidice and Harriett Barrineau.

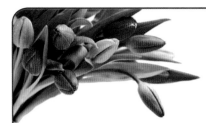

Earnestine's Story

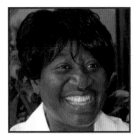

Earnestine Brown

Earnestine was in her late forties in June of 2007 when she was diagnosed with infiltrating ductal carcinoma. She had seen cancer in her extended family, so she says that her diagnosis didn't come as a complete surprise. She was, though, concerned about how her family would cope with the changes cancer would bring. Her three children, Shannon, Krystle and Amber, needed her. Her aging mother needed her. She was the head of her household and, at the time of her diagnosis, held two jobs to pay the bills.

She didn't have time for cancer, but once she was diagnosed, she was anxious to learn what could be done. She underwent lumpectomy with lymph node dissection, chemotherapy and radiation therapy.

Now that cancer treatment is behind her, Earnestine has a new focus on taking care of herself and enjoying her children and grandson. She demonstrates the best of survivorship when she says, *"For me, cancer had its ups and downs—but I'm still here."*

Her commentary throughout the book explains how she learned to slow down and take care of her health. During her treatment, she also learned to depend on her family for support. Her daughter, Krystle, provides commentary in the companion volume to this book, the *Breast Cancer Support Partner Handbook*.

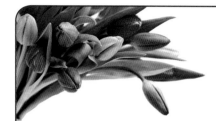

Anna's Story

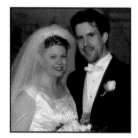

Anna Cluxton

Anna was 32 years old and single when she noticed a flattened area below her left nipple. She performed monthly breast self-exams, but she had never felt anything different in this area. Gradually, she noticed that the area would flatten out more when she raised her arm. Anna mentally dismissed it as hormonal changes or recent weight loss, but continued to keep her eye on it. She had other important things to do—she was planning her wedding.

The wedding went as planned without any problems. She and her new husband, Brian, went to Jamaica for their honeymoon. During the trip, she noticed that she could now feel a lump under the flattened area of her breast. When they arrived home, she called her OB/GYN, who performed an ultrasound. The doctor immediately decided a mammogram was needed. Anna saw a surgeon and had a fine needle biopsy seven days after she had been sitting on the beach in Jamaica. Twenty minutes after the biopsy, she was told that it looked positive for cancer. *"Brian and I were completely shocked,"* Anna told me. *"I can't even remember what else the doctor said to us after those words."*

One month after the wedding, Anna underwent seven hours of surgery for a mastectomy with an immediate TRAM flap reconstruction. All 16 lymph nodes removed during the surgery came back negative. Anna had chemotherapy. The day of her first chemo treatment, Brian shaved his head to show his support. *"When other couples are supposed to be starting their new life together, Brian was sitting on the bathroom floor holding me as I was throwing up."*

Anna recalls the experience: *"Cancer changed our lives as individuals and as a couple. I was young—too young for breast cancer, some would think. But I learned from experience that breast cancer does happen to young women. I also learned that having cancer at an early age brings different types of problems to a woman and her spouse. Because of this, I became involved in the Young Survival Coalition, an organization focused on supporting young women with breast cancer. I went on to get my MBA in healthcare administration and work in breast health. I served as President of the Young Survival Coalition during 2010 – 2011. I feel like I am making a difference every day so that no one, in particular a young woman, has to feel alone when she is diagnosed with cancer."*

Anna and Brian's life changed quickly. They were a very young couple facing a breast cancer diagnosis, but they allowed an unexpected visitor to turn their lives into a mission to help others. I asked Anna to share how a young woman thinks and responds to the different decisions that have to be made. Throughout this book, you will read Anna's response to her cancer diagnosis as a young woman. Brian provides the same type of commentary in the companion book, *Breast Cancer Support Partner Handbook.*

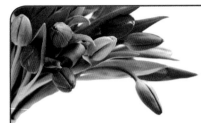

Lisa's Story

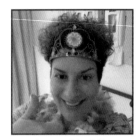

Lisa DelGuidice

Lisa was single, working as a software designer and teaching fitness classes when she was diagnosed with breast cancer in 2015. After a routine mammogram showed microcalcifications, a biopsy confirmed she had ductal carcinoma in situ (DCIS). *"I left the surgeon's office in shock because I had no lump, no symptoms, nothing to make me think I had breast cancer. I had taken good care of myself. Yet, my reality was that I had breast cancer. I had to pick myself up, dust myself off and make a plan for what I needed to do."*

After the surgeon explained her surgical options, Lisa evaluated them and decided that a double mastectomy with immediate implant reconstruction was the best option for her. *"You never know what choices you will make until you are forced to make them."* Being a single, professional woman, Lisa wanted cancer to be history and eliminate a lot of "what ifs" from her mind. *"I wanted a clean slate. There was no easy way out, but I did have choices."*

"Many people approach their cancer surgery with fear, apprehension and tears, but I did not want to be that person. I wanted to approach my surgery with a positive attitude. On the day of my surgery, I walked into the hospital with my pink tiara and my pink boa ready to show my cancer that I was tougher and stronger than it was. As I walked down the hall, everyone chuckled and they called me the 'Cancer Princess.' No denying it, surgery was tough physically, but I kept my focus on the goal of being cancer-free."

"Personally, breast cancer was definitely a wake-up call. My work life and my personal life were way out of balance. Seventy-hour work weeks left little time for me. Cancer caused me to make major changes. I reduced my hours at work and now I take time for me—not in a selfish way, but a positive way. I am fortunate that breast cancer opened my eyes. Today, I am ALIVE, happy, healthy and living a wonderful, new chapter of my life."

I asked Lisa to join us as a commentator for *Voices of Experience* in this edition after receiving a letter from her recounting her cancer experience. I knew she had valuable insight about approaching cancer with a *victor*, rather than a *victim*, attitude. She had a unique approach, but one that had underlying principles of regaining control and facing the future with an attitude of *"I will survive."* Her perspective as a professional, single woman was needed to serve as an inspiration to other women.

Lisa's sister, Rosemary, provides commentary in the companion volume to this book, the *Breast Cancer Support Partner Handbook*.

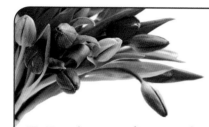

Harriett's Story

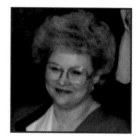

Harriet Barrineau

Harriett was diagnosed with breast cancer in 1991 at the age of 44. At the time of diagnosis, she was married and had four sons. Today she also has four daughters-in-law and eight grandchildren. Harriett says, *"This is what survival means."*

Because of the characteristics of her tumor, she had a modified radical mastectomy and followed her surgery with chemotherapy. Over a year later, the resulting posture shift caused back pain and spurred Harriet's decision to have a prophylactic second mastectomy and immediate bilateral reconstruction.

As a Breast Health Navigator, I had the opportunity to work with Harriett. She often shared her fears, feelings, failures and triumphs during her breast cancer experience. Her honest and insightful reflections during her diagnosis, treatment and recovery are a source of comfort to other women who are just beginning their journeys. Harriett openly shares with other women what she has experienced. She tells them that they will not always feel hopeless and that there are going to be problems, but that with determination, they, too, can make it. She is the epitome of survivorship—the quality of using present coping skills and learning new skills to triumph over a seemingly insurmountable task.

Today, Harriett works with her husband's accounting firm. Harriett remembers how after her diagnosis, she searched for people who would share with her the ins and outs of the experience. To help other women in their search for answers, she has volunteered with Reach to Recovery through the American Cancer Society.

Harriett's quotes in this book serve as the voice of one who personally knows the perils of the journey you are undertaking; she is a woman who has been where you are and where you are going—a woman who has survived! Al, her husband, provides the same type of commentary in the *Breast Cancer Support Partner Handbook*.

The storms of life cause the oak trees to develop deeper roots.
Life's problems cause us to become stronger and more
sensitive human beings, if we take the opportunity
to grow and learn from our experiences.

—Judy Kneece

Table of Contents

Opening Pages

Chapter Titles

Appendix

Reference

Tear-Out Worksheets

As Survivors, we learn that survivorship is an attitude we adopt.
It is the one component of recovery that no one else can do for us.
We have to decide for ourselves how we intend to respond
to our illness and how we will approach our recovery.
We, alone, decide to become Survivors.

— Judy Kneece

Using This Handbook

The *Breast Cancer Treatment Handbook* is a comprehensive guide designed to help you understand breast cancer treatment and work as an informed patient with your healthcare team. This partnership helps you make decisions that are best suited for you.

Because all patients do not receive the same treatment after surgery, not all chapters in this book will apply to your care. To help customize your learning and to keep you from being overwhelmed, we have listed major treatment categories and their relevant chapters below. Rather than reading all the information at one time, you may wish to select the category that applies to you when you need to understand a specific treatment or make a treatment decision. To assist you in custom managing your care, tear-out worksheets are located at the back of this book.

CHAPTER 1

The Emotional Impact of Breast Cancer

"My emotions were on a constant roller coaster ride. One minute I was grateful I had a good prognosis; then anger, fear and depression would take over. I realized I was going to need help working through my emotions."

—*Harriett Barrineau*

"I made peace with my diagnosis—and then I asked for strength . . . I had a child who was in college. It was important for me to be there for my child's graduation."

—*Earnestine Brown*

Shocked. Scared. Angry. Disappointed. Numb. Irate. Crushed. Disarmed. Brokenhearted. Furious. Speechless. Overwhelmed. These are all terms women have used to describe their emotions after hearing the words, *"You have breast cancer."* Most women report that they heard or remembered little after hearing the diagnosis. Their fears took control as they recalled all that they knew about breast cancer. Most wondered, *"Will I die?"* Often, they remembered someone who had gone through a similar diagnosis, and they mentally substituted themselves into the role. In the midst of this mind-boggling experience, the physician informed them of surgical options and possible treatments. "Overwhelmed" is usually an inadequate word for the experience. Most women feel a complete loss of control over their lives at this point.

If this is where you find yourself today, the first thing you need to realize is that breast cancer is usually a very treatable disease and survival rates are at an all-time high. You also need to know that strong emotions and fears are normal. It is also important to understand that breast cancer is most often not a medical emergency; you can usually take several weeks to sort through your emotions and seek answers to your questions without endangering your health. Your physician will discuss the appropriate decision-making time frame with you. Use this time to understand your

"I didn't process everything for a few days after hearing I had breast cancer. Then several days later, at six o'clock in the morning, I had an emotional meltdown. Having my husband there to comfort me helped. But I also needed time by myself to reflect on what was happening to me. I had an unplanned future to consider."

—*Anna Cluxton*

treatment options. It will be best for you, both emotionally and physically, to take the time needed to make informed, rational decisions about your treatments.

What Is a Normal Response?

Women experience an array of emotions and respond to the diagnosis according to their basic personalities and previous life experiences. The one thing that most patients have in common is that a cancer diagnosis is usually a new experience, one that demands a great deal of physical and emotional energy. Most women cry and feel depressed as they sort through their potential losses. Tears are a very natural and appropriate response to deal with loss and confirm that you are dealing with reality. Do not deny yourself the right to cry. Grieving and tears are signs that your emotional healing has begun.

Some women experience great anger. They may direct this anger toward themselves for not taking steps toward an earlier diagnosis, toward a physician or even a family member. Anger is an emotion people use to try to regain control over a situation in which control has been lost. Usually, it is not a productive way to solve problems; however, it is a natural response. Anger will diminish and a sense of control will return as you begin to learn about and understand the disease and how you can participate in your recovery.

Communicating With Family

Cancer is a family affair. It emotionally affects every member of the family. A cancer diagnosis is similar to throwing a stone into a body of water. The stone causes ripples that are greatest to those closest to you and diminish in intensity as they reach those further away emotionally.

Family members share in your emotional pain. The diagnosis is also a shock to them. Like you, they have a need to express their feelings, usually by crying, feeling sad and questioning what is ahead as they grieve with you over your news. This is a necessary and natural part of the family's emotional adjustment to your diagnosis.

You can play a vital part in facilitating their emotional healing by talking openly about your feelings and allowing them to ask questions and express their thoughts. This is probably one of the hardest parts of the breast cancer experience—open, honest communication. If honest communication begins at the time of diagnosis, it will help both you and your family. Often, we think that if we say nothing or do not let anyone see us crying or feeling depressed, we are making it easier for other people. The opposite is true. Hiding and not talking about feelings creates an atmosphere of uncertainty. People don't know what to say or do, and this uncertainty results in increased anxiety among family members.

Positive attitudes are needed. However, attitudes that seem overly optimistic may block communication in families because they set the stage for everyone to be in denial and mask their feelings. Your family needs to see you express a full range of emotions and to be able to do so themselves. Begin to share as soon as you can, and ask them to share with you. They may need your permission before they talk because they don't want to upset you. They want to help you through this time. When you talk openly about your feelings and needs, they can know how to best help you. Let them be a part of your recovery by allowing them to do things for you. For example, when they offer to do a chore, accompany you to the doctor or do something special for you, accept the offer. Feeling useful helps to facilitate their emotional healing.

Communicating With Friends

After a diagnosis of cancer, many people are concerned about you and want to know how you are doing. This is encouraging, but answering numerous phone calls, texts and emails in the midst of making decisions and undergoing treatment can become burdensome. Technology can help ease the burden of keeping friends and family informed. A website service called CaringBridge® offers anyone going through a health crisis a free online communication site. Setting up a hub at CaringBridge® allows you to update your health status online and for your friends to access the site at any time to follow your recovery. Friends can communicate by leaving a message that you can access at your convenience. Setting up your own communication hub at www.caringbridge.org is a simple process that takes just a few minutes.

When Communication Is Difficult

The reality is, a cancer diagnosis doesn't change one's basic personality or emotional responses to life. If you, your partner or other family members found it difficult to communicate before the diagnosis, it may still be difficult during this time. If this is the case, you will need to find someone with whom you can share your thoughts and fears in an understanding, non-judgmental atmosphere. It is essential that you find someone with whom you feel free to communicate. You need a safe place to talk, where your feelings, thoughts and fears will not be criticized but will be listened to instead.

Studies have shown that women who have good support systems adjust and respond to treatment more effectively. Ask your healthcare team, or check with the American Cancer Society, for names of counselors or support groups for breast cancer patients in your area. Breast cancer support groups provide a safe and helpful environment where you can share, learn and receive support from women who know exactly how you feel and what you are facing. The goal is to find somewhere to communicate your feelings. Communicating openly will set the stage for a successful recovery.

Getting the Facts Straight

Learning about your disease, surgery and treatment is important for regaining a sense of control. Breast cancer is a disease with many variables. There are approximately 15 types of breast cancer, many that require different surgical management and treatment. For this reason, you cannot compare notes with a friend who had breast cancer or listen to well-meaning family or friends because there are too many differences in treatments. You also need to use reliable sources, such as those listed in the Reference section of this book, if you search the Internet for information. Your information needs to come from someone who knows your exact diagnosis and has up-to-date information on the medical management of your disease. Your healthcare team will be the best source for accurate information.

Decisions, Decisions, Decisions!

Beginning the day you are diagnosed, you will need to work with your treatment team to make multiple treatment decisions. Making decisions can be overwhelming because you are often required to make them in a short period of time.

There seem to be two extremes in decision making. One extreme is being so fearful that a person refuses to learn about treatment options. The other extreme is a never-enough, never-ending search for information. Either extreme in decision making can lead to increased stress. Letting your fear cause you to avoid examining options and wanting to leave decisions completely up to others leaves you feeling powerless. On the other hand, incessant over-analysis in search of the perfect answer is emotionally exhausting. There must be a balance.

If you lean toward fear-based decision making, thinking, *"I'm afraid of what I may find out, so I'd rather not know,"* I encourage you to face your fears and find out all you can. Remember that knowledge is power. The more you understand about something, the less power it has over you. Most often, you will find that even unpleasant news is better than a lurking fear. When you know the facts, you can take appropriate steps of action. The old saying "forewarned is forearmed" is true because it allows you time to prepare for the experience. In Chapter Four, we will discuss facing your fears in more detail.

If you tend to be a person who cannot get enough information to make a decision, this can also hamper your ability to cope. Incessant searches on the Internet or multiple physicians' opinions can serve as a way of avoiding making a decision altogether. "Paralysis of analysis" is certainly true; it will immobilize you. Have you ever noticed how much better you feel once you make a decision about how you are going to deal with something? You should take the time to carefully study your options—but set a time limit on your search so that you can make a decision and reduce your anxiety.

Emotional Challenges

As you are communicating, actively learning about your disease and making decisions, you will find yourself experiencing mood swings. There will be periods when you feel that you are doing well. Then, you may find that you once again feel overwhelmed, asking, *"Why?"* and *"What did I do to deserve this?"* or saying, *"I don't think I can go through this."* These are normal responses while you are working through a crisis. You won't always feel in control. Feelings of depression, with periods of crying, may be dispersed throughout your recovery. When these times occur, don't be too hard on yourself for not being brave. Acknowledge them as normal and then take steps to restore your positive mood. For some, it helps to get out of the house for a special outing, to spend time with friends or to work on a hobby.

Physical Challenges

A crisis can also drain you of normal energy and require that you get more rest. Listen to your body and get adequate rest. Most women need seven to eight hours of uninterrupted sleep daily. This may mean that you have to ask family members to assume some of your household duties for a time.

Managing the Unexpected Challenges

Breast cancer has unexpectedly caused you to put many of your plans and dreams on pause. At this time, you may be feeling overwhelmed as you deal with the changes that breast cancer is forcing you to make in your life. Admittedly, the changes are difficult. However, I encourage you to keep in mind that these changes are time-limited and will only last for a season. The surgery and treatments you undergo, though difficult, are the tools that give you hope for a disease-free tomorrow.

During this time, give yourself permission to step out of the hero role and seek the support you need. Being self-sufficient and not asking for help will only slow down your recovery. Take advantage of the support, either emotionally or physically, that your family, friends and healthcare team offer and can provide. Plan to participate with your healthcare team in making treatment decisions, but don't allow yourself to make a career out of your cancer. Try to seek balance between receiving treatment and living your life.

Managing the breast cancer experience requires information, support and a plan. This is what this book is all about—encouraging you while helping you master the information needed to meet this unexpected challenge.

"When I heard the words, 'You have breast cancer,' a million emotions ran through my mind. Was it found early enough? Has my cancer spread? Will I need chemo and radiation? How will I look after surgery? I was living in the 'world of unknowns.' Sure, I was scared because I didn't know what was ahead of me, but I also knew I needed to put my 'Let's Beat Breast Cancer' plan into action."

—Lisa DelGuidice

CHAPTER 2

Relationship With Your Partner

"I needed reassurance from my husband. I needed to hear, 'I love you.' I needed attention from him. His faith had to be strong enough for both of us for a short time. But, later, I realized he also needed support. He, too, was hurting. He found this unique source of understanding in a mates' support group."

—*Harriett Barrineau*

At diagnosis, your partner is confronted with the same surprise and faces the same overwhelming emotions as you. In the midst of all of this, most partners strive to be strong, understanding and supportive. The way your partner responds to your diagnosis is determined by your partner's basic personality and previous coping experiences. Behaviors may vary among people, but under it all are the basic emotions of fear, loss and uncertainty. A partner's love for you causes a strong emotional response and an extreme feeling of helplessness when you are diagnosed with breast cancer. This is one thing they cannot fix. In an interview concerning support partners, Dr. Marilyn T. Oberst stated:

> *Learning to live with cancer is no easy task. Learning to live with **someone else's** cancer may be even **more difficult**, precisely because no one recognizes just how hard it is to deal with someone else's cancer.*

Communicating With Your Partner

For your partner, it is difficult to see you, the one they love, suffering emotionally and physically. Some partners may emotionally withdraw as they mentally sort out the situation. They may say very little. Others may be very verbal. Remember, this is also a new experience for them. They, too, are hurting emotionally and often feel inadequate in their responses. You can help by sharing your needs verbally. Do not wait, hoping that they will know what you need or how you wish for them to help you.

Recent studies by Dr. Oberst show that during the first six months after a diagnosis, some partners may experience a greater degree of emotional

"I was so afraid of what having 'damaged goods' for a wife would do to our young marriage. It became very important to both of us to know when to reach out to each other and when to let go."
—*Anna Cluxton*

stress than the patient. This is because their personal fears and anxiety are created by not knowing what is expected of them in their new role as a support partner. You can help by expressing your needs and encouraging them to talk to others who understand the role of a support partner. Call your cancer treatment center or local American Cancer Society office for the name of support groups for partners, or ask for the name of a peer volunteer. Chaplains working in cancer treatment centers are an excellent resource because they understand the unique stressors that families face with a cancer diagnosis. Encourage your partner to reach out to others to meet their own personal needs.

Intimate Relationship Changes

"What effect will my diagnosis and surgery have on my intimate relationship?" "Will I still be loved?" "How will my new body image affect our sexual relationship?" These thoughts are in the back of most women's minds. They are valid questions that need to be explored and understood. Intimate relationships are built on mutual love, trust, attraction, shared interests and common experiences in life. Breast cancer will not change these shared feelings.

What may change is how you view your body, and that can affect your sexual intimacy. The physical aspect of lovemaking may temporarily change because of loss of energy resulting from your treatments. However, you can resume your sexual relationship as soon as you feel able. You are still the same person your partner selected and loves. You can bring a new dimension to this relationship by openly discussing your feelings about the changes in your body image. Try to communicate these concerns honestly.

Often, you will need to be the one to initiate the discussion about their fears or needs. Your partner may feel these issues are too personal or too sensitive. It is helpful to address these concerns as soon as you are diagnosed. Allowing time to pass only makes the conversation more difficult and walls of silence easier to build.

Another issue that needs to be addressed early to prevent future changes in the physical relationship is allowing your partner to see your surgical incision. Often, this is difficult because you may feel embarrassed about the change in your physical appearance. Some patients fear that their partner may reject them as a sexual partner. May I assure you that I have never observed this response in my twenty-five years of experience. Instead, overwhelmingly, patients report that when their partner saw their scars, they expressed great compassion and empathy. When you allow your partner to see your surgical scar, it helps them to share your experience. It can help increase the emotional bond between the two of you. It also reduces the future embarrassment of being seen nude, which can cause problems in the sexual relationship. Agreeing to view your new body image early after surgery is the best approach. Although it may seem easier to postpone this step, it only becomes more difficult with time.

Partners often fear that their physical closeness by hugging, holding or resuming the sexual relationship may cause pain or injury to the incision site. Many times what women mistakenly sense as sexual rejection after breast surgery is an effort on the part of the partner to protect them from any pain or discomfort. Stating your desire for continued physical contact and letting your partner know what is pleasurable will reduce their unspoken fear of causing you physical pain.

Open communication will decrease anxiety for both you and your partner, which will enable your personal and sexual relationship to grow even stronger. There is usually a period of adjustment, but most couples put their fears behind them and reestablish a satisfying and loving relationship. By sharing both the troubles and triumphs of cancer openly, you and your partner will have the opportunity to strengthen bonds of affection, trust and commitment.

Support Partner's Guide Available

A companion to this book, the *Breast Cancer Support Partner Handbook*, is available for your support partner. The book is designed as a guide to help support partners understand how to best help you while understanding their own emotional responses to the diagnosis. The book addresses the unique emotional issues that a person faces during a partner's breast cancer diagnosis and explains what your partner can do to help. You may order the book from www.EduCareInc.com.

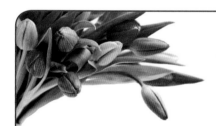

Remember...

- *Your partner suffers emotionally from the diagnosis, just as you do.*

- *Most support partners are unsure about the best way to help. Helping them adapt to the role of support partner requires open communication. You must let your partner know how to best help during the experience by verbalizing your needs and expressing your desires.*

- *Encourage your support partner to reach out for support from others who understand the unique needs of a support partner.*

- *Intimate relationships are based on love, trust, shared interests and common experiences; breast cancer does not change this.*

- *Sexual intimacy after surgery is dependent upon open communication. Discuss the change in your body image, view the incision early and verbalize your need for continued intimacy.*

- *Breast cancer can bring a couple closer and strengthen the bonds of affection, trust and commitment.*

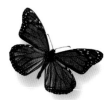

Thoughts To Ponder...

Loss has a way of changing our lives dramatically. We become transformed. However, the idea that learning and personal growth could come from our loss when we are in the middle of our pain is an almost disgusting idea. This is how most people feel the first six months or longer. It takes time, and we have to move past our crisis to see the changes that have occurred.

—Anne Kaiser Stearns

Our natural inclination may be to run from emotional pain, to avoid the feelings, to ignore the circumstance that hurts us. However, it's when we stay, sit in the feelings, and face what's happening that we cope best and heal most quickly. Facing pain empowers us and strengthens us. Denying it or running away does not. Hang in—don't run away!

—Judy Tatelbaum, LCSW

As survivors, we take a misfortune in life and change it into something that produces personal growth and somehow benefits others.

As survivors, we choose hope after loss. We choose to look at what we can do now that cancer has invaded our lives. We acknowledge our loss and nurse our pain, but we move on to make the diagnosis a source of motivation for a new direction in our lives.

—Judy Kneece

This may be the toughest, but also the most important step we take, after we face a painful life experience. It's not unusual to want to quit because we hurt, because this loss or trauma or disappointment is so hard to face. Personal power comes not from quitting, but from having the courage to go on with life. We must remember pain eventually ends, and life goes on. And so must we. We may not be able to control life's adversities. We cannot prevent illness or dying, or stop accidents or danger, but we can have power over how we confront the painful times in our lives. Use these secrets to heal yourself, to recover and to live a wonderful life.

—Judy Tatelbaum, LCSW

Helping Your Children Cope

"When I told my children I had cancer, I found out that they handled it the way I handled it."
—Earnestine Brown

"My young cousins asked questions about my cancer. We were open and honest with them— after checking with their parents."
—Anna Cluxton

Children react to a parent's illness in a variety of ways according to their ages, developmental stages and personalities. As a parent, you want your illness to create as little negative effect as possible on their lives. How do you handle this situation so that it causes the least amount of emotional distress for your children? From the beginning, tell your children the truth and answer their questions honestly. Often, it may appear that keeping the facts from them would be more helpful, but this is not wise. Children are very perceptive; they instinctively sense when something is wrong in the family. Not knowing what is wrong will often cause them to imagine things, which can result in more anxiety than knowing the truth. It is also important that they hear the news first from you or a family member, not from strangers. When information is presented truthfully, on their level of understanding, they can interact with you and receive answers to their questions and fears. It may be helpful to ask your medical team if they have information about how to talk with children about cancer.

In the *Journal of Psychosocial Oncology*, Karen Greening, MSW, LCSW, summarizes a child's five basic needs during a parent's diagnosis:

- A need for clear information on what is happening
- A need to be involved and to help out
- A need for realistic reassurance
- An opportunity to express thoughts and feelings
- A need to maintain normal interests and activities

"Having always been the caretaker in my family, I found it difficult to let my four sons know I needed anything. I finally told them that I needed to talk about my fears and feelings, even though talking about Mom's breasts was not the most comfortable subject. Our love for one another and deep faith in God brought us closer together during this crisis."
—Harriett Barrineau

Impact of Diagnosis on Children

In his book, *How Do We Tell The Children?*, David Pertz, M.D., explains:

> *A child's first questions about illness and death are an attempt to gain mastery over their frightening images of abandonment, separation, loneliness, pain and bodily damage. If we err on the side of overprotecting them from emotional pain and grief with 'kind lies,' we risk weakening their coping capacities.*

Tips for Telling Your Children:

- Wait until you and your partner have some control of your emotions, if possible. For some, this may take a day or two; others may be able to share on the first day.

- Plan, along with your partner or family member, what you will say to the children. Select a time when both of you can share without interruptions. Turn off the television and hold telephone calls to prevent distractions.

- Begin by sharing something similar to the following: *"Mommy has found a lump in her breast. The doctor says that the lump is cancer (call it by the right name). The doctors say that they need to take this lump out because these are not good cells and they grow fast. The doctors and nurses can also help by giving me medicine."* Continue to share the facts truthfully and simply. If you have an example of medicine making a difference, such as antibiotics healing an infection, it may be helpful.

- Be aware that a young child's greatest concern is often of themselves—*"Who will take care of me?" "Where will I stay?"*

- Explain to your children that their thoughts or actions did not cause your cancer and that they cannot catch your cancer.

- Assure your children, if you begin to cry, that tears are normal. It is okay to be sad and to cry.

- Allow the children to ask questions. Answer questions to the best of your ability. If you do not know the answers, be honest and say you do not know. Keep your answers age-appropriate.

- Reassure them that you will continue to tell them what is happening.

- Involve them in the process of helping you adjust to surgery and possible treatments. Help them feel as if they are part of the solution to the problem by sharing chores that contribute to the well-being of the family.

- Children need to communicate openly and honestly. However, don't be surprised if they don't seem to be overly concerned and quickly return to their normal duties and interests. Take this as a compliment; your openness has assured them that, as a family, you can cope with your new situation.

Telling Your Child's Teachers

Inform your child's teachers and coaches that your child is dealing with a cancer diagnosis (or family crisis) at home. This alerts them to identify potential changes in a child's behavior as stress reactions to the change in the home environment. They will be able to recognize if the child is suffering from overwhelming sadness and needs emotional support. They can also offer additional help with schoolwork if stress makes it hard for your child to concentrate.

Older children and teens may feel more comfortable sharing their feelings with adults outside the home rather than with their parents. Knowing that there is a health concern at home allows these trusted adults to offer valuable emotional support to your child.

Teachers are often in a position to request assistance from other school personnel, such as guidance counselors and school psychologists, in order to offer additional professional emotional support to a child.

Other Parenting Tips:

- Allow your child time for active or aggressive play as an outlet for frustration and anxiety. For a young child, this may include pounding on a hammering toy, banging on a drum or playing with fierce toys (sharks, dinosaurs, etc.). Older children may enjoy basketball or video games.
- Arrange for a little extra love and attention to be shown to your children during this stressful time. Fathers, family members and friends may be willing to devote extra time to the children.
- Plan family time every day, if possible.
- Guard against the tendency to make a teen your only source of emotional support.
- Ask other family members to help teens maintain their social activities as much as possible.
- Be aware of teens' social concerns and possible embarrassment if you use breast humor as a coping mechanism.

Seek Professional Help If You Notice:

- Marked change in school performance; poor grades despite trying very hard
- Younger child reverts back to bed wetting
- Extreme worry or anxiety manifested by refusing to go to school, go to sleep or take part in age-appropriate activities
- Frequent angry outbursts or anger expressed in destructive ways
- Hyperactive behavior of fidgeting or constant movement beyond normal
- Persistent anxiety or phobias
- Persistent nightmares or sleeping difficulties
- Stealing, promiscuity, vandalism or illegal behavior (drug/alcohol use)
- Persistent disobedience or aggression; violations of the rights of others
- Opposition to authority figures

Families often worry about the effect the illness will have on their children. The most important factor in how children respond is how they see you and your partner respond to the illness. If they see you communicating openly and honestly while sharing with a positive attitude, they will be more likely to respond the same way. The family can value this time as one of growth and maturity in problem solving. If you find it difficult to know what to say or realize problems are developing in the family with your children, contact your cancer treatment center and ask for a referral to a children's counselor.

Children's Support Resource

An excellent resource for children is **Kids Konnected**. For the cost of postage, they will send care packages to families experiencing cancer. Packages are individually tailored to each family, depending on the ages of the children, who has cancer and what stage the cancer is in. Packages contain books, workbooks, brochures and additional information to help the child or teen better cope with what cancer brings. Every package includes a "Hope" teddy bear for each child and a security blanket for children under five.

Kids Konnected

26071 Merit Circle, Suite 103, Laguna Hills, CA 92653
949-582-5443 | www.kidskonnected.org

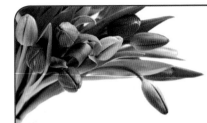

Remember...

- *Children are resilient. They respond to life the way they see those in their environment responding.*

- *Your cancer diagnosis can serve as a child's life lesson on how a family deals with an unexpected crisis.*

- *Children need to be told the truth about your cancer diagnosis, at the level of their understanding, by you or a close family member.*

- *Children need all of their questions answered honestly.*

- *Truthfulness, coupled with love, will enable your child to grow stronger through this family crisis.*

- *Children need to feel a part of the family by assisting with household chores.*

- *Teens need to maintain their social life as much as possible and not become the only source of communication or support for the parent.*

- *Telling your child's teachers and coaches allows them to monitor for changes in your child's behavior and performance. Understanding the new family stress allows them to offer support and, if needed, provide you a referral to a professional who can help.*

- *Monitor your child's behavior for clues that they may need help in coping. Reach out to professionals if you see your child struggling emotionally.*

- *A parent's breast cancer does not have to be a negative experience for children. It can serve as a time when families grow stronger.*

CHAPTER 4

Calming Your Fears

"My husband's first reaction to my diagnosis was that we had been given a death sentence. Mine was just the opposite. I saw death as the easy choice. My greatest fear was having to live with the aftermath of breast cancer."

—Harriett Barrineau

"My greatest fear about breast cancer was all of the unknowns. Fear of the unknown is a tough obstacle to overcome. To deal with my fears, I did my research about my options, questioned my doctors, read books and talked to other breast cancer survivors."

—Lisa DelGuidice

At diagnosis, the struggle with cancer is often more difficult mentally than physically. Most women feel physically well when diagnosed, but they emotionally struggle after they hear the word cancer. Many patients feel paralyzed and isolated by their fear. In support groups, women are often surprised to hear other women express exactly the same fears. In fact, most fears women have are common to everyone coping with a diagnosis. Your personality, previous coping experiences and your present support system may change your fear's intensity, but the underlying concerns are often the same.

The Most Commonly Expressed Fears After a Cancer Diagnosis:
- Will I die?
- How do I need to plan for the future?
- Are they telling me the truth?
- Will I still be able to have children?
- Will I live to see my children grow up?
- How can I protect my loved ones from the pain this causes?
- What will I look like after surgery?
- Can I cope with my new body image?
- Will treatment be painful?
- Will treatment work?
- How will I know if cancer recurs?
- I feel helpless. What can I do about cancer?

"I remember coming across a website about a young woman who died from breast cancer and it scared me to death. Until that moment I don't think I had made the actual connection in my mind that I could die from this. Talking to my doctors and getting honest answers helped me put everything into perspective."
—Anna Cluxton

First, know that fear is natural. In fact, women who do not express fear are the most at-risk psychologically. Disarming fear begins with recognizing its presence, expressing the fear to the appropriate person and taking steps of action. Do not hold on to your fears in silence. Identify your fears and express them. Often, when fears are expressed, strategies can be developed to help you deal with your fear.

Where Do You Start?

Continuing to live in a state of fear is like sitting in a dark room, imagining what might be there, while refusing to turn on the light to see what really surrounds you. The same principle is true with a cancer diagnosis. If you don't take the steps to turn on the light, you will be trapped by your uncertainties and will not be able to feel the sense of power that comes from knowing exactly what you are dealing with. Addressing your fears about cancer eliminates the clutter that consumes a lot of mental and physical energy. Make the decision not to waste your energy on the unknown—identify your fears, get answers to your questions and take appropriate action steps.

Remember that turning on the light does not mean that you will not feel fearful. You will still feel a sense of fear. That's normal. You have simply ruled out imagined fears by knowing what you are dealing with.

To address your fears, it is important to understand the facts about your cancer diagnosis. Ask your physician about your breast cancer's stage. Breast cancer is staged on a scale from 0 through 4. Stage 0 is the least aggressive and stage 4 means that your cancer has spread to other organs in your body and has the greatest potential to be life-threatening.

In any stage, breast cancer most often requires learning to live with cancer rather than dying from it. Learning the facts about your own cancer frees you to make appropriate decisions about living your life with cancer and alleviates many unfounded fears. If you do not ask questions and understand the facts, your fear will become an inner source of tension that drains your energy—precious energy that could be better used in living life to the fullest.

Plan To Address Fears

Make a list of the fears that are clouding your mind. Be honest. You do not have to show anyone the list. After you have made your list, list the people or person that the fear involves. If another person is involved, such as your partner or physician, express your fear to that person. Think about the fear and plan actions you can take to understand or change it.

A worksheet for listing your fears and your planned strategies to disarm them is located on page 259. When you are ready to express your fears to the appropriate person, state your fear questions using "I" language. Example: *"I am very concerned about the effect of my surgery on our sexual relationship. I don't want it to change."* You may say to your physician, *"I want to know all of the details about my disease and the side effects of treatment."*

Fear	Person(s) Involved	Things I Can Do
Will I still be sexually attractive?	Partner	■ Express fear ■ Express desire for closeness ■ Purchase attractive lingerie ■ Plan for special times
Are they telling me the truth?	Physician/ Nurses	■ Ask for honesty and all of the facts ■ Read about my disease
What can I do about living with cancer?	Support Group	■ Attend a support group ■ Ask for name of a counselor

Fear can be a great obstacle to recovery. Expressing the fear, determining your resources and developing a plan of action will cause the fear to be less of a threat. Communicate openly with your healthcare team to clear up any misinformation. Verbalizing your fears to the team allows them to help you seek a strategy to deal with your anxieties. Not all uncertainty will be alleviated, but the fears can certainly be brought to a manageable level.

Support groups, professional counseling and spiritual faith have all been proven to assist in the management of fear. These sources offer a wealth of strength for dealing with a cancer diagnosis. As your physician and healthcare team are working to eradicate the cancer from your body, you can help them by keeping your mind as free from stress and fear as possible.

Support Groups

Support groups are a safe place to express your fears and have your questions answered by those who truly understand. You may have loving support from your family and friends, but often they do not seem quite able to understand what you really feel. In a breast cancer support group, the shared experiences of other women can help you to adapt and to re-engage your fighting spirit. It is helpful to see those who are months ahead of you living full, productive lives after mastering the crisis of breast cancer. They have tips and encouragement to share with you. Take advantage of this source of strength and understanding. Most patients feel that support groups were helpful to their recovery.

For support group recommendations, ask your treatment team or call your local American Cancer Society. When you have identified a support group, you may wish to call and ask about the structure and goals of the group. Select a group that is affiliated with a medical facility, if possible. These groups are usually facilitated by professionals who have an understanding of breast cancer and are able to provide accurate answers to your questions.

Visit the group at least twice before making a decision. If you do not feel that the group meets your needs, visit another group. Try to avoid a group that is allowed to become a pity party. Select one which offers education, allows sharing among participants and promotes an optimistic approach to recovery.

Support can also be found on the Internet. The advantage to online support groups is that they are easily accessible and do not require travel to connect with other patients. Online support groups also provide an opportunity for patients to find specific types of support such as, pregnant with cancer or hereditary breast cancer.

Women who participate in groups or seek support from professionals have been proven to adjust more quickly both physically and emotionally than non-participants. Support groups are a way to reduce your fears and get answers to your questions.

It is helpful if your partner can also attend a support group. Often, partners have very few people in whom they can confide and receive helpful support. Ask about local support groups for your partner.

Professional Counseling

Some women do not feel comfortable in a large group or do not have access to a support group because of time or distance. If you are unable to find a support group that meets your needs, ask your healthcare team for the name of a specialized counselor, therapist, psychiatrist or online support. Asking for help is not a sign of weakness; but is a sign of strength. Seeking appropriate support is as necessary as seeking appropriate medical treatment. The difference is that you may have to express your need for this service.

Individual counseling allows you to express your feelings and fears in an atmosphere of trust and support. Your selected counselor helps you plan strategies to make this crisis a manageable event in your life. This is usually short-term crisis counseling.

Spiritual Faith

Inherent in each of us is a deep need to understand our existence and our future. Cancer causes a real threat to our sense of safety and forces these issues to be foremost in the mind. Answers to your struggles, understanding why, how and what about tomorrow, are found in your faith. It will be helpful if you reach out and seek the help of your spiritual counselor during this time. If you do not have a pastor, priest, rabbi or spiritual leader, ask your hospital for the name and number of their chaplaincy service. Chaplains are trained in dealing with the adjustment to the crisis of cancer. Take advantage of this valuable service.

In the book *Cancervive*, Susan Nessim shares her feelings as a cancer survivor:

> *Cancer has taken us on an amazing journey. When we look in the mirror we may see our faces as unchanged, but the person they belong to has undergone a spiritual metamorphosis. We have shed our old skins. Now we must assess who we've become and where we're headed. We've gained new insights into the depths of our spiritual strength, physical resiliency and courage.*

Looking at the cancer experience through the eyes of spiritual faith gives the experience meaning and purpose. Susan continues:

> *In the school of life, cancer survivors feel as if they've just completed an accelerated course—not that anyone, given the choice, would sign up for that course again. But for those fortunate enough to have gained a new perspective, the lessons learned are as precious as life itself.*

Why Do I Keep Losing It Emotionally?

Feelings and fears are a lot like holding on to Jell-O®—just when we think we have them in our hands and under our control, they slip right out of our grasp.

This is the natural course of dealing with a crisis. We are not always in control of our feelings. We may think we are doing well and handling our emotions. Then, seemingly without warning, new problems arise, fears of the future return, tears begin to flow and depression comes to visit. Dealing with a cancer diagnosis is not an easy task. It keeps bringing new problems and fears as you progress through treatment and recovery. If you feel that your emotions slip out from under your control at times, you are normal. Most people dealing with a cancer diagnosis have this happen. When it does, you just have to start all over and look at the underlying cause of your present fears and see what, if anything, you can do. Don't be too hard on yourself. You don't have to be a superwoman.

> *"My best advice to newly-diagnosed women is, 'Don't be fearful.' Fear can ruin you. Trust your doctors—they're going to do everything they can for you, and if they don't, get someone else. Demand the best out of whoever is taking care of you. Ask hard questions. Never stop learning. This is your life we're talking about."*
>
> —*Earnestine Brown*

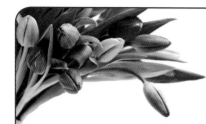

Remember...

- *Fear is not a sign of weakness. It is common to all women diagnosed with breast cancer. If you feel fearful, relax—you are normal.*

- *Fears vary in intensity according to an individual's personality, previous coping experiences and support system.*

- *Fears lose their power when they are expressed openly and when steps are taken to disarm them.*

- *The first step is to name the fears and questions that cloud your mind. Write them down.*

- *Support groups offer emotional help and can answer many fears and questions.*

- *Some women are not comfortable in a large group and can benefit greatly from individual professional counseling.*

- *Spiritual faith is a strong component in giving meaning to fear and providing a sense of strength to surmount the crisis of diagnosis. Reach out for spiritual understanding.*

- *Keeping control of our emotions is often like holding on to Jell-O®—sometimes they ooze out or slip from our control for a while. This is normal.*

Additional Information

Tear-out Worksheet
Managing My Fears - page 259

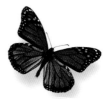

Thoughts To Ponder...

Each of us must confront our own fears, must come face to face with them. How we handle our fears will determine where we go with the rest of our lives. To experience adventure or to be limited by the fear of it.

—Judy Blume, Cancer Survivor

Many of our fears are tissue-paper thin, and a single courageous step would carry us right through them.

—Brendan Francis

You gain strength, courage and confidence by every experience in which you really stop to look your fear in the face. You are able to say to yourself, "I have lived through this horror. I can take the next thing that comes along." You must do the thing you think you cannot do.

—Eleanor Roosevelt

Nothing in life is to be feared, it is only to be understood. Now is the time to understand more, so that we may fear less.

—Marie Curie

Almost always when we're afraid of something we're talking to ourselves that something bad is going to happen. Unconsciously, we are forcing our minds and bodies into a stress mode, preparing to meet the imagined disaster. To reduce the fear, say something positive to yourself, something like, "I know I can do this because other women have already gone through it."

—University of Florida Counseling Center

Courage is not the lack of fear. It is acting in spite of it.

—Mark Twain

I have a lot of things to prove to myself. One is that I can live life fearlessly.

—Oprah Winfrey

Partnering With Your Treatment Team

"I bought and kept a journal where I wrote down every question that would pop into my head between physician visits. I did not want to forget my questions; getting them answered was too important. I took my journal to all of my appointments. It became a funny thing because the physicians would say, 'Okay, so now on to the Lisa Book!' I wanted to be involved in, and understand, every step of the process, and for that reason, I had to ask questions, understand my options and not be afraid to speak up."

—*Lisa DelGuidice*

During the next few months, many decisions will need to be made about your healthcare. As a patient, it is to your advantage to understand and participate in these decisions. This is your life. It is not a dress rehearsal. Decisions made about the type of treatment you receive are long-lasting. There are no retakes on decisions. Because of this, it is extremely important that these decisions are made with your input and that they meet your needs when possible. To ensure this, physicians and nurses need you to ask any questions you may have and express any fears or desires to them about treatment decisions. Only with your honest input can decisions be made that are best for you.

Many patients report that communicating with their healthcare team was often a challenging task. Communication can be a challenge because breast cancer is a totally new experience for most patients. Breast cancer treatment involves many different physician specialties, and each specialty has its own medical language. This can often make communication difficult and overwhelming. The goal of this chapter is to help you understand how to effectively communicate your needs so that you can be involved in your treatment and receive the care you deserve.

"Invite a family member or friend to go with you to appointments. Having another 'set of ears' is invaluable. They not only listen, but come up with questions that you may not have thought about."
—*Lisa DelGuidice*

Physicians Involved in Breast Cancer Care

During breast cancer treatment, a variety of physicians will be involved in your care. Each physician has a special expertise in treating breast cancer.

- **Radiologist**: Uses diagnostic techniques such as mammography, ultrasound, breast MRI and minimally invasive biopsy to diagnose cancer.
- **Pathologist:** Analyzes body tissues or cells under a microscope to determine if disease is present and diagnoses the type of disease, along with its unique characteristics.
- **Surgeon:** Surgically removes the identified area of suspicion from the body.
- **Reconstructive (Plastic) Surgeon:** Reconstructs an altered or removed breast using body tissues or implants.
- **Medical Oncologist:** Treats cancer using a variety of methods, including chemotherapy, immunotherapy and hormonal therapy.
- **Radiation Oncologist:** Treats cancer by using radiation therapy to destroy cancer cells.

To assist you in communicating effectively with each physician, refer to the physician-specific worksheets located at the back of this book.

Communicating With Your Physician Between Visits

When meeting with a new physician, ask about their preferred method of patient communication for questions, non-emergency requests and emergencies. Some physicians prefer that you call their office and leave a message for non-emergency communication, while others prefer that you communicate through your Breast Health Navigator. Today, some physicians and Breast Health Navigators have email services that allow them to communicate with their patients through a secure transfer of information. Ask if email communication is an option.

Reporting Obstacles That Could Impact Your Care

Often, there may be a personal situation or obstacle unrelated to your cancer that could prevent you from receiving the treatment you need. The Patient Treatment Barriers Assessment Sheet, on page 257, lists potential obstacles. Read through the assessment list and check the boxes that apply. If you identify any potential obstacles, take the sheet to your healthcare provider on your next visit. These issues are usually reviewed by a social worker or a patient navigator and referred to the most appropriate professional to help solve the problem. Anything that could prevent you from receiving the best care possible is of interest to your healthcare team.

Learning the Meaning of Medical Terms

Understanding the meaning of medical terms is helpful in communicating accurately with your healthcare team. You can prepare for your appointments by looking up any term you do not understand in the glossary at the back of this book. Understanding the meaning of a term will help you understand and communicate more clearly.

How To Best Report Symptoms

During treatment, your key role as a patient is to be a good reporter of symptoms, not to determine whether a symptom is important or not. Let your physician determine the significance of a symptom. You report; the physician will diagnose.

Reporting Symptom Levels (Scale of 0 - 10)

The best way to report many symptoms is on a scale of 0 – 10. Reporting pain, fatigue, headaches, depression, anxiety and

Rating	Symptom Level
0	**Normal**
1 – 3	**Mild** *(annoying)*; *doesn't interfere with daily activities*
4 – 6	**Moderate** *(nagging)*; *interferes with daily activities*
7 – 10	**Severe** *(disabling)*; *stops daily activities*

any other symptom on the scale of 0 – 10 allows your physician to more accurately understand how it is interfering with your quality of life. Understanding the degree to which a symptom is causing problems helps a physician determine what treatment or medication may be needed. Example: *"I have a headache that rates a seven. I have taken two Tylenol® every six hours for the past two days, and it has not helped."*

Number of Episodes

Some symptoms, such as nausea, vomiting or diarrhea, need to be reported as the number of episodes experienced within 12 – 24 hours. Report what you have done to control the symptom(s). Example: *"Yesterday, I had five episodes of diarrhea within 24 hours. I took two anti-diarrheal tablets yesterday afternoon. I have had three episodes of diarrhea today."*

Reporting Fever

Report fever in degrees, when it occurred, how long it lasted and what you did to relieve the fever. Example: *"I had a fever of 102° F yesterday. After I took two Tylenol®, it came down to 100° F but went back up to 102° after four hours. It continues to do the same today. I have not had any other symptoms."*

Reporting a Combination of Symptoms

It is also important to tell your physician if you had a combination of symptoms. Knowing this information assists the physician in more accurately determining a diagnosis. Example: *"I have been experiencing nausea, vomiting, body aches and a fever of 101.5° F since yesterday at 7:00 p.m. Today, I am unable to keep Tylenol® or nausea medication down."*

Reporting Quality of Life Issues

Tell your physician about issues that impact your ability to enjoy day-to-day activities. These issues are not life-threatening, but they are important and can impede your recovery. Report the symptom(s) in terms that describe the degree of impact on your life.

- **Physical energy:** Report level in understandable terms, like *"I am unable to stay up over three hours without rest,"* or *"I am unable to work."*
- **Depression or feeling blue most of the time:** *"I feel too depressed to participate in everyday activities with my family. I find myself crying frequently."*
- **Anxiety or nervousness:** *"I feel anxious and shaky most of the day. It interferes with my ability to concentrate and interact with my family."*
- **Sleep:** Report an inability to go to sleep or stay asleep and how long you are able to sleep uninterrupted. *"I have problems going to sleep and sleep only (amount in hours) before I wake up. I then find it difficult to go back to sleep. I wake up the next morning exhausted and I feel sleepy during the day."*

Reporting Health Changes During an Office Visit

As a patient, you can maximize your appointment time with your healthcare providers by reporting any area of your health that has changed since your last visit. Remember, a new symptom needs to be reported early in the appointment to allow the physician time to consider whether any action is needed. If a symptom is reported late in the appointment, it may require that you return for another office visit.

Healthcare Decision Reminders

- When you are diagnosed with breast cancer, many people will offer you treatment advice. This is well-meaning advice, of course, but because they do not have all of the information on your specific cancer, the information may not apply to you. Women's magazines and the media will also recommend treatments, but they may be experimental or not apply to the type of cancer you have and may confuse you. It is best to rely on the information your healthcare team provides to avoid becoming distracted by information that does not apply to your cancer.

- Know that you deserve to have your questions answered by your healthcare team. This is not unreasonable; getting answers to your questions is an important part of your recovery.

- Do not be embarrassed to ask any question. There are no silly or stupid questions. There are many other people who have asked the same questions.

- Realize that physicians and other healthcare team members are on a working schedule that allows only a certain amount of time for each patient. If they appear rushed, it is not because they do not care or want to take the time; instead, it is because they have a schedule to meet.

- Understand that calling and asking to speak to a physician immediately is difficult due to other scheduled patients. Physicians usually have a certain time of day when they, or a nurse, return calls.

- If you do not understand what a physician is explaining to you, simply say, *"I'm not sure I understand what you are telling me. Can you please explain it again?"* You can also ask, *"Can you please spell the word you just used for me?"* If you need more information, do not hesitate to ask.

- Make the most of your allotted appointment time. Skip the small talk to ensure that you are using your time to report and get the medical information you need.

- When going to an appointment with your healthcare provider, prepare a list of what you need to discuss for your physical and mental recovery to progress as smoothly as possible. Often, patients think they will remember what to report or ask during the appointment, but they leave with important questions unasked and unanswered. As you are well aware, appointment times are short, and many things have to be checked by your provider. It is normal for healthcare providers to concentrate on your physical disease and treatment; however, your questions about quality of life and side effects deserve to be brought to their attention as well.

Actively communicating your needs and symptoms makes you a partner in your healthcare. This is the patient every physician dreams of having—one who comes prepared to report her physical status and needs, one who is educated on the basics of her cancer and one who understands the time constraints in a medical practice.

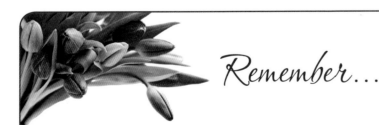

Remember…

- *Recovery is a partnership between you and your healthcare team.*

- *Take an active role by preparing for your appointment.*

- *Maximize your appointment time by reporting any changes in your health and asking any questions you may have early in your exam.*

CHAPTER 6

What Is Breast Cancer?

"When I was told I had to have breast surgery, I didn't focus on what I was losing but what I was gaining. Yes, my breasts are a big part of being a woman, but they DON'T define me. They DON'T make me feel passion. They DON'T fuel my self-esteem. My breasts are only body tissue. I am MORE than breast tissue. I decided to approach my need for breast surgery very logically—if my appendix was diseased, I would have it removed; if my gallbladder was diseased, I would have it removed. I felt the same way about my breasts; they were diseased, and they had to be removed to save ME. When I thought about it that way, I had no choice!"

—Lisa DelGuidice

"Breast cancer saved my life … I had spent my whole life taking care of people—my mother for twenty years, getting my kids through college. My husband left me with a mess, and I took care of that. Now, I had to learn to take care of myself."

—Earnestine Brown

After a breast cancer diagnosis, it is helpful to understand the basic factors of the disease. Understanding these factors will help explain why women with breast cancer receive different types of treatment for the same disease. Breast cancer is an umbrella term which describes a group of approximately 15 different types of cancerous tumors occurring in the breast. There are many variables, which make your breast cancer as unique as your fingerprint. After surgery, your final pathology report will reveal all of the specific details about your cancer.

What Causes Breast Cancer?

No one knows the exact causes of breast cancer. Doctors seldom know why one woman develops breast cancer and another does not. Most women will never be able to pinpoint an exact cause. What we do know is that breast cancer is always caused by damage to the DNA of a cell, called a mutation. The DNA is the pattern for all of your body's characteristics. When a healthy cell undergoes damage, it loses its ability to repair itself and greatly increases its ability to convert into a cancerous cell.

One known cause of breast cancer is hereditary breast cancer. Hereditary breast cancer occurs when a person inherits a gene mutation (damaged gene) from either a mother or father at conception. It is estimated that up to ten percent of breast cancers are caused by a hereditary mutation.

"Breast cancer is not the unconquerable enemy I thought it was."
—Harriett Barrineau

"'Know thy enemy'—what an understatement. I learned so much about cancer in the first few weeks after my diagnosis. And I continue to learn as much as possible, as this is an unending battle!"
—Anna Cluxton

The other ninety percent of cancers are sporadic (not inherited) breast cancers with the gene damage occurring at some point after birth. One of the first steps your physicians will take in developing your personalized treatment plan is to determine whether you have hereditary or sporadic breast cancer.

Comparison of Sporadic and Hereditary Breast Cancers:

- **Sporadic Breast Cancer:** Damage to the genes in breast cancer cells occurs **after** a person is born; it occurs at some point during their lifetime. Most causes of gene mutations are unknown. The accumulation of damage to a breast gene causes cancer. Patients who receive their genetic damage after birth usually have breast cancer that occurs at an **older** age and is found as one cancer in one breast. Gene damage is present only in the breast where the damage occurred. Hereditary genetic testing cannot identify sporadic breast cancer.

- **Hereditary Breast Cancer:** Women **inherit** a gene mutation from either their mother or father. Patients with an inherited mutation usually have breast cancer that occurs at a **younger** age. Cancer may occur as more than one tumor in a breast and may also occur in the opposite breast (bilateral). These women have a much higher increased risk of developing ovarian cancer and other cancers. Hereditary mutations are identified by testing a person's blood or saliva for a genetic mutation since the mutation is found in every cell in the body. The most common mutations are BRCA1 and BRCA2.

Identifying Patients With Hereditary Breast Cancer

Determining whether a gene mutation caused your breast cancer is crucial because hereditary breast cancer patients require a different approach to treatment. Therefore, it is essential to determine whether your breast cancer may be caused by an inherited mutated gene **before** treatment begins.

To determine whether your cancer may be hereditary, your physician will begin by evaluating your personal and family cancer history. Several generations of your family history are carefully reviewed to determine if diagnosed cancers follow a pattern indicating genetic inheritance. Your personal cancer characteristics are combined with your family history to determine whether you meet the criteria for genetic testing. If you are adopted and do not know your family history, your personal cancer characteristics can provide an indicator for a testing decision or you may be eligible for testing based on the absence of family information.

Hereditary Genetic Testing Criteria May Include:
- **Personal History**
  - Breast cancer diagnosed before age 50
  - Triple negative (estrogen, progesterone, HER2) breast cancer
  - Ovarian cancer previously diagnosed
  - Two primary breast cancers
- **Family History**
  - One breast cancer, under age 50
  - One invasive ovarian cancer, at any age
  - Two breast cancers, at any age
  - Pancreatic cancer, at any age
  - Male breast cancer
  - Ashkenazi Jewish ancestry with breast cancer
  - Identified BRCA mutation in the family

Source: National Comprehensive Cancer Network Guidelines; Version 1.2017

If you are having genetic testing, refer to *Appendix A: Understanding Diagnostic Tests; Breast Cancer Genetic Testing* on page 196 for additional information.

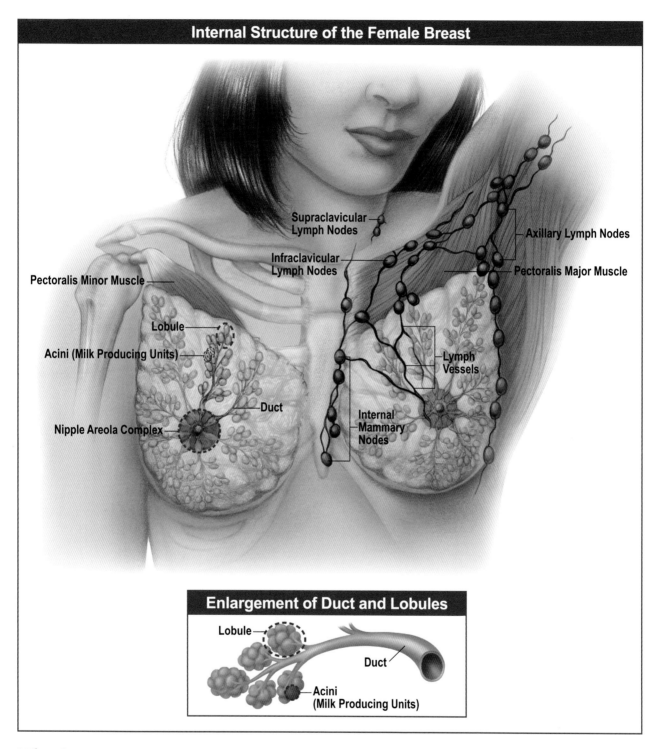

Internal Structure of the Female Breast

Supraclavicular Lymph Nodes

Infraclavicular Lymph Nodes

Axillary Lymph Nodes

Pectoralis Major Muscle

Pectoralis Minor Muscle

Lobule

Acini (Milk Producing Units)

Lymph Vessels

Duct

Internal Mammary Nodes

Nipple Areola Complex

Enlargement of Duct and Lobules

Lobule

Duct

Acini (Milk Producing Units)

Why Cancer Treatment Is Necessary

When diagnosed with breast cancer, most women feel fine physically. Because they don't feel ill, it is often difficult to understand why they need aggressive treatment. Understanding the characteristics of cancer can help remove the question of why seeking treatment is necessary.

Characteristics of Cancer Cells:

- Cancer cells exhibit uncontrolled growth. Compared to normal cells, they divide rapidly and grow at an accelerated rate. Unlike normal cells, cancer cells do not stop dividing and do not die; they are immortal.

- Cancer cells are aggressive. They will leave their site of origin and invade nearby cells, growing into and through them. Normal cells never leave their site of origin.

- Cancer cells, when large enough, will invade the lymphatic and blood vessel systems. Cancer cells will then enter into the blood or lymph fluid and travel to distant parts of the body where the cells can set up new sites; this is called metastatic cancer.

All cancer cells have qualities that can allow them to become life-threatening. This threat requires interventions to stop them. For this reason, your treatment team will recommend surgery to remove the cancerous tumor. According to your tumor characteristics, additional treatments of chemotherapy, targeted therapy, radiation therapy, immunotherapy or hormonal therapy may also be recommended. Each of these additional treatments will be thoroughly discussed in later chapters.

Types of Breast Cancer

Each of the 15 types of breast cancer has a unique pattern of cellular structure (histology) when a pathologist views the specimen under a microscope. Not only do they look different, but they also have distinct characteristics of how they behave in the body.

Cancers are first classified according to where they begin in the breast—either a duct or lobule. The term **breast carcinoma** refers to cancer that develops in the cells that line either a duct or a lobule.

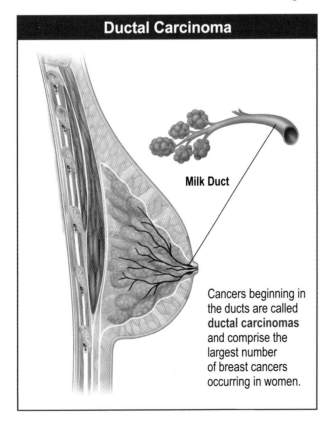

Ductal Carcinoma

Milk Duct

Cancers beginning in the ducts are called **ductal carcinomas** and comprise the largest number of breast cancers occurring in women.

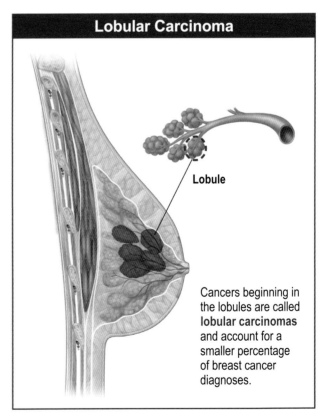

Lobular Carcinoma

Lobule

Cancers beginning in the lobules are called **lobular carcinomas** and account for a smaller percentage of breast cancer diagnoses.

Cancers are then classified as being in situ or invasive (infiltrating). In situ means the cancer is still inside the walls of where it began. Invasive means the cancer has grown through the walls of where it began.

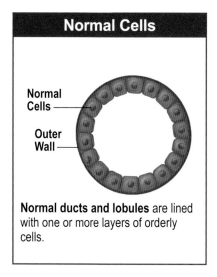

Normal Cells

Normal Cells

Outer Wall

Normal ducts and lobules are lined with one or more layers of orderly cells.

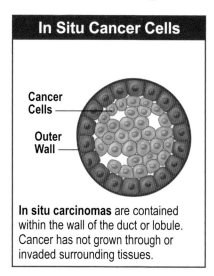

In Situ Cancer Cells

Cancer Cells

Outer Wall

In situ carcinomas are contained within the wall of the duct or lobule. Cancer has not grown through or invaded surrounding tissues.

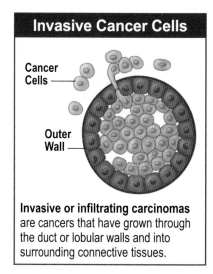

Invasive Cancer Cells

Cancer Cells

Outer Wall

Invasive or infiltrating carcinomas are cancers that have grown through the duct or lobular walls and into surrounding connective tissues.

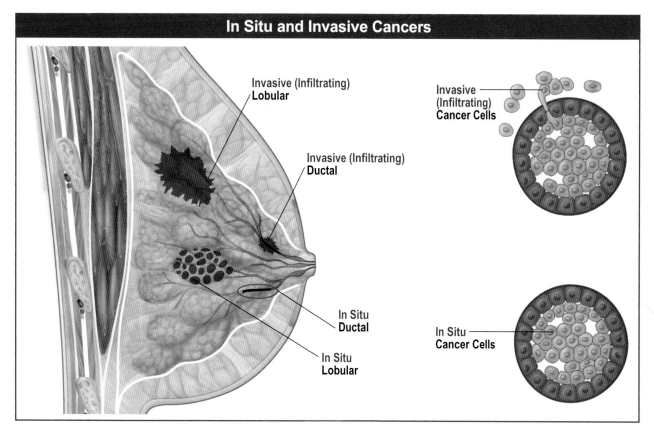

In Situ and Invasive Cancers

Invasive (Infiltrating) **Lobular**

Invasive (Infiltrating) **Ductal**

In Situ **Ductal**

In Situ **Lobular**

Invasive (Infiltrating) **Cancer Cells**

In Situ **Cancer Cells**

Cancer Growth Rate

Cancer begins with one damaged cell and continues to double until it is discovered. Breast cancers may double in size every 23 to 209 days. If we take an estimated doubling time of 100 days, a tumor would have been in your body approximately eight to ten years when it reaches one centimeter in size (⅜ inch)—the size of the tip of your smallest finger. Some cancers grow rapidly, while others grow slowly. Cancers may grow in spurts, and the doubling time may vary at different times. However, by the time a one-centimeter tumor is found, the tumor has already grown from one cell to approximately 100 billion cells.

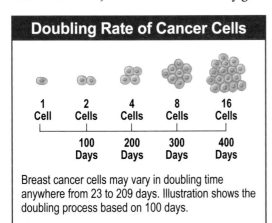

Doubling Rate of Cancer Cells

1 Cell	2 Cells	4 Cells	8 Cells	16 Cells
	100 Days	200 Days	300 Days	400 Days

Breast cancer cells may vary in doubling time anywhere from 23 to 209 days. Illustration shows the doubling process based on 100 days.

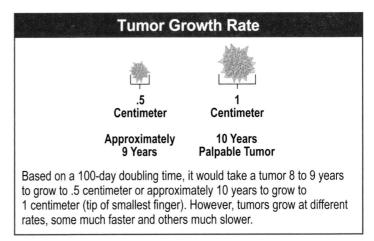

Tumor Growth Rate

.5 Centimeter — Approximately 9 Years

1 Centimeter — 10 Years Palpable Tumor

Based on a 100-day doubling time, it would take a tumor 8 to 9 years to grow to .5 centimeter or approximately 10 years to grow to 1 centimeter (tip of smallest finger). However, tumors grow at different rates, some much faster and others much slower.

Summary

Breast cancer is not a sudden occurrence but is a process that has been developing for an extended period of time. Therefore, when a biopsy confirms a cancerous tumor, most often you are not facing an immediate medical emergency. You have time to learn about your particular disease and treatment options. Most physicians recommend surgery within several weeks of biopsy. There are exceptions; for example, inflammatory carcinoma requires immediate treatment with chemotherapy for maximum control.

Additional Information

Appendix

Appendix A: Understanding Diagnostic Tests;
Breast Cancer Genetic Testing - page 196

Special Breast Cancer Diagnoses

Bilateral Breast Cancer

Bilateral breast cancer means that cancer was found in both breasts. Evaluation may include:

- After a biopsy of each tumor, your pathology report will reveal if the cancers are of the same cell type or if they are of two different cell types.
- MRI may be ordered to evaluate your breasts further.
- Genetic testing is usually recommended if you are premenopausal or perimenopausal to determine if you have a mutated gene.
  - Patients testing positive are usually recommended to undergo bilateral mastectomies.
  - Patients with a negative genetic test have surgical options, including:
    » Bilateral mastectomies, with or without reconstruction
    » Bilateral lumpectomies, if tumors meet the criteria for size
    » Lumpectomy on one side and mastectomy, with or without reconstruction, on the opposite side
- Staging is based on the largest-sized tumor

Occult Breast Cancer

Occult breast cancer means that a cancerous lymph node was identified by biopsy but mammography did **not** find a cancerous tumor in your breast. An MRI may be ordered to study the breast further for an abnormality. If an abnormality is not identified, a mastectomy is recommended. Additional treatment recommendations are based on the pathology of the removed positive node.

Inflammatory Breast Cancer

Inflammatory breast cancer is a very aggressive cancer that involves cancerous cells that block the lymph vessels in the breast, causing redness, swelling and eventually pain. Inflammatory breast cancer requires immediate chemotherapy before surgery. After the disease is controlled with chemotherapy, mastectomy is recommended.

Paget Disease

Paget disease is cancer that occurs on the surface of the nipple and in the underlying ducts. Cancer in the ducts may be contained within the ducts (DCIS) or it may be invasive (invasive ductal). MRI is usually performed to study the extent of the cancer. After biopsy, the pathology report describes histological characteristics of the cancer. The two surgical options are:

- Central lumpectomy that removes the nipple/areola and underlying ducts
- Total mastectomy

Mastectomy is the surgery most often chosen because lumpectomy removes the nipple/areola and the ducts under the nipple, which leaves a concave center similar to a doughnut.

Pregnant With Breast Cancer

If you are pregnant and discover that you have breast cancer, it can be emotionally overwhelming. At a time when you were preparing to bring a new life into the world, you now find yourself forced to fight to protect your own life. The good news is that you can receive treatment for your breast cancer while you are pregnant. When comparing women diagnosed in the same stage, treatment during pregnancy produces survival outcomes similar to the treatment of women who are not pregnant. After the first trimester (three months) of the pregnancy, cancer treatment can be adapted so that your baby will not suffer ill-effects from your treatments. Breast cancer does not appear to harm a baby.

In the past, women were often advised to end their pregnancies when they were diagnosed, but now this advice is rare. Pregnancy termination is only recommended if your cancer requires that you receive chemotherapy during the first three months of your pregnancy. The National Cancer Institute states, *"Ending the pregnancy does not seem to improve the mother's chance of survival and is not usually a treatment option."* Most treatment options can be adapted to allow you to continue with your pregnancy.

Surgery and Radiation Therapy During Pregnancy

Breast surgery during pregnancy may require a mastectomy since radiation therapy is not considered safe during pregnancy. A lumpectomy may be an option if surgery can be scheduled within six weeks of expected delivery. This allows radiation to be delayed until after delivery. A lumpectomy usually requires postoperative radiation therapy as a part of treatment.

Chemotherapy and Pregnancy

Chemotherapy can cause birth defects if given during the first trimester of your pregnancy, when the embryo's vital organs are forming. If you are diagnosed in the first few weeks of pregnancy and your stage of disease requires immediate chemotherapy (for example, you are diagnosed with inflammatory breast cancer), your doctor may recommend that you end the pregnancy. However, if the stage of your cancer is favorable and you are further along in your first trimester, your doctors will likely delay any recommended chemotherapy until the start of the second trimester (starting the fourth month of pregnancy). Each woman has to be individually evaluated as to the best treatment option for her diagnosis.

Male Breast Cancer

Breast cancer may occur in men at any age, but it occurs most often between 60 and 70 years of age. Male breast cancer accounts for about one percent of breast cancers diagnosed yearly.

Since there is no routine screening for men, male breast cancer is usually discovered when the patient notices a change in his breast. Male breast cancer presents with the same symptoms as in a woman—most often a hard lump or a bloody nipple discharge. Diagnostic and biopsy procedures are the same. Surgery and treatment are also very similar to female breast cancer.

Most Common Types of Cancer Diagnosed in Men:

- Infiltrating or invasive ductal carcinoma (also most common female breast cancer)
- Inflammatory breast cancer
- Paget disease of the nipple

Survival rates when compared to women diagnosed at the same stage are very similar. However, because of the higher incidence of BRCA2 mutations, men diagnosed with breast cancer are recommended to undergo genetic testing so that the information can be passed on to female relatives. (Refer to *Appendix A: Understanding Diagnostic Tests; Breast Cancer Genetic Testing* on page 196.)

Comprehensive information on male breast cancer can be located online: www.cancer.gov/cancertopics/pdq/treatment/malebreast.

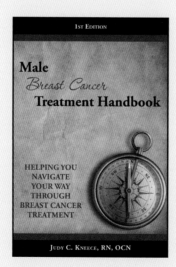

**Male
Breast Cancer
Treatment Handbook**

Available Fall 2018

www.EduCareInc.com

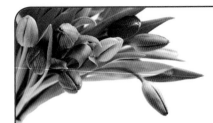

Remember...

■ Breast cancer is not a sudden occurrence; it has been developing for years. The average breast cancer has been in the body for 8 – 10 years when it is discovered.

■ The vast majority, 90 percent, of breast cancers that occur are considered sporadic. Sporadic breast cancer means that the damage to a person's breast gene, which caused their cancer, occurred after the person was born. Women with sporadic breast cancer usually have their cancer occur at an older age. Cancer appears as only one tumor in one breast.

■ A smaller percentage of cancers, 10 percent, are caused by a hereditary genetic mutation. These patients inherited a damaged breast gene from either their mother or father at conception. The most commonly inherited breast cancer mutations are BRCA1 and BRCA2 (BR=Breast; CA=Cancer). Hereditary breast cancer patients usually have their breast cancer occur at a younger age. Cancer may occur as single or multiple tumors in one breast or tumors may occur in both breasts (bilateral). When tumors are tested in pathology for tumor receptors, they may also be triple negative (negative for estrogen, progesterone and HER2 receptors).

■ When a patient is diagnosed with breast cancer, characteristics of their tumor and their age, along with their personal and family history, serve as indicators of which type of cancer, either sporadic or hereditary, they may have. If the characteristics appear to be hereditary, genetic testing can determine if a hereditary mutation is present. Determining the type of cancer is essential because treatment options differ for hereditary and sporadic breast cancers.

■ The nature of cancer cells is that they divide rapidly and uncontrollably. They possess the ability to invade surrounding tissues and move to distant parts of the body where they can become life-threatening. Cancer, when contained within the breast only, is NOT life-threatening.

■ Cancer requires prompt and appropriate treatment to stop its growth and spread.

■ Breast cancer is usually not a medical emergency. Most often you have time to gather information and get answers to your questions before surgery or treatments begin.

■ Don't compare your breast cancer diagnosis with the diagnoses of others. There are approximately 15 different types of breast cancer. Treatment options will vary.

■ Breast cancer has many characteristic variables. Your breast cancer is as unique as your fingerprint.

■ Breast cancer is not a cookie-cutter disease but is a disease with many individual variables.

■ Because there are many variables that make up your cancer, it is important to rely on your healthcare team, who is familiar with your final pathology report, when you are seeking treatment advice.

Surgical Treatment Decisions

"I had a limited amount of time to make my surgical decisions. I had to push to meet with a plastic surgeon to fully explore my options. I made my decisions after talking with my healthcare team and based my decision on what I felt was the best choice for me. I couldn't look back and have regrets."

—*Anna Cluxton*

"I was frightened by how fast things were happening. I felt totally ignorant about breast cancer and had no idea where to turn for information or education."

—*Harriett Barrineau*

Facing breast cancer surgery is emotionally difficult for most women. When you learn that it is necessary to alter or lose a breast, it is normal for many unexpected emotions to occur. In the midst of these strong emotions, it is helpful to remind yourself that surgery is a necessary step to protect your future health. As we discussed earlier, breast cancer will continue to grow, divide and move to other parts of the body if it is not removed. The goal of surgery is to stop this process. Surgery, though it may be difficult to accept, is a vital step to reclaiming your health.

Breast Surgery
Different stages of breast cancer require different surgical treatment to ensure maximum control of the disease. There are two basic types of breast surgery:

- **Lumpectomy/Breast Conservation** removes the tumor and a small amount of surrounding tissue from the breast.
- **Mastectomy** removes the entire breast. There are several types of mastectomy procedures which will be explained in this chapter.

Some tumors, based on their characteristics, require mastectomy, while other tumors qualify for either lumpectomy or mastectomy.

Factors Evaluated When Determining Surgical Options:
- **Tumor Type:** Diagnosed after pathology study of the biopsy specimen.
- **Tumor Size:** Size may determine whether lumpectomy is an option.
- **Lymph Nodes:** Possible involvement of cancer in the lymph nodes may determine surgical options.

"I left the surgeon's office in a state of shock. I had no lump, no symptoms . . . nothing to make me think I had cancer. But the reality was, I DID have cancer and there was no easy way out. The surgeon informed me that I had surgical and reconstructive options and gave me a book explaining the options. Just knowing that I had choices made me feel so much more in control of my future health."

—*Lisa DelGuidice*

- **Breast Size:** Breast size compared to tumor size may determine if lumpectomy surgery will be cosmetically acceptable.

- **Tumor Location:** A tumor located under the nipple or two tumors in the same breast may not give a suitable cosmetic look if removed by lumpectomy.

- **Mammogram:** Mammography films show whether cancer is multifocal (multiple cancers in one quadrant of the breast) or multicentric (multiple cancers in more than one quadrant). This may be evidenced by microcalcifications (small calcium deposits) or other mammographic abnormalities.

- **Involvement of Other Local Body Parts:** Spread of cancer to the skin, muscle or chest wall may determine the type of surgical procedure.

- **BRCA1 or BRCA2 Status:** An identified positive carrier of a BRCA1 or BRCA2 mutation is usually better served by a bilateral mastectomy, although this must be determined on an individual basis.

- **Other Gene Mutations:** Testing may include other genes with varying levels of breast cancer risk.

- **Reconstruction:** Your desire for reconstruction, now or later, influences the surgical decision.

- **Health:** Your current health or health history may limit surgical options.

- **Disease Control:** Surgery that will provide the best chance for disease control is recommended.

- **Cosmetic Results:** Surgery that will provide the best cosmetic result is recommended.

- **Personal Desire:** Your preference regarding the type of surgery is considered.

Making Surgical Decisions

If your breast and tumor are within certain size limits, your surgeon may offer you the option of choosing between lumpectomy or mastectomy. If you are given this option, making a decision may be challenging. The decision should be made after a careful review of the advantages and disadvantages of both surgeries. Remember, the option to choose between surgical procedures is not available for some breast cancers.

To help with the process of determining the type of surgery that you would prefer, refer to the *Surgical Decision Evaluation* on page 265. It is suggested that you answer the questions on the worksheet as an initial step. Next, carefully review the advantages and disadvantages of lumpectomy and mastectomy listed below. It is imperative that you feel comfortable with your final surgical decision.

Advantages of Lumpectomy:

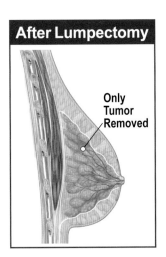

After Lumpectomy

Only Tumor Removed

- Saves a large portion of the breast, usually including the nipple and areola
- Preserves your body image
- Allows you to wear your regular bras
- Avoids the need for a prosthesis
- Decreases surgical recovery time; usually several weeks shorter than mastectomy
- Increases psychological acceptance, unless monitoring remaining breast tissue for recurrence creates high levels of anxiety
- Usually an outpatient procedure

Disadvantages of Lumpectomy:

- Increases potential for additional surgery if positive tumor margins are identified after initial surgery
- Requires time for radiation therapy to the remaining breast tissue (up to six weeks).

- Changes in texture (lumpiness) or color (suntanned appearance), along with decreased sensations (feeling) occur in the breast, after radiation therapy
- Decreases the size of the remaining breast tissues when swelling subsides after radiation treatments
- Increases difficulty of breast exam because of increased lumpiness from radiation therapy
- Increases potential for chronic swelling or lymphedema in either the breast or the arm if radiation therapy is administered to the underarm area
- Increases risk of future breast surgery if cancer recurs (low risk)
- Radiation may limit surgical options in the future

Advantages of Mastectomy:

- Removes approximately 95 percent of the breast gland, reducing local recurrence to the lowest degree possible
- Allows breast reconstruction using your own body tissue or a synthetic implant

Disadvantages of Mastectomy:

- Changes in body image due to breast removal
- Requires a breast prosthesis or reconstructive surgery to restore body image
- Increases surgical recovery time by several weeks compared to lumpectomy

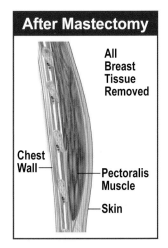

After Mastectomy

All Breast Tissue Removed

Chest Wall

Pectoralis Muscle

Skin

In situ disease patients with no scheduled lymph node evaluation may skip the following section and continue reading on page 38.

Invasive Breast Cancer Treatment

The major treatment differences between invasive and in situ breast cancer include:

- **Lymph Node Evaluation:** Most patients with an invasive tumor require evaluation of their lymph nodes to see if cancer has spread outside of the breast.
- **Chemotherapy Timing:** Neoadjuvant chemotherapy may be given before surgery for an aggressive cancer, such as inflammatory breast cancer or triple negative breast cancer. It may also be given to shrink a large tumor to a size that allows a lumpectomy to be performed.

The Role of Lymph Nodes

If you have invasive cancer, it is helpful to understand how the lymphatic system functions, why lymph nodes are evaluated and how cancer-positive nodes affect treatment decisions.

The lymphatic system is a network of thin, tube-like vessels that carry clear lymph fluid to all parts of the body to pick up cellular waste. The walls of the lymphatics are permeable and allow body waste to flow into the vessels for removal from the body. The lymph vessels are located next to the vascular (blood) vessels throughout the body. After the lymphatic fluid picks up cellular waste from tissues, it then filters the fluid through rounded areas of the lymph system, referred to as **lymph nodes**. Lymph nodes look like small, round capsules that vary from pinhead to olive size. Lymphocytes and monocytes, which fight infection, are produced in the lymph nodes. The lymph nodes also act as filters to stop bacteria, cellular waste and cancer cells from entering the blood stream.

Breast Lymph Nodes

The breast has its own network of lymph vessels and lymph nodes. The majority of the lymph nodes draining the breasts are located near the armpits, called the axillary nodes. Lymph fluid may also exit the breast through other lymph node chains, such as the infraclavicular (below the collarbone), supraclavicular (above the collarbone) or internal mammary (next to the breastbone).

Lymphatic drainage is a major route by which breast cancer cells leave the breast and spread to other parts of the body. Cancerous cells may enter the lymph fluid and become trapped as the fluid is filtered through the nodes and multiply. The nodes draining the breast tumor are often the first site of cancer growing outside of the breast. Determining whether cancer has spread to the nodes is an important factor needed to stage your cancer. Lymph node status also remains the most powerful predictor of the potential for recurrence of breast cancer.

How Lymph Nodes Are Evaluated

Evaluation of your axillary lymph nodes is performed by a breast surgeon. The nodes may be screened before surgery with ultrasound biopsy to guide the surgeon in planning the method of node evaluation during surgery (sentinel lymph node biopsy or axillary lymph node dissection). Lymph node evaluation may not be required for older women or for women whose node status would not impact their treatment decisions or extend their survival.

Lymph Node Levels

Level 1: Axillary

Level 2: Mid Axillary
(Under Pectoralis Minor Muscle)

Level 3: Infraclavicular
(Below Collarbone)

Level 4: Supraclavicular
(Above Collarbone)

Level 5: Internal Mammary
(Next to the Breastbone)

- **Ultrasound Screening:** Before surgery, your surgeon may evaluate your lymph nodes using ultrasound. During ultrasound, if a node shows certain characteristics, the surgeon will perform a biopsy of the nodes using fine needle aspiration (FNA) or core biopsy. With FNA, a fine needle, attached to an empty syringe, is inserted into the nodes, and a sample of cells is withdrawn into the syringe. With core biopsy, a hand-held instrument with a larger needle is inserted into the breast to remove cores of tissue. The biopsy specimen is sent for evaluation. If the specimen is negative for cancer, the surgeon will plan to perform a **sentinel lymph node biopsy** during surgery. If the specimen is positive for cancer, the surgeon may plan an **axillary lymph node dissection** during surgery.

- **Sentinel Lymph Node Biopsy (SLNB):** Sentinel lymph node biopsy removes the first (sentinel) node that drains the tumor for an initial evaluation to see if it is positive for cancer. Tumors may have one or more sentinel nodes. The sentinel nodes are the gatekeepers to the rest of the lymphatic nodes. Sentinel lymph node biopsy removes the node most likely to indicate whether cancer has spread from the breast. During mastectomy, sentinel lymph node biopsy can be performed through the same surgical incision. During lumpectomy, it usually requires a second incision.

- **Axillary Lymph Node Dissection (ALND):** Axillary lymph node dissection is a procedure in which the nodes under the arm are surgically removed, usually from levels one and two. For identification purposes, nodes are divided into three levels in the underarm and chest area. The number of nodes in each level varies from person to person. Axillary lymph node dissection removes from 10 – 40 nodes. During mastectomy, axillary lymph node dissection can sometimes be performed through the same surgical incision. During lumpectomy, it usually requires a second incision.

Sentinel Lymph Node Biopsy

Sentinel lymph node biopsy is the preferred procedure to evaluate lymph nodes in patients with early stage breast cancer. Benefits of sentinel lymph node biopsy include:

- Improves the accuracy of selecting the correct nodes to be surgically removed
- Prevents unnecessary node removal outside the lymphatic drainage field of the tumor
- Reduces the number of nodes removed, which greatly decreases the potential for future lymphedema (swelling caused by accumulation of lymphatic fluid in the arm)

Factors That May Exclude a Patient as a Candidate for Sentinel Lymph Node Biopsy:

- Pregnancy
- Suspicious palpable lymph nodes or known positive nodes
- Tumors with involvement in chest wall or skin
- Inflammatory breast cancer

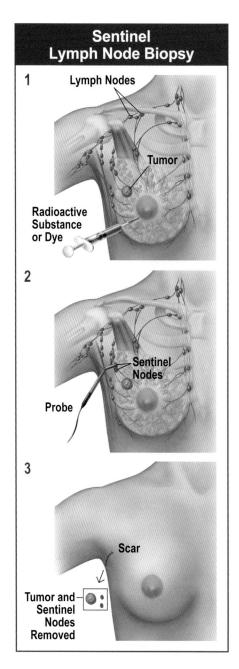

Sentinel Lymph Node Biopsy

1 — Lymph Nodes, Tumor, Radioactive Substance or Dye

2 — Sentinel Nodes, Probe

3 — Scar, Tumor and Sentinel Nodes Removed

Sentinel Lymph Node Biopsy Procedure

1. The sentinel lymph node procedure begins with an injection of a radioactive substance (technetium) into the breast before going to surgery. The injection is most often given around the areola, but may also be given directly into the tumor or around the tumor. Blue dye may be injected just prior to surgery. The radioactive substance or dye is carried by the lymphatic system to the first node(s) draining the tumor.

2. To locate the sentinel node before an incision is made, the surgeon uses a hand-held gamma-detection probe to scan the nodal areas of the breast. When the probe locates a high level of radioactive concentration, the instrument emits an audible sound, and the equipment registers a numerical value. After the entire area is scanned, the surgeon marks the area with the highest numerical value to make the incision for node removal. If blue dye was injected, it helps the surgeon visually identify the nodes for removal.

3. The removed node(s) and tumor are sent to pathology to determine whether they are positive or negative for cancer cells. If the sentinel node was negative for cancer, no additional node surgery is required because it is unlikely that cancer has spread to other nodes. If one of the sentinel nodes is positive for cancer, additional node removal is sometimes necessary to determine whether other nodes may have cancer. Lumpectomy patients scheduled for whole breast radiation may not require additional surgery if the nodal area is included in the area of treatment. Some surgeons prefer to send the removed nodes to pathology, get the results and, if necessary, remove additional nodes during the surgery. Other surgeons prefer to complete the surgery and, if necessary, bring the patient back at a later

date for additional node removal. Because of the variables in additional node removal, it may be helpful to ask your surgeon, *"If cancer is found in my sentinel node(s) will I require additional node removal?"* and *"When will additional nodes be removed?"*

Potential Side Effects of Sentinel Lymph Node Biopsy:

- Pain during injection
- Bruising at the injection sites

Potential Side Effects of Blue Dye:

- Allergic reaction to the blue dye
- Bluish tint of your breast, temporary and not harmful
- Bluish tint of your urine, temporary and not harmful

Lymph Node Evaluation Results

Status of the lymph nodes is important because future treatment decisions are often based on the number of nodes in which cancer cells are found. Your surgeon will tell you how many nodes were removed during your surgery. The pathology report will describe your node status as:

- **Negative nodes** indicate that your lymph nodes did **not** have any evidence of cancer.
- **Positive nodes** indicate that cancer **was found** in the lymph nodes. The pathology report will also report the number of positive nodes.

> **In situ disease patients with no scheduled lymph node evaluation may resume reading at this point.**

Lumpectomy: Breast-Conserving Surgery

Breast-conserving surgery preserves the breast and is commonly called a lumpectomy. Lumpectomy is a surgical option for women with early stage breast cancer who desire to preserve their breast. The good news about lumpectomy is that survival rates are equal when compared to mastectomy. However, there are some characteristics that may disqualify a patient from lumpectomy as an option. Potential disqualifying factors include:

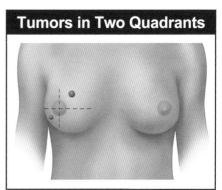

Tumors in Two Quadrants

- Pregnancy, if radiation therapy is required before delivery (lumpectomy is possible in the third trimester as long as radiation can be postponed until after delivery)
- More than one primary tumor in different quadrants of the breast *(see illustration)*
- Mammogram showing evidence of widespread, suspicious microcalcifications (extensive DCIS), indicating high potential for recurrence
- Location of the tumor (under the nipple or multiple tumors usually have poor cosmetic results)
- Size of the tumor (a large tumor in a small breast causes poor cosmetic results)
- Prior radiation therapy to the breast or chest area
- Collagen vascular disease (lupus, scleroderma, etc.), if radiation therapy is required after lumpectomy
- Severe chronic lung disease, if radiation therapy is required after lumpectomy

- Obese women requiring radiation therapy (most radiation tables have a weight limit)
- Positive margins showing remaining cancer after second surgery indicates a high risk for recurrence
- Positive BRCA1 or BRCA2 gene mutation is present (treatment team decision)
- Inflammatory breast cancer
- Restrictions on travel or transportation for radiation therapy treatments

If you are considering a lumpectomy, a consultation with a radiation oncologist to discuss radiation treatments will give you additional insight that may help you make a more informed decision.

Options for Women With Larger Tumors

The cosmetic appearance of the breast after lumpectomy surgery depends on the size of the tumor compared to the size of the breast. There are options for women with a large tumor who prefer to preserve their breast. Neoadjuvant chemotherapy may be given prior to surgery to shrink the tumor to a smaller size, making lumpectomy cosmetically acceptable. Partial reconstruction with a small implant or your own tissues may also be an option for women with larger tumors. If your goal is to keep your breast, discuss these options with your surgeon.

Locating the Tumor Before Lumpectomy

During a lumpectomy, the surgeon needs to be able to feel the tumor for accurate surgical removal. If a tumor cannot be felt, it is necessary that the cancerous area be marked for the surgeon. Methods to mark a non-palpable cancer for surgical removal by lumpectomy may include:

- **Biopsy Clip:** During a core biopsy, the area is often marked by the placement of a small clip that can be visualized under ultrasound. During surgery, ultrasound can accurately locate the clip which identifies the area for surgical removal.

- **Wire Localization:** Shortly before surgery, a radiologist places a thin wire (or wires) to mark the tumor while it is visualized under imaging guidance (mammography, ultrasound or MRI). The wire is taped to your breast, and you are transferred to surgery. Images of the wire placement are sent to surgery for the surgeon's visual reference for accurate removal. The wire is removed during surgery. *Note: More than one wire is often needed to mark the area for DCIS removal because the cancer follows the path of a duct(s) and may be extensive.*

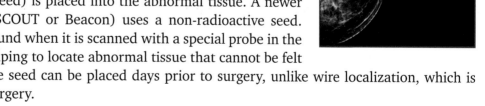

Wire Localization

Wire Placed in Area of Abnormality

- **Seed Localization:** Before surgery, a tiny radioactive seed (the size of a small sesame seed) is placed into the abnormal tissue. A newer technology (SAVI SCOUT or Beacon) uses a non-radioactive seed. The seed emits a sound when it is scanned with a special probe in the operating room, helping to locate abnormal tissue that cannot be felt by the surgeon. The seed can be placed days prior to surgery, unlike wire localization, which is placed the day of surgery.

Surgical Procedure Descriptions

On the following pages are graphics and information that describe lumpectomy surgery and the different types of mastectomy surgeries. Each procedure is illustrated showing the area of tissue removed and how your body will appear after the surgery. Lumpectomy scars vary according to where the tumor is located in the breast and whether lymph nodes were also removed. Mastectomy scars vary among surgeons. To determine the position of your post surgery scar(s), ask your surgeon to mark the planned position of your scar(s) on the *Appearance After Surgery* worksheet on page 264.

Lumpectomy Surgical Procedure

Lumpectomy surgery allows a woman to keep her breast, including her nipple and areola. Lumpectomy removes only the tumor and a small amount of surrounding tissue. If your tumor is invasive, sentinel node biopsy is performed during surgery, most often requiring a second incision. DCIS tumors usually do not require sentinel node biopsy. Radiation therapy is usually recommended after lumpectomy surgery.

Lumpectomy Scars

The location of the tumor in the breast determines scar placement. The surgeon's goal is to completely remove the tumor and to position the scar so that it has the best cosmetic appearance. Lumpectomy scars may be located:

- Directly over the tumor
- Partially around the areola (illustrated)
- Under the arm (axillary)
- In the crease under the breast (inframammary)

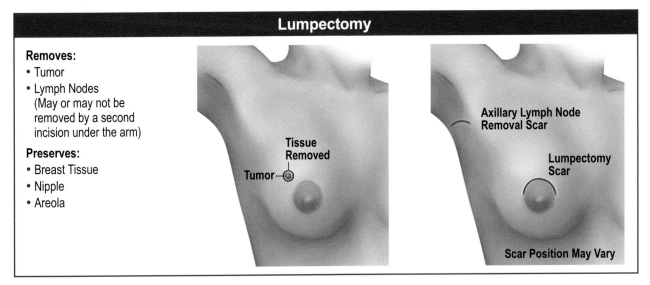

Lumpectomy

Removes:
- Tumor
- Lymph Nodes (May or may not be removed by a second incision under the arm)

Preserves:
- Breast Tissue
- Nipple
- Areola

Tumor
Tissue Removed

Axillary Lymph Node Removal Scar
Lumpectomy Scar
Scar Position May Vary

Oncoplastic Lumpectomy Procedure

A newer method of lumpectomy surgery, called oncoplastic surgery, removes the tumor using plastic surgery techniques. These techniques can eliminate the visible tissue indentation often seen at the lumpectomy incision site. It can also allow women with large or sagging breasts to undergo a breast lift during their cancer surgery. Oncoplastic surgery can be performed by a trained breast surgeon or with a plastic surgeon working along with your cancer surgeon.

Mastectomy Procedures

There are four basic types of mastectomy procedures. Ask your surgeon which procedure will be performed and how your lymph nodes will be evaluated.

During mastectomy, breast skin and breast tissue are both removed but in differing amounts. More breast tissue is removed because it has the potential to develop breast cancer. In the following illustrations, the area of breast skin that may be removed is outlined in burgundy and shaded in pink. The area of breast tissue under the skin that may be removed is outlined with a black dotted line.

Mastectomy Scar

The goal of the surgeon during mastectomy is to remove the overlying skin of a tumor along with any biopsy scarring, which causes scar placement to vary.

Four Different Types of Mastectomy

1. Modified Radical Mastectomy

A modified radical mastectomy is the most commonly performed type of mastectomy.

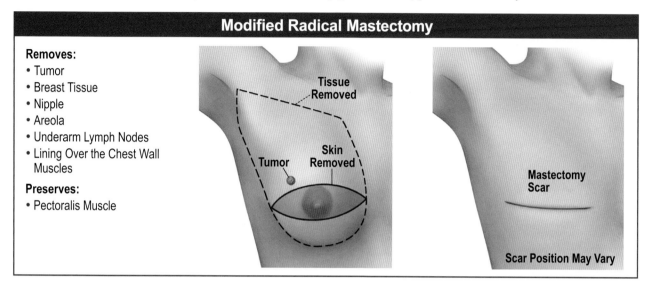

Modified Radical Mastectomy

Removes:
- Tumor
- Breast Tissue
- Nipple
- Areola
- Underarm Lymph Nodes
- Lining Over the Chest Wall Muscles

Preserves:
- Pectoralis Muscle

Tissue Removed

Tumor Skin Removed

Mastectomy Scar

Scar Position May Vary

2. Total, Simple or Prophylactic Mastectomy

A prophylactic mastectomy is a total or simple mastectomy performed **before** cancer has been found. This is an elective surgery and is a decision made collaboratively between the patient, surgeon and oncologist. Reasons for prophylactic mastectomy may include:

- Desire for bilateral reconstruction after cancer surgery; non-cancerous breast is removed
- Diagnosis of cancer that has a high rate of occurring in the opposite breast; non-cancerous breast is removed
- Strong family history of breast cancer; both breasts are removed in selected instances
- Identified positive carrier of a BRCA1 or BRCA2 gene mutation or certain other high-risk genes; both breasts are removed

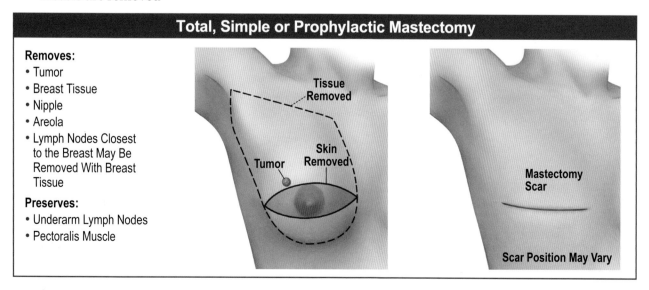

Total, Simple or Prophylactic Mastectomy

Removes:
- Tumor
- Breast Tissue
- Nipple
- Areola
- Lymph Nodes Closest to the Breast May Be Removed With Breast Tissue

Preserves:
- Underarm Lymph Nodes
- Pectoralis Muscle

Tissue Removed

Tumor Skin Removed

Mastectomy Scar

Scar Position May Vary

3. Skin-Sparing Mastectomy

Skin-sparing mastectomy preserves the breast skin when performing a simple or modified mastectomy. The surgery removes the breast tissues from a circular incision around the areola (dark colored circle). The nipple and areola are later reconstructed, which conceals the surgical scar on the breast.

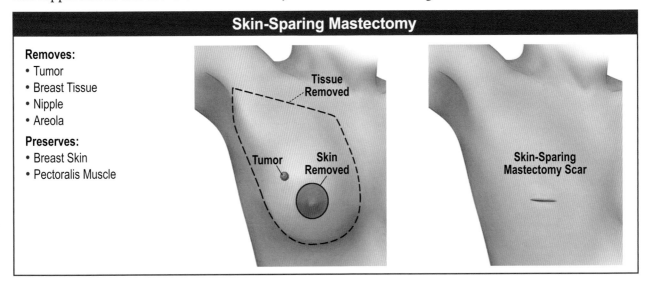

Skin-Sparing Mastectomy

Removes:
• Tumor
• Breast Tissue
• Nipple
• Areola

Preserves:
• Breast Skin
• Pectoralis Muscle

Tissue Removed

Tumor

Skin Removed

Skin-Sparing Mastectomy Scar

The sparing of the breast skin greatly reduces or eliminates the need to stretch the skin and provides a perfect envelope for an implant or autologous reconstruction. This procedure may preserve the sensitivity of the skin over the reconstructed breast. Skin-sparing mastectomy is the recommended surgery for most women who plan to have reconstructive surgery.

4. Nipple-Sparing Mastectomy

Nipple-sparing mastectomy is a surgical technique that spares the nipple and areola during mastectomy. The key is to remove as little breast skin as possible for the best cosmetic result after reconstruction.

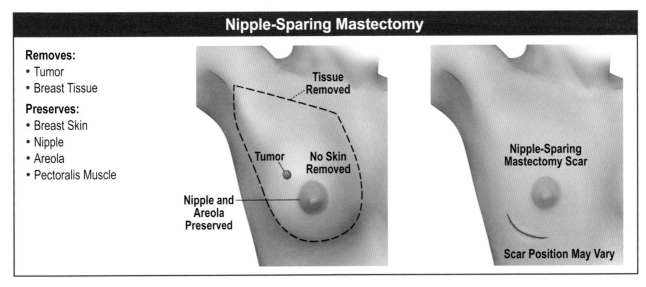

Nipple-Sparing Mastectomy

Removes:
• Tumor
• Breast Tissue

Preserves:
• Breast Skin
• Nipple
• Areola
• Pectoralis Muscle

Tissue Removed

Tumor

No Skin Removed

Nipple and Areola Preserved

Nipple-Sparing Mastectomy Scar

Scar Position May Vary

Nipple-Sparing Scar

Nipple-sparing mastectomy scar positioning varies among surgeons. The position of the surgical incision may be located at:

- Bottom of the crease of the breast (inframammary fold)
- Partially around the areola and extending outward toward the arm
- Partially around the areola and extending downward toward the inframammary fold
- Partially around the areola (periareolar)

Suitable candidates are women who have a small cancer that is not located close to the nipple, has no skin involvement and has negative axillary lymph nodes. BRCA positive and DCIS women who choose prophylactic mastectomy are usually candidates for nipple-sparing mastectomy.

After the breast is reconstructed, it looks nearly cosmetically identical to the other breast since the nipple and areola are the most distinguishing characteristic of a woman's breast appearance.

Concerns About the Contralateral (Non-Surgical) Breast

After cancer is diagnosed in one breast and you are facing surgery, you may be concerned about the other breast. Be assured that the mammography film of the contralateral breast will be evaluated carefully to be sure there are no suspicious areas that need further evaluation before cancer surgery. Discuss your options with your physician.

Contralateral Breast Mastectomy

The decision to remove your contralateral breast during breast cancer surgery, or at a later date, should be made **only** after careful evaluation of the facts to ensure that you make an informed decision.

Important Facts To Consider:

- The risk of cancer occurring in your contralateral breast is low. It is estimated that only 3 – 9 percent of patients will have cancer occur in the contralateral breast before they reach the age of 85.
- The removal of the contralateral breast does **not** improve the survival rate from breast cancer.
- The contralateral breast will be closely monitored for breast cancer in the future. Any cancer occurrence would most likely be detected at a very early stage.

Disadvantages of Contralateral Prophylactic Mastectomy:

- Removes healthy, non-cancerous breast tissue
- Eliminates future natural breast sexual stimulation that increases sexual arousal and pleasure

Advantages of Contralateral Prophylactic Mastectomy:

- Eliminates potential cancer occurrence in contralateral breast
- May reduce anxiety for some women who worry about future occurrence in the contralateral breast
- Allows bilateral reconstruction to closely match breast symmetry
- Avoids future cost and inconvenience of cancer screening

Final Surgery Decision

You may find it helpful to speak with a patient who has already had the procedure you are considering. Ask your physician if there is a patient who would be willing to talk with you. You may also call your local American Cancer Society's Reach to Recovery program coordinator and ask if she can provide the name of a volunteer who will be willing to share her lumpectomy/mastectomy experience.

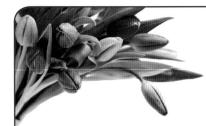

Remember...

- *Breast surgery, though difficult to undergo physically and mentally, is a necessary step to rid your body of a life-threatening disease and protect your future health.*

- *Make the surgical decision that you feel most comfortable with—not your spouse, friend or doctor's preference. This is a decision about your body, you need to decide. This is an essential step toward regaining your sense of control.*

- *If lumpectomy is your choice, remember that survival rates are equal with mastectomy. You don't have to lose your breast to save your life.*

- *If mastectomy is your choice, review your breast reconstruction options before your breast cancer surgery even if you want to delay your reconstruction to a later time. This allows your surgeon to place your incisions in a location most suitable for future reconstruction.*

- *Reconstruction can be performed with implants or with your own body tissues. Reconstructing your breast restores your body image and allows most women to better adjust to the loss of their breast.*

- *Reconstruction can be performed at the time of your cancer surgery or delayed until a later time. Timing depends on your choice and the type of treatments you are scheduled to undergo after surgery.*

- *Implants are the least invasive reconstructive procedure. However, they are not a lifetime device and will require future replacement.*

- *Although autologous (tissues from your own body) reconstruction is a more invasive procedure and requires a longer recovery time, it is a lifetime procedure.*

- *When you look at your surgical scars, remind yourself that they are evidence that you were blessed to have a disease for which there was treatment—making you a Survivor and not a statistic.*

Additional Information

Tear-out Worksheets
Appearance After Surgery - page 264
Surgical Decision Evaluation - page 265

CHAPTER 8

Reconstructive Surgery

"When I studied my reconstruction options after bilateral mastectomies, I decided that immediate reconstruction with breast implants was my choice. I went regularly for expander 'pump up' sessions and eventually had my final implants placed, followed by nipple reconstruction and areola tattooing. Reconstruction helped restore the confidence mastectomy had taken away from me."

—*Lisa DelGuidice*

Women diagnosed with breast cancer are confronted with many decisions about their care. For women planning mastectomy, the decision whether or not to have breast reconstruction to restore their body image is a major decision. For the majority of women, losing a breast causes a lowered perception of body image. The good news is that even though you are losing a breast to surgery, you have the option to restore your body image through breast reconstruction.

Breast reconstruction has made a big difference for many women who have undergone breast cancer surgery. Some women choose to have immediate reconstruction to maintain their feminine silhouette and alleviate the necessity of wearing a prosthesis. Other women prefer to wait until all of their cancer treatment is completed to have their breast reconstructed.

The decision to have breast reconstruction requires a lot of personal thought, research and discussion. Remember, part of gaining control over your cancer is understanding the options that are available to you and choosing those that best meet your needs. As you research your choices, keep asking yourself, *"How would I like to look a year from now?"*

The time to make the decision about immediate reconstructive surgery is short, and there are many types of procedures to consider. Making a decision at this time may seem overwhelming. However, it is an important decision to evaluate carefully. It is highly recommended that you consider consulting a reconstructive surgeon **before** your cancer surgery even if you do not think that breast reconstruction is an option you will choose. Only after getting all of the facts can you make a fully informed decision. Your surgeon can provide you with names of experienced plastic surgeons who offer a consultation at no charge.

"I had immediate reconstruction—a TRAM (used my stomach muscle, skin and fatty tissue to construct a new breast). When I woke up, even though I was bandaged up, I really almost couldn't believe they had removed the breast because the TRAM turned out so well."
—*Anna Cluxton*

"I had delayed reconstruction about a year after my mastectomy. I chose to have a prophylactic mastectomy on the opposite breast followed by tissue expanders and saline breast implants."
—*Harriett Barrineau*

In this chapter, we will discuss the different reconstructive procedures and explain the advantages and disadvantages of each in order to help you make an informed decision. Even though you may think reconstruction is not a decision you will choose, I encourage you to read this chapter before making a final decision.

Advantages of Breast Reconstruction:

- Restores your feminine body image
- Eliminates need to purchase and wear a prosthesis or special bras
- Allows you to wear any clothing, including swimsuits and low-cut attire
- Eliminates the daily reminder of breast surgery by not having to wear a prosthesis
- Increases the psychological adjustment to breast surgery for most women

Disadvantages of Breast Reconstruction:

- Increases surgical pain and recovery time
- Increases potential for infection or surgical complications due to the more complicated surgery

Breast Reconstruction Terms

To effectively explore breast reconstruction options, it is necessary to understand the meaning of some medical terms. To help you, we have listed definitions of commonly used terms below:

- **Acellular Dermal Matrix:** A tissue substitute that may be used during reconstruction
- **Autologous:** Tissue from your own body
- **Breast Mastopexy:** Surgery to lift the opposite breast to match contour of the reconstructed breast
- **Breast Reduction:** Surgery to reduce and lift the opposite breast to match the reconstructed breast
- **Capsular Contracture:** Scar tissue that forms around an implant distorts its shape, causes pain and may potentially require implant removal
- **Contour:** Shape of a breast
- **Contralateral Breast:** Opposite, non-surgical breast
- **Cosmesis:** Final appearance of a breast
- **Donor Tissue:** Selected tissue from one's own body that creates the new breast mound
- **Flap:** Donor tissue moved to the breast area
- **Hernia:** Abdominal bulge of tissues where muscle is removed
- **Mastectomy Site:** Mastectomy scar area
- **Microsurgeon:** Surgeon trained to perform surgery under a microscope
- **Necrosis:** Death of tissues from lack of blood supply
- **Ptosis:** Normal drooping or sagging caused by aging
- **Seroma:** Collection of fluid under skin or around implant
- **Symmetry:** Similar shape of the breasts

Breast Reconstruction Consultation

Today, there are numerous types of procedures available to reconstruct your breast. Deciding on the type of reconstruction is a joint decision made between you and the plastic surgeon after a consultation. During your consultation, the surgeon carefully reviews your health history for potential limiting factors and, along with your personal desires, recommends the most appropriate type of procedure for you.

Reconstructive Evaluation Includes:

- Physical makeup (body size, breast size, degree of sagging)
- Current physical health and past health history
- Breast cancer history (type of cancer; positive for BRCA1 or BRCA2 mutation)
  - Some cancer types may require bilateral mastectomy
- Radiation therapy planned
- Reconstruction type you prefer (implant or autologous)

Factors That May Limit Reconstruction Options:

- Obesity (especially more than 25 – 35% over ideal body weight)
- History of radiation therapy to the chest wall
- Smoker, or recent history of smoking
- Autoimmune disease (lupus, multiple sclerosis, insulin dependent diabetes mellitus, scleroderma, Hashimoto's thyroiditis, fibromyalgia)
- Blood-clotting disorders
- Current or previous history of asthma or chronic lung disease
- Current cardiovascular disease
- Psychiatric disorder
- Previous substance abuse
- Inflammatory breast cancer

Concerns About Reconstructive Surgery

Women often fear that reconstruction may hide or prevent the detection of cancer recurrence in the breast area. There is no evidence that breast reconstruction, with your body tissues or with an implant, causes cancer to grow or recur. There is little difficulty in detecting an early local recurrence after reconstruction. These issues should not be a concern when making your decision.

Women frequently think they may be too old for reconstruction. If you would like to restore your body image, age is not a limiting factor. Whether you are 18 or 80, if you are in good health, you may be a candidate for breast reconstruction.

Cost is another concern patients have about reconstructive surgery. The good news for patients is that in 1998, The Women's Health and Cancer Rights Act (WHCRA) was signed into law, providing coverage of the cost of reconstruction for women who elect to have a mastectomy. This law requires insurance providers to cover not only reconstruction of the surgical breast but also surgery, if needed, to the opposite breast to achieve symmetry between them. It also includes coverage of any complications resulting from a mastectomy, including lymphedema (swelling of the surgical arm). This law allows women to choose a mastectomy, knowing that their reconstruction costs are covered with the exception of any required insurance deductibles.

Timing of Reconstruction Surgery

Reconstruction can be done immediately following your cancer surgery or at a later time. There is no time limit after cancer surgery for reconstruction as an option to restore your body image. However, if your future cancer treatment includes radiation therapy, the best time for reconstruction requires a review of your individual case by your treatment team. After review of the type of procedure you prefer, a decision of timing for surgery will be recommended.

Advantages of Immediate Reconstruction:

- Requires only one surgery, which lowers cost
- Reduces recovery time in comparison to two separate surgeries
- Maintains body image because you awake with a breast mound (exception: tissue expander placed prior to implant)

Disadvantages of Immediate Reconstruction:

- Increases surgical pain and recovery time
- Increases potential for infection or surgical complications

Advantages of Delayed Reconstruction:

- Allows time to investigate your reconstruction options carefully
- Allows time to seek several consultations and carefully select surgeon
- Causes no delay in cancer treatments because of potential surgical complications

Disadvantages of Delayed Reconstruction:

- Requires second surgery
- Increases potential that surgery may occur in another calendar year, requiring you to pay a second deductible
- Requires you to purchase and wear a prosthesis and special bras until reconstructive surgery; you cannot go braless or wear low-cut clothing
- Increases psychological distress from having to deal with an altered body image while waiting for reconstructive surgery

Breast Reconstruction Procedures

Options available for women desiring breast reconstruction have greatly increased during the past decade. Traditional procedures have undergone refinement and new techniques have been developed, which have greatly improved the cosmetic outcome of reconstruction. In this section, we will discuss the types of procedures and techniques that may be options to restore your breast.

Breast Reconstruction Technique Innovations

One of the new techniques that may be used to improve the cosmetic outcome of your surgery is the addition of acellular dermal matrix. This is an option when additional tissue is needed. Dermal matrix is a soft-tissue substitute created from donated human skin that has been processed to remove all of the cells. It is the same type of tissue used for skin grafts in burn patients. After placement in the body, dermal matrix acts as a lattice that allows your own cells to grow into the matrix, transforming it into living skin that functions as your own. Brand names include AlloDerm®, FlexHD® and DermaMatrix®.

Another emerging technique to improve cosmetic outcome is the use of body-fat grafting. The surgeon removes fat cells from other parts of your body—usually the thighs, abdomen or buttocks—by liposuction. The removed fat cells are then processed into a liquid and injected into the area of the breast needing additional soft tissues.

Dermal matrix or fat-grafting may be used during implant or autologous reconstruction when extra tissue is needed to achieve better cosmetic outcomes.

Two Basic Types of Breast Reconstruction

- **Breast Implant:** A flexible sac is placed under the chest muscle, filled with either saline (sterile salt water) or silicone gel.
- **Autologous Reconstruction:** Skin and fat, with or without the muscle, is moved from your abdomen, back, buttocks, inner thighs or upper thighs to reconstruct a new breast mound.

Breast Implants

Breast implants are a breast-shaped, synthetic shell filled with either saline or silicone gel. Implants come in a variety of shapes and fillings to meet your reconstructive needs. Reconstructing the breast with an implant is the least surgically invasive of all reconstructive surgeries. However, implants are not a lifetime device and will require future surgery to replace them when they wear out. Immediate reconstruction with an implant extends your cancer surgery approximately one hour for each breast.

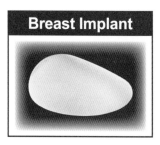

Breast Implant

Candidates for Implant Reconstruction:

- Women with small to medium-sized breasts
- Women who are not candidates for autologous reconstruction
- Women desiring bilateral reconstruction with increase or decrease in size
- Women who do not want additional surgical scars
- Women who do not want a longer, more complicated surgery

Implant Advantages Compared to Autologous Reconstruction:

- Decreases surgical time and pain after surgery
- Decreases recovery time because it is a less complicated surgery

Implant Disadvantages Compared to Autologous Reconstruction:

- Difficult to match a remaining large or drooping breast
- Potential of tissues around the implant to harden, called capsular contracture, which may cause pain and change the implant shape; severe capsular contracture may require surgical removal and implant replacement
- Difficult to get implant reconstructed breast to hang symmetrically and match opposite breast
- Implant stays the same size with weight gain or weight loss, unlike autologous tissues, which follow body weight changes
- Implant may leak or rupture, requiring surgical removal and replacement
- Implant has a limited lifespan of 10 to 15 years because of aging and deterioration; requires future surgical replacement (not a lifetime procedure)

Three Variations of Implant Procedures:

1. Tissue expander followed by fixed-volume implant placement
2. Combination implant and expander
3. Fixed-volume implant

1. Tissue Expander Before Implant Placement

Implants are usually placed under the chest muscle, which requires stretching the muscle and skin to create a pocket to hold the final fixed-volume implant. To stretch the tissues, a temporary deflated implant, called a tissue expander, is placed under the muscle during surgery. Occasionally, dermal matrix may be attached to the bottom of the chest muscle to accommodate a larger size expander.

When you wake up from breast surgery, you will not have a breast mound. You will need some type of filling in your bra that can be easily adjusted to match the size of your opposite breast. Starting a few weeks after placement, the expander is gradually filled through a valve located under the skin with an injection of saline (sterile salt water) solution. At each filling, the surgeon injects about 50 cc of saline. This may cause slight discomfort for about 24 hours after each filling as the body adjusts to the new size. This gradual filling stretches the muscle and skin to the size needed for the final fixed-volume implant placement. In approximately 4 – 6 months, the expander is removed, and the final fixed-volume implant is placed during a second outpatient surgery.

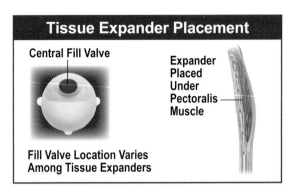

Tissue Expander Placement

Central Fill Valve

Expander Placed Under Pectoralis Muscle

Fill Valve Location Varies Among Tissue Expanders

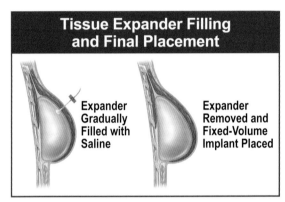

Tissue Expander Filling and Final Placement

Expander Gradually Filled with Saline

Expander Removed and Fixed-Volume Implant Placed

2. Combination Implant and Expander

A newer type of saline implant serves as both an expander and an implant. After the implant is surgically placed, the surgeon can adjust the size for up to six months with saline injections. This combination model allows the gradual expansion of the muscle and skin and does not require a separate surgery for removal when the desired size is reached. The valve used to fill the implant is removed in the surgeon's office.

3. Fixed-Volume Implant

A fixed-volume implant is prefilled to the desired size and shape of the breast and may be placed at the time of mastectomy surgery. This procedure is often referred to as "direct-to-implant." Initial placement of a fixed-volume implant does not require a second surgery. Direct-to-implant is often made possible by the surgeon using dermal matrix. Patients who want a smaller size breast and patients who have had skin-sparing or nipple-sparing mastectomy are usually candidates.

Saline Implants Compared to Silicone Implants

After deciding that an implant is your choice for reconstruction, you need to decide if you prefer a saline implant or a silicone implant.

Saline Implants

Saline implants are filled with sterile salt water that has the same concentration of salt as most body fluids, causing it to have no adverse impact on the body if it leaks or ruptures. If a saline implant ruptures, it deflates within hours, causing your chest to appear flat. Surgery is required to remove and replace the implant. Saline implants feel firmer when touched than silicone implants.

Silicone Implants

Silicone implants are filled with a very thick silicone gel, similar to uncooked egg whites, which causes the implant to feel soft and more like the natural breast. The most recent advancement in silicone implants is a model often referred to as the "gummy bear" implant because of the stiff consistency of the silicone. The consistency makes it less likely to leak but also causes the implant to feel firmer than other silicone implants. The gummy bear implant has a teardrop shape, which provides more fullness to the bottom of the breast, causing it to look more natural. This implant requires a longer incision for placement because it is not as flexible.

Implant Leaks and Ruptures

If a silicone implant ruptures, it can go undetected for years because the thick filling leaks very slowly—unlike a saline leak, which is immediate. For this reason, the FDA recommends magnetic resonance imaging (MRI) three years after placement of a silicone implant and then every two years after that to detect any ruptures. (MRI is not covered by insurance.) Leaking implants require surgical removal and replacement.

Radiation Therapy After Implants

Breast implants are not recommended for women who are planning to undergo radiation therapy. However, some physicians place the expander during cancer surgery but do not begin filling it until after the completion of radiation therapy. Ask your surgeon about their preference.

Autologous Reconstruction

Autologous breast reconstruction uses a woman's own body tissues. Body skin and fat, with or without muscle, is taken from the abdomen, back, buttocks, inner thighs or upper thighs to reconstruct the breast mound. During the past decade, many advancements and refinements have been made in the types of procedures available. The goal of autologous reconstruction is to create a breast mound that has a natural shape and matches the size and contour of the opposite breast—a natural looking breast. Today, most patients qualify for one of the autologous procedures. As you are making your decision, be aware that not all plastic surgeons perform some of the autologous procedures discussed in this book.

Autologous Reconstruction Advantages Compared to Implant:

- Avoids many breast implant related complications; does not require future surgical replacement
- Feels warm and soft like natural breast tissue
- Allows surgeon to match the normal drooping and contour of opposite breast
- Allows surgeon to add additional skin flap to avoid stretching the skin if a mastectomy scar is tight
- Improves contour of donor site (abdomen or buttock) due to the reduction of body fat
- Allows volume and shape of autologous tissues to follow body weight changes

Autologous Reconstruction Disadvantages Compared to Implant:

- Requires sacrificing tissues from another body part to reconstruct your breast
- Increases surgical and recovery time when compared to implant reconstruction
- Increases pain after surgery when compared to implant reconstruction
- Increases potential for tissue necrosis (cell death) of reconstructed breast from lack of blood supply to newly transplanted tissues, which requires surgical removal of transplanted body tissues

Autologous Reconstruction Tissue Selection

Tissue selected for autologous reconstruction may come from a patient's abdomen, back, buttocks, inner thighs or upper thighs. The tissue selected and moved to the breast area is called a **flap**. There are two major distinctions between flap types: blood supply and muscle.

Flap Blood Supply Types:

- **Pedicle Flap:** Donor tissues are left **connected** to the blood supply (not cut free) and moved to the breast area.
- **Free Flap:** Donor tissues are **cut free** from the local blood supply, transferred to the breast area and reattached using a microscope (*illustration 1*). Free flaps are the most complex of all reconstructive procedures, requiring a plastic surgeon with expertise in microsurgery.

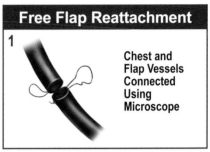

Free Flap Reattachment

1 Chest and Flap Vessels Connected Using Microscope

Flap Muscle Types:

- **Muscle-Containing Flap:** The underlying muscle and tissue are cut and transferred to the mastectomy site (*illustration 2*). Donor flaps that contain muscle may cause increased post-surgical pain and future donor site weakness (abdomen or back).
- **Muscle-Sparing Flap:** Flap does not include the underlying muscle for transfer. A small incision is made into the muscle, but the muscle is spared (*illustration 3*). Procedures that do not use the muscle are less painful, have a shorter recovery time and do not cause future donor site weakness.

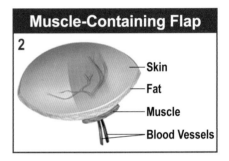

Muscle-Containing Flap

2 Skin — Fat — Muscle — Blood Vessels

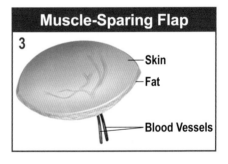

Muscle-Sparing Flap

3 Skin — Fat — Blood Vessels

Autologous Reconstruction Procedure Names

The names of autologous reconstructive surgeries describe the site of donor tissues. Free flap surgeries include the name of the blood vessels that reattach the tissues to the breast blood supply.

- **Abdomen:**
  - **TRAM** (Transverse Rectus Abdominis Myocutaneous muscle)*
  - **DIEP** (Deep Inferior Epigastric Perforator)+
  - **SIEA** (Superficial Inferior Epigastric Artery)+
- **Back:**
  - **LD** (Latissimus Dorsi)*
  - **TAP** (Thoracodorsal Artery Perforator)+

- **Buttock:**
  - **SGAP** (Superior Gluteal Artery Perforator)+
  - **IGAP** (Inferior Gluteal Artery Perforator)+
- **Thigh:**
  - **TUG** (Transverse Upper Gracilis) Flap+
  - **PAP** (Profunda Artery Perforator) Flap+

*Uses underlying muscle
+Free flap requires surgeon skilled in microsurgery

Autologous Abdominal Procedures

The abdomen is the most frequently selected donor site for autologous breast reconstruction because most women have adequate abdominal fat.

Evaluation of Abdominal Donor Site

For abdominal procedures, the surgeon assesses if previous procedures such as surgery, laparoscopy or liposuction have caused scarring or damage to the tissues or blood supply. If scarring is found in the abdominal flap area, another type of reconstruction is recommended. Individual assessment is necessary because some surgeries cause scarring, and others do not. For this reason, women with previous C-sections or a hysterectomy may be candidates if the muscle or blood supply was not damaged.

TRAM (Transverse Rectus Abdominis Myocutaneous Muscle) Flap: Pedicle Flap

- **Candidates:** Mastectomy patients with adequate abdominal fat and no previous scarring in flap area.
- **Procedure:** Transfers abdominal skin, fat and muscle, still connected to local blood supply (pedicle flap), by tunneling the flap under the skin to the mastectomy site. Donor flap is sutured to the mastectomy site.

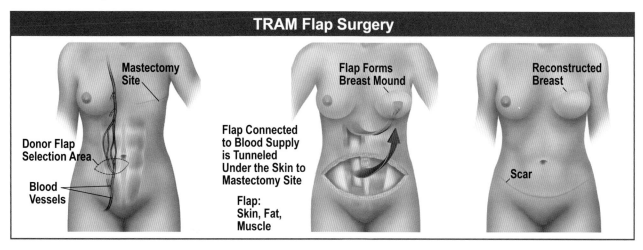

TRAM Flap Surgery

- **Advantages:** Improves abdominal contour—tummy tuck. Creates an instant breast mound after surgery. No microsurgery required because blood vessels are not cut. TRAM can closely match the size and sagging of the other breast. Breast tissues are warm, feel soft and follow changes in body weight—loss or gain. Shorter surgical time than abdominal procedures which cut blood vessels.
- **Disadvantages:** Scar on abdomen. Cuts and transfers abdominal muscle, which increases pain after surgery and causes difficulty standing up straight for several days. Longer recovery time than procedures that do not cut and transfer muscle.
- **Risks:** Loss of donor flap due to necrosis. Future abdominal weakness and potential for a hernia.

Free TRAM (Transverse Rectus Abdominis Myocutaneous muscle): Free Flap

- **Candidates:** Mastectomy patients with adequate abdominal fat and no previous scarring in flap area.
- **Procedure:** Cuts and transfers abdominal skin, fat, muscle and local vessels. Requires microsurgery to reattach flap vessels to the breast blood supply. Donor flap is sutured to mastectomy site.

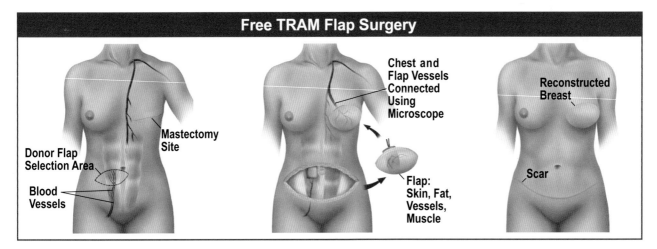

Free TRAM Flap Surgery

- **Advantages:** Improves abdominal contour—tummy tuck. Creates an instant breast mound after surgery. Closely matches the size and sagging of the other breast. Breast tissues are warm, feel soft and follow changes in body weight—loss or gain.

- **Disadvantages:** Scar on abdomen. Requires microsurgery to reconnect cut donor flap blood vessels to breast blood vessels. Cuts and transfers abdominal muscle, which increases pain after surgery and causes difficulty standing up straight for several days. Longer recovery time than procedures that do not cut and transfer muscle.

- **Risks:** Abdominal hernia or loss of donor flap due to necrosis.

Muscle-Sparing TRAM: Free Flap

- **Candidates:** Mastectomy patients with adequate abdominal fat and no previous scarring in flap area.

- **Procedure:** Transfers abdominal skin and fat with a very small section of muscle, but cuts local blood vessels (free flap). Requires microsurgery to reattach the blood supply. Donor flap is sutured to mastectomy site.

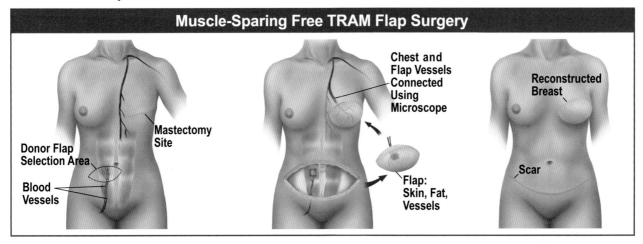

Muscle-Sparing Free TRAM Flap Surgery

- **Advantages:** Improves abdominal contour—tummy tuck. Creates instant breast mound after surgery. Closely matches the size and sagging of the other breast. Breast tissues are warm, feel soft and follow changes in body weight—loss or gain. Shorter recovery time than TRAM or free TRAM flaps which cut and move muscle.

- **Disadvantages:** Scar on abdomen. Requires microsurgery to reconnect donor flap blood vessels to breast blood vessels, which increases the surgical time over TRAM but shortens recovery time.
- **Risks:** Loss of donor flap due to necrosis.

DIEP (Deep Inferior Epigastric Perforator): Free Flap

- **Candidates:** Mastectomy patients with adequate abdominal fat and no previous scarring in flap area.
- **Procedure:** Transfers abdominal skin, fat and blood vessels with **no** muscle. Small incision made into muscle to harvest vessels. Cuts flap blood supply (free flap). Requires microsurgery to reattach the flap artery and vein to breast blood vessels. Donor flap is sutured to the mastectomy site.

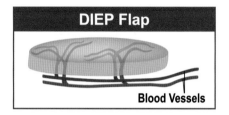

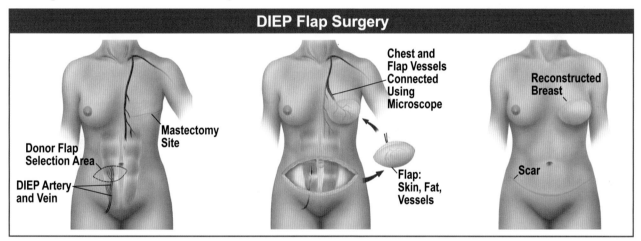

- **Advantages:** Improves abdominal contour—tummy tuck. Creates an instant breast mound after surgery. Closely matches the size and sagging of the other breast. Breast tissues are warm, feel soft and follow changes in body weight—loss or gain. Shorter recovery time than TRAM or free TRAM flaps which cut and move muscle.
- **Disadvantages:** Scar on abdomen. Requires microsurgery to reattach donor flap deep inferior epigastric artery and vein to breast blood supply, which increases surgical time over TRAM but shortens recovery time over TRAM or Free TRAM.
- **Risks:** Loss of donor flap due to necrosis.

SIEA (Superficial Inferior Epigastric Artery): Free Flap

SIEA is identical to the DIEP procedure described above, with the exception of the vessels selected to restore the blood supply to the flap. The superficial inferior epigastric artery and vein are selected. These vessels are located closer to the skin. Approximately 30 percent of women have adequate blood to these vessels. A SIEA procedure is less invasive than a DIEP procedure.

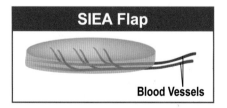

Autologous Back Procedures

Latissimus Dorsi: Pedicle Flap

- **Candidates:**
  - Patient with small to medium-sized breast. (Implant may be required.)
  - Patient who requires additional tissue after a lumpectomy.
  - Patient who has skin damage from previous radiation therapy and needs additional skin.
  - Patient who is not a candidate for abdominal flap (previous surgical scarring or lack of fatty tissues).
- **Procedure:** Transfers back skin, fat and muscle. Flap remains connected to its local blood supply (pedicle flap). Flap is tunneled under the skin to the mastectomy site and sutured in place. For a patient needing more volume, a fixed-volume implant is placed under the flap.

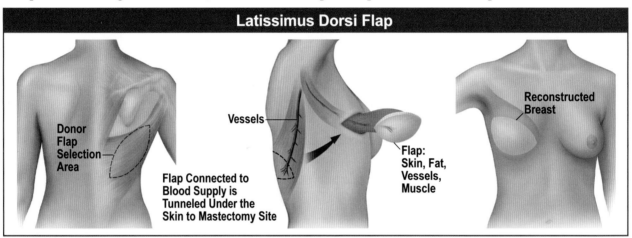

- **Advantages:** No microsurgery required. Back tissues are usually healthy with adequate skin.
- **Disadvantages:** Scar on back. May affect range of motion in shoulder area.
- **Risks:** Potential seroma (collection of fluid) or loss of donor flap due to necrosis.

TAP (Thoracodorsal Artery Perforator): Pedicle Flap

- **Candidates:** Patient who requires additional tissue after a lumpectomy or cosmetic procedure.
- **Procedure:** Transfers back skin, fat and blood vessels with **no** muscle. Blood vessels are left connected to the flap. Flap is tunneled under the skin to mastectomy site and sutured in place.

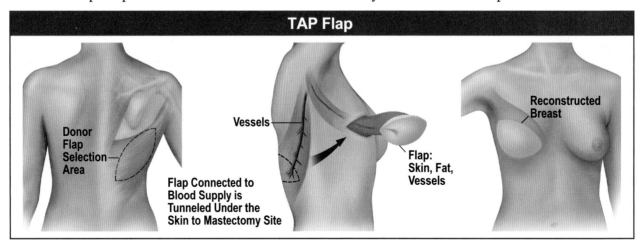

- **Advantages:** Does not cut and move muscle. Reduces shoulder weakness.
- **Disadvantages:** Scar on back.
- **Risks:** Potential seroma or loss of donor flap due to necrosis.

Autologous Buttock Procedures

SGAP (Superior Gluteal Artery Perforator): Free Flap
IGAP (Inferior Gluteal Artery Perforator): Free Flap

- **Candidates:**
  - Patient who is thin or of normal weight.
  - Patient who is not a candidate for an abdominal flap because of previous surgical scarring.
  - Patient needing bilateral reconstruction.
- **Procedure:** Transfers buttock skin, fat and blood vessels with **no** muscle. Flap blood vessels are cut and require microsurgery to reconnect to the breast blood vessels. Donor flap is sutured to mastectomy site.

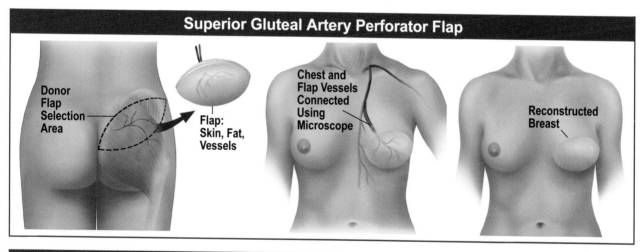

Superior Gluteal Artery Perforator Flap

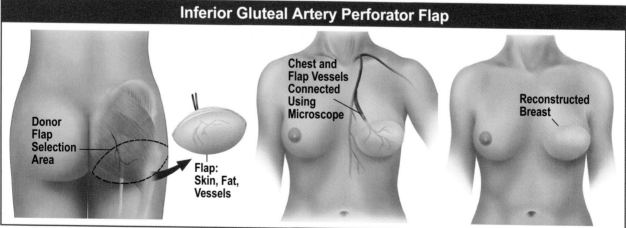

Inferior Gluteal Artery Perforator Flap

- **Advantages:** Most women have a healthy, adequate amount of buttock fat. SGAP scar hidden by underwear. IGAP scar hidden in lower buttock crease.
- **Disadvantages:** Scar on buttock.
- **Risks:** Potential seroma or loss of donor flap due to necrosis.

Autologous Thigh Procedures

TUG (Transverse Upper Gracilis) Flap: Free Flap

- **Candidates:**
  - Patient with adequate inner thigh fat.
  - Patient who is not a candidate for abdominal flaps because of previous surgical scarring.
  - Patient who has small breasts and does not require a large amount of fatty tissue.
  - Patient needing bilateral reconstruction.
- **Procedure:** Transfers inner thigh skin, fat and a small amount of muscle. Flap vessels are cut and require microsurgery to reconnect to the breast blood vessels. Donor flap is sutured to mastectomy site.

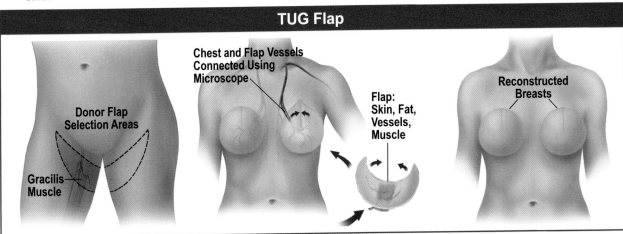

TUG Flap

- **Advantages:** Gracilis muscle pulls legs inward. Using the gracilis muscle causes minimal post-surgical problems for patients. Most women have a healthy, adequate amount of inner thigh fat. Eliminates additional visible scars.
- **Disadvantages:** Scar on inner thigh.
- **Risks:** Potential seroma or loss of donor flap due to necrosis.

PAP (Profunda Artery Perforator) Flap: Free Flap

- **Candidates:**
  - Patient with adequate upper thigh fat.
  - Patient who is not a candidate for abdominal flaps because of previous surgical scarring.
  - Patient who has small breasts and does not require a large amount of fatty tissue.
  - Patient needing bilateral reconstruction.
- **Procedure:** Transfers skin, fat and blood vessels from the upper thigh, below the buttock. Flap vessels are cut and require microsurgery to reconnect to the breast blood vessels. Donor flap is sutured to mastectomy site.

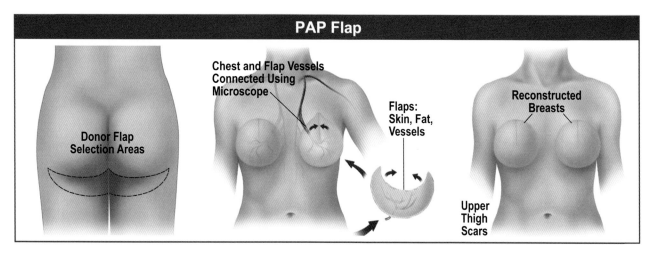

PAP Flap

Donor Flap Selection Areas

Chest and Flap Vessels Connected Using Microscope

Flaps: Skin, Fat, Vessels

Reconstructed Breasts

Upper Thigh Scars

- **Advantages:** Bilateral reconstruction improves thigh contour—thigh lift. Most women have a healthy, adequate amount of upper thigh fat. Eliminates additional visible scars.
- **Disadvantages:** Scar on upper thigh.
- **Risks:** Potential seroma or loss of donor flap due to necrosis.

Selecting an Autologous Reconstruction Procedure

Autologous reconstruction has many options. If you are considering using your own tissues, your surgeon will review your health history and physical makeup; then, along with your personal desire, recommend the surgery most appropriate for you. Autologous procedures require additional hospitalization time, and recovery is longer than with implants; but, unlike implants, after the procedure is successfully completed, your new breast will not require special imaging and will last a lifetime.

Autologous Reconstruction Recovery:

- Requires assistance for several days when you return home
- Requires returning home with 3 – 4 bulb drains that require emptying for 4 – 10 days
- Requires 6 weeks of healing before returning to strenuous activities
- Requires 4 – 6 weeks before returning to work (extra time needed for a job requiring physical exertion)
- Causes bruising that may last up to six weeks
- Causes swelling in the reconstructed breast and donor site for several months
- Causes numbness in the reconstructed breast and donor site that may persist for 6 – 12 months
- Causes most women to feel emotionally down during early stages of recovery; this subsides when mobility returns

Report to Physician Immediately:

- Body temperature elevation above 100.5°
- Reconstructed breast or flap donor site that feels warm or has skin color changes
- Breast or flap donor site that begins to swell quickly or has a sudden increase in pain
- Infection (redness or colored drainage) in the area of an incision or drain insertion site

Self-Care After Reconstruction:

- Take sponge baths for several days. Ask your surgeon when you can shower. Tub baths are not recommended for the first two weeks.
- Use a mild soap when bathing. Do not scrub the surgical incisions with a washcloth.
- Pat your skin dry after bathing with a towel around the surgical incisions before applying a bandage or clothing. A hairdryer set on cool can speed the drying process.
- Change your bandage as directed to keep the area(s) clean and dry.
- Take prescribed antibiotics until **all** tablets have been taken.
- Take prescribed pain medication as needed; do not drive while using prescription medication.
- Avoid alcohol while on prescription medication.
- Switch to extra strength Tylenol® or ibuprofen as soon as possible.
- Do not smoke.
- Do not lift objects weighing over 5 pounds for three weeks.
- Do not sleep on the reconstructed breast for three weeks.
- Get out of bed on the opposite side of your reconstruction.
- Begin exercises to restore your range of motion by stretching, when given permission.
- Plan to remain physically active by taking daily walks.

Balancing and Touch Up

Several months after reconstructive surgery, the surgeon will decide if some minor balancing or touch-up procedures will improve the cosmetic appearance of the breast. This is also the time that the contralateral (remaining) breast can be surgically repaired to match the reconstructed breast. For women who prefer not to undergo additional surgery, an adhesive nipple prosthesis is available to provide the appearance of a nipple under clothing.

Nipple and Areola Reconstruction

The nipple is usually reconstructed from existing skin on the breast, or occasionally from tissues removed from other areas of the body, such as the thigh. The skin is cut and molded to form the shape of the nipple and sutured to the breast mound. Nipple reconstruction is usually performed approximately six months after reconstruction or when breast symmetry is satisfactory. Surgery is outpatient, and the procedure has minimal pain.

Nipple and Areola Reconstruction

1. SKIN FLAP
Surgeon cuts some of the skin and soft tissue on the breast mound to form a new nipple.

2. NIPPLE FORMED
Surgeon wraps tissues around each other to form reconstructed nipple.

3. SUTURES
Surgeon sutures new nipple into place.

4. TATTOOING
After the nipple heals, the areola is added by tattooing to match the opposite breast.

Various other techniques, including skin grafts from other parts of the body, may be used. Most often, though, surgeons use a local skin flap. Ask your surgeon which technique will be used.

Several months after nipple reconstruction, the areola is most often added by tattooing a dark pigmented color around the nipple to match the other areola.

Nipple-Sharing Reconstruction

Nipple-sharing is a breast reconstruction procedure that may be an option if the non-surgical breast nipple is of adequate size to divide. The procedure removes half of the nipple on the non-surgical, healthy breast and grafts it to the reconstructed breast to create a nipple. Nipple-sharing allows a reconstructive surgeon to match the size, shape, color, texture and projection of the opposite breast. This is a safe, reliable technique that provides the best possible match for the newly reconstructed breast.

3D Nipple and Areola Tattooing

A new method of restoring the nipple and areola is 3D tattooing. A skilled tattoo artist creates a three-dimensional nipple by using shading to create the illusion of a protruding nipple, which eliminates the need for surgical reconstruction. An Internet search will help you locate a tattoo artist in your area who specializes in 3D tattooing.

Reconstruction Limitations

Breast reconstruction restores the shape of the breast and increases self-image for most women. However, it does not restore normal breast sensation; your reconstructed breast will not provide you the same kind of pleasure as before surgery. For most women, breast reconstruction helps them to feel more attractive and enjoy sex more because they are not self-conscious about a missing breast.

A year after autologous surgery, approximately half of patients may begin to experience some feeling in their breast—changes in temperature and pressure. The feeling returns because the nerves on the chest wall have grown into the new flap tissues. This does not restore sexual sensations, but the tissues begin to have some feeling.

Making Your Final Decision

Choosing to have breast reconstruction is an individual decision that only you can make. Carefully consider all of your reconstructive options while keeping your mind focused on the question, *"How do I want my body to look a year from now?"* You deserve every opportunity to feel completely whole again. Patients often share that it was the toughest decision to make—facing additional surgery—but one that they do not regret. Seize the opportunity to restore your body image.

Reconstruction Procedures Comparison Charts

There are many breast reconstruction options available. Each procedure has advantages and disadvantages. The wide selection of procedures available often causes confusion when a patient tries to decide which procedure best suits her needs. To help with your decision-making process, please refer to the *Comparison of Breast Reconstruction Procedures* charts beginning on page 62.

Reconstruction Timelines

Patients often ask about the timing of reconstruction procedures in regard to breast cancer treatment. The *Breast Reconstruction Timeline Estimates* chart on page 64 provides estimated reconstruction timelines for patients having:

- Mastectomy with no planned chemotherapy or radiation
- Mastectomy with planned chemotherapy and/or radiation

Comparison of Breast Reconstruction Procedures

Type	Procedure	Advantages	Disadvantages	Recommended	Not Recommended
Implant Procedures					

Tissue Expander
 	
Followed By
 	
Saline or Silicone Fixed-Volume Implant
	▪ Expander placed under muscle
	▪ Saline fillings for 4-6 months to expand
	▪ 2nd surgery required for fixed-volume implant placement
		▪ Shorter surgical and recovery time compared to autologous reconstruction	▪ No immediate breast mound
			▪ Multiple saline fillings required
			▪ 2nd surgery for implant
			▪ MRI surveillance (silicone)
			▪ Replacement: 10–15 years
			▪ Risks:
			  • Capsular contracture
			  • Leakage or rupture
				▪ Medium-sized breast
				▪ Bilateral reconstruction
				▪ Women not wanting major reconstructive surgery
					▪ Future radiation therapy planned
					▪ Some physicians may place expander during breast surgery but not fill until radiation is completed

Direct-to-Implant
 	
Saline or Silicone Fixed-Volume Implant Only
	▪ Fixed-volume implant placed at surgery	▪ Immediate breast mound
		▪ One surgical procedure
		▪ No filling of expander required
			▪ Replacement: 10–15 years
			▪ Potential revisions needed
			▪ MRI surveillance (silicone)
			▪ Risks:
			  • Capsular contracture
			  • Leakage or rupture
				▪ Skin-sparing mastectomy
				▪ Nipple-sparing mastectomy
				▪ Bilateral reconstruction
					▪ Future radiation therapy planned

Abdominal Procedures					

TRAM Flap
 	
Transverse **R**ectus **A**bdominis **M**yocutaneous
 	
Pedicle Flap
	▪ Abdominal: skin, fat, muscle
	▪ Flap blood vessels remain connected
	▪ Flap tunnelled under skin to mastectomy site
		▪ Instant breast mound
		▪ Microsurgery not required
		▪ Improves abdominal contour
		▪ Can match larger opposite breast in size and drooping
			▪ Scar on abdomen
			▪ Difficulty standing up straight for a few days because of muscle transfer
			▪ Abdominal weakness
			▪ Risks:
			  • Seroma
			  • Hernia
			  • Flap necrosis
				▪ Mastectomy
				▪ Women with extra abdominal fat
					▪ Previous scarring from surgical procedures in area of flap
					▪ Women requiring strong abdominal muscle, if muscle is used
					▪ Smokers
					▪ Certain medical conditions

Free TRAM
 	
Transverse **R**ectus **A**bdominis **M**yocutaneous
 	
Free Flap With or Without Muscle
	▪ Abdominal: skin, fat, with or without muscle
	▪ Flap blood vessels cut
	▪ Free flap moved to mastectomy site
	▪ Microsurgery to reattach blood vessels required
		▪ Instant breast mound
		▪ Improves abdominal contour
		▪ Can match larger opposite breast in size and drooping
			▪ Scar on abdomen
			▪ Difficulty standing up straight for a few days because of muscle transfer
			▪ Requires microsurgery
			▪ Abdominal weakness
			▪ Risks:
			  • Hernia
			  • Flap necrosis
				▪ Mastectomy
				▪ Women with extra abdominal fat
					▪ Previous scarring from surgical procedures in area of flap
					▪ Women requiring strong abdominal muscle for activities
					▪ Smokers
					▪ Certain medical conditions

DIEP
 	
Deep **I**nferior **E**pigastric **P**erforator
 	
Free Flap
	▪ Abdominal: skin, fat
	▪ Flap blood vessels cut
	▪ Free flap moved to mastectomy site
	▪ Microsurgery to reattach blood vessels required
		▪ Instant breast mound
		▪ Abdominal muscle cut, but not moved
		▪ Improves abdominal contour
			▪ Scar on abdomen
			▪ Requires microsurgery
			▪ Risks:
			  • Seroma
			  • Flap necrosis
				▪ Mastectomy
				▪ Women with extra abdominal fat
					▪ Previous scarring from surgical procedures in area of flap
					▪ Smokers
					▪ Certain medical conditions

SIEA
 	
Superficial **I**nferior **E**pigastric **A**rtery
 	
Free Flap
	▪ Abdominal: skin, fat
	▪ Flap blood vessels cut
	▪ Free flap moved to mastectomy site
	▪ Microsurgery to reattach blood vessels required
		▪ Instant breast mound
		▪ Abdominal muscle not moved
		▪ Improves abdominal contour
			▪ Scar on abdomen
			▪ Requires microsurgery
			▪ Risks:
			  • Seroma
			  • Flap necrosis
				▪ Mastectomy
				▪ Women with extra abdominal fat
					▪ Previous scarring from surgical procedures in area of flap
					▪ Smokers
					▪ Certain physical conditions

Comparison of Breast Reconstruction Procedures

Type	Procedure	Advantages	Disadvantages	Recommended	Not Recommended
Back Procedures					
LD Latissimus Dorsi **Pedicle Flap**	■ Back: skin, fat, muscle ■ Flap blood vessels remain connected ■ Flap tunnelled under skin to mastectomy site and sutured	■ Potential option for a smoker ■ Low capsular contracture rate ■ Microsurgery not required	■ Scar on back ■ Muscle cut and transferred, causing shoulder weakness ■ Implant may be needed for volume ■ Risks: • Seroma • Flap necrosis	■ Small to medium-sized breast ■ Lumpectomy defect ■ Cosmetic surgery defect ■ Previous abdominal scarring ■ Previous radiation therapy	■ Women requiring strong shoulder muscles for activities (golf, swimming, tennis)
TAP Thoracodorsal Artery Perforator **Pedicle Flap**	■ Back: skin and fat only ■ Blood vessels remain connected ■ Flap tunnelled under skin to mastectomy site and sutured	■ No muscle removed from back	■ Scar on back ■ Risks: • Minor shoulder weakness • Seroma • Flap necrosis	■ Women needing additional skin or fat tissue ■ Lumpectomy site ■ Cosmetic surgery defect	■ Extremely thin, limited body fat
Buttocks Procedures					
SGAP Superior Gluteal Artery Perforator **Free Flap**	■ Buttock: skin, fat ■ Flap blood vessels cut ■ Flap moved to mastectomy site ■ Microsurgery to reattach blood vessels	■ Instant breast mound ■ Most women have adequate fatty buttock tissue ■ Scar hidden by underwear	■ Scar at donor site ■ Risks: • Seroma • Flap necrosis	■ Mastectomy ■ Women not candidates for abdominal procedures ■ Bilateral reconstruction	■ Smokers ■ Certain medical conditions
IGAP Inferior Gluteal Artery Perforator **Free Flap**	■ Buttock: skin, fat ■ Flap blood vessels cut ■ Free flap moved to mastectomy site ■ Microsurgery to reattach blood vessels	■ Instant breast mound ■ Most women have adequate fatty buttock tissue ■ Scar located in lower buttock crease	■ Scar at donor site ■ Risks: • Seroma • Flap necrosis	■ Mastectomy ■ Women not candidates for abdominal procedures ■ No abdominal fat ■ Bilateral reconstruction	■ Smokers ■ Certain medical conditions
Thigh Procedures					
TUG Transverse Upper Gracilis **Free Flap With Muscle**	■ Inner thigh: skin, fat, small amount of muscle ■ Flap blood vessels cut ■ Free flap moved to mastectomy site ■ Microsurgery to reattach blood vessels	■ Instant breast mound ■ Thigh tissues are rarely damaged from previous surgical procedures	■ Scar at donor site ■ Risks: • Seroma • Flap necrosis	■ Bilateral mastectomy ■ Women not candidates for abdominal procedures ■ Bilateral reconstruction	■ Smokers ■ Certain medical conditions
PAP Profunda Artery Perforator **Free Flap With Muscle**	■ Upper thigh: skin, fat ■ Flap blood vessels cut ■ Free flap moved to mastectomy site ■ Microsurgery to reattach blood vessels	■ Instant breast mound ■ Thigh tissues are rarely damaged from previous surgical procedures	■ Scar at donor site ■ Risks: • Seroma • Flap necrosis	■ Bilateral mastectomy ■ Women not candidates for abdominal procedures ■ Bilateral reconstruction	■ Smokers ■ Certain medical conditions

Breast Reconstruction Timeline Estimates
(Timelines vary according to each individual patient, as well as surgeon's preference.)

Mastectomy With No Chemotherapy or Radiation Planned		
Mastectomy + Tissue Expander	**Nipple Sparing Mastectomy *** **+ Direct-to-Implant**	**Mastectomy + Autologous Flap**
4 to 6 Months Later ↓	3 to 6 Months Later ↓	3 to 6 Months Later ↓
Expander Removed / Implant Placed	**Balancing & Touch-up Procedures**** *(If wanted/needed)*	**Balancing & Touch-up Procedures **** *(If wanted/needed)*
3 Months Later ↓		3 - 4 Months Later ↓
Balancing & Touch-up Procedures ** *(If wanted/needed)*		**Nipple Reconstruction**
3 Months Later ↓		6 - 8 Weeks Later ↓
Nipple Reconstruction		**Areola Reconstruction**
6 - 8 Weeks Later ↓		
Areola Reconstruction		

* Direct-to-implant surgery performed with mastectomy that removes nipple and areola; requires reconstruction of the nipple and areola.
** Opposite breast: breast lift, reduction or augmentation; reconstructed breast repositioning; fat transfers for contour correction.

Mastectomy With Chemotherapy and/or Radiation Planned	
Mastectomy + Chemotherapy	**Mastectomy + Chemotherapy + Radiation**
Mastectomy + Tissue Expander	**Mastectomy + Tissue Expander**
4 to 8 Weeks Later ↓	4 to 8 Weeks Later ↓
Chemotherapy (8 to 18 Weeks) *	**Chemotherapy (8 to 18 Weeks) ***
2 to 6 Months Later ↓	4 to 8 Weeks Later ↓
Implant Exchange(s) **	**Radiation (5 to 7 Weeks)**
3 to 6 Months Later ↓	3 to 12 Months Later ↓
Balancing & Touch-up Procedures **** *(If wanted/needed)*	**Flap Procedure ***** *DIEP, SIEA, TRAM, Latissimus Dorsi, PAP, TUG*
3 Months Later ↓	3 to 6 Months Later ↓
Nipple Reconstruction	**Balancing & Touch-up Procedures ****** *(If wanted/needed)*
6 to 8 Weeks Later ↓	3 Months Later ↓
Areola Reconstruction (with Tattoo)	**Nipple Reconstruction**
	6 to 8 Weeks Later ↓
	Areola Reconstruction (With Tattoo)

* Reconstruction can usually proceed with long-term therapies like Tamoxifen or Herceptin.
** An autologous flap can be used instead of an implant.
*** Occasionally an implant may still be an option.
**** Opposite breast: breast lift, reduction or augmentation; reconstructed breast repositioning; fat transfers for contour correction.

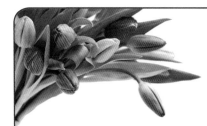

Remember...

- *Breast reconstruction can be performed using synthetic implants placed under the chest muscle, or by using your own body tissues.*

- *Each type of breast reconstruction procedure has advantages and disadvantages. Timing of reconstruction can be immediate, performed at the time of your cancer surgery, or delayed to a later time.*

- *If you are scheduled for a mastectomy, a consultation with a reconstructive surgeon **prior** to your cancer surgery is recommended, even if you are planning delayed reconstruction. A consultation allows the surgeon to evaluate your personal medical history, cancer history and physical makeup to offer recommended options for reconstruction.*

- *If you are feeling overwhelmed after reviewing your reconstructive options, you do not have to make a decision now. Reconstruction can be performed at a later date, even years later.*

Additional Information

Tear-out Worksheets
Reconstructive Decision Evaluation - page 266
Reconstructive Surgery Questions - page 267

Reconstruction Information
To read explanations of DIEP and SGAP procedures, check timelines and see
before and after photos, visit:www.mauricenahabedian.com or www.diepflap.com.

Thoughts to Ponder...

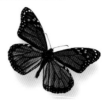

Appreciating all of life, we can see painful events as opportunities, for those are the moments that truly stretch us and expand us to grow and deepen beyond who we think ourselves to be.

In what may seem the worst of times, when we face loss, or tragedy, we discover our heroism, our courage, our love, our creativity, and our power.

These seemingly catastrophic experiences are occasions to stretch ourselves beyond whoever we have been up to now and to play life full-out. These are profound challenges.

—Judy Tatelbaum

Loss in our lives causes us to stop and review what we have and where we are. At this point, we can learn how we can grow and how we can make our lives more rewarding as a result of the experience.

—Judy Kneece

The storms of life cause the oak trees to develop deeper roots. Life's problems cause us to become stronger and more sensitive human beings, if we take the opportunity to grow and learn from our experiences.

—Judy Kneece

If you insist on seeing with perfect clarity before you make a decision, you'll never decide. The future always looks like fog; only when you are on the other side can you see what was previously hidden from view.

—Judy Kneece

Plan to monitor your self-talk. Be careful about what your mind is saying to you. Your thoughts become a self-fulfilling prophecy. When we think "I just can't cope with this situation," we lose our energy to even try. When we tell ourself "I can get through this" or "I will survive this," we find our energy return and we are ready to take on the challenge. You can become your own survival coach by saying encouraging words to yourself. Try monitoring your self-talk and see what happens.

—Judy Kneece

CHAPTER 9

The Surgical Experience

"I wanted to approach my surgery for double mastectomies and immediate reconstruction with a positive attitude. I didn't want to go into a seven-hour surgery afraid and crying. I decided to turn my emotional state around and not focus on what I was losing, but rather, what I was gaining. So, on the day of surgery, I walked into the hospital with a pink tiara and a pink boa . . . ready to show this cancer that I was tougher and stronger than it was. I had everyone smiling and chuckling and I heard shouts of, 'You go girl!' as I passed by. I was determined to kick cancer's booty."

—*Lisa DelGuidice*

Preparation for surgery begins with your first visit to the breast surgeon. During this visit, your surgeon will carefully review all previous reports, including your diagnostic mammography report, biopsy pathology report and any other studies performed. A careful personal and family history will be taken. A physical exam, including a breast exam, will be performed. After gathering all of this information, the surgeon will ask about your personal preferences for surgery and determine whether you desire reconstruction. Surgical recommendations will then be discussed by the surgeon.

It is helpful to prepare for this visit by having all needed personal and family history information readily available. Some patients find it helpful to write this information down before the visit. Information your surgeon will need includes:

- **Medical History**: Dates of major illnesses and surgeries; allergies; family history of breast cancer.

- **Current Medical Providers**: Names and contact information of other specialists treating you, such as a cardiologist or pulmonologist.

- **Self-Care Limitations**: Physical limitations that would prevent you from being able to care for yourself at home after surgery. If you have limitations, a home health service may need to be ordered to assist you for a short period of time after you return home.

- **Current Medications**: List of all prescription and over-the-counter medications, vitamins, minerals and herbal products you currently take. This is essential because some medications increase the potential for bleeding and need to be discontinued before surgery.

"Probably the most alone I have ever felt was the five minutes after my husband left my side before I went into surgery. Alone, scared of the unknown, so afraid. I felt like my heart was going to beat out of my chest. But then the anesthesia took effect and I went to sleep, and what seemed like minutes later, my surgeon was waking me up. In reality it was 8 hours later! Brian also says this was the hardest time for him."
—*Anna Cluxton*

- Over-the-counter medications that increase bleeding include:
  - » Aspirin (Check labels for commonly used terms for aspirin which include ASA, acetylsalicylic acid or salicylates.)
  - » Ibuprofen (Advil®, Motrin®)
  - » Naproxen (Aleve®, Midol®)
  - » Gingko biloba
  - » Garlic
  - » Ginseng
  - » Fish oil
  - » Dong quai
  - » Feverfew

Pre-Admission Assessment

Shortly before surgery, you will be scheduled for a pre-admission physical assessment. A nurse will ask you about your physical and medical history. Pre-admission testing will include a blood test, urinalysis, possibly an electrocardiogram and any other tests your physician may think are necessary. Remember to take your insurance card when going for this assessment.

It is now customary for everyone entering a hospital to be asked if they have a living will before being admitted. If you have a living will, healthcare directives or any special instructions, take them with you to be attached to your chart the day of surgery.

During the assessment, you will be given instructions about any special preparations before surgery. For example, you will be told not to eat or drink after midnight before your surgery and to stop smoking as early before surgery as possible. Ask the nurse if you should take any of your regular medications the morning of surgery. If instructed to take a medication in pill form before surgery, take it with a small swallow of water. If you take insulin, you may want to contact the physician who normally manages your insulin dosage for instructions on dosage the morning of the surgery.

You will be told what time you need to arrive before your surgery and the scheduled time of your surgery. Ask if there are any restrictions on the number of people allowed to wait in the surgical waiting room. Your next step is to prepare for the day of surgery.

Hospitalization Packing Suggestions:

- Personal hygiene items: comb, brush, toothbrush, toothpaste, deodorant, makeup and shampoo
- Robe and pajamas (front-opening); undergarments (2 - 3 changes); bedroom shoes
- Reading material
- Cell phone and charger
- Pencil and note paper
- Small travel pillow (to elevate your arm while in the hospital and to place under your seat belt)
- Clothes to wear home (a large, soft sweatshirt or loose-fitting, front-opening top is most comfortable; flat, comfortable shoes are also recommended)
- Bra: Ask your surgeon if they will supply a post-operative surgical bra. If not, you may wish to bring your own bra.
  - **Lumpectomy Patients** need a soft, well-fitting, front-closing bra to wear after surgery to reduce post-surgical pain. Many women find a cotton sports bra is a good choice. It is suggested that you purchase two or more because you will be wearing a bra 24 hours a day during your recovery.
  - **Mastectomy Patients** have several options. Some women prefer not to wear a bra until all of their surgical dressings are removed. A loose sweatshirt or front-opening, dark-colored blouse is a good option during this time. Others prefer to wear a bra and insert a light fiber filling into the bra cup to

match the other breast. After the bandages are removed, a soft bra with no underwires is needed so that the bra will not rub the incision. A cotton sports bra is a good choice. Soft cotton camisoles, designed with a pocket for the fiber filling and pockets to hold your surgical drain bulbs, can be purchased online or at a prosthesis shop. These camisoles are also recommended for women undergoing radiation therapy.

- **Reconstructive Patients** need to ask their surgeon for a recommendation.

Surgery Day Support

It will be helpful to have someone with you. A family member or friend will be able to assist you and make this time more comfortable by providing emotional and psychological support and helping you as needed.

Reporting for Surgery

On the day of surgery you will need to report to the surgery area at the assigned time. Leave your money, credit cards and checkbook at home or with a family member. Do not wear jewelry (watches, rings, earrings) or contact lenses. Wear eyeglasses, if needed, because you will need to read and sign admission and consent forms. Dental devices can be worn and removed just prior to your surgery. The nurse will place them in a special storage container during surgery and they will be made available to you as soon as you wake up.

Informed Consent

Shortly before surgery, you will be asked to sign an informed consent form. Your physician or an assistant will explain the information contained in the consent form. This explanation will occur before you are given any sedating medications. Read the consent form carefully before signing. Signing the form means that you understand the information. Consent forms will also be presented for your signature before chemotherapy, radiation therapy or reconstructive surgery. Information on the informed consent form will include:

- Type of surgery or treatment you will receive
- Name of the doctor who will perform the surgery or provide treatment
- Risks and benefits of the surgery or treatment
- Identification of any experimental treatments

Events Prior to Surgery

Your medical history will be reviewed again before surgery. Inform your nurse if any changes in your health have occurred since the initial assessment (cold, fever, diarrhea, etc.).

After changing into a hospital gown, an intravenous (I.V.) needle will be inserted into the arm opposite of the surgical site for medication and fluid administration. If the anesthesiologist (a physician who puts you to sleep) has not talked to you previously, they will talk to you before you go into surgery. Medication will be administered through the I.V. port to relax you. A family member will be allowed to stay with you until you are taken to the operating room.

After you are positioned on the surgical table, a blood pressure cuff will be placed on your arm to monitor your blood pressure, a device will be placed on your finger to measure the oxygen in your blood, and adhesive pads connected to an electrocardiogram machine will be placed on your chest to monitor your heart rate.

Anesthesia will be administered through your I.V. during this process. After you go to sleep, a tube will be placed in your throat to help you breathe.

The surgeon will then cleanse a large area surrounding the surgical incision site, and the surgery will be performed.

Events Immediately After Surgery

When the surgical procedure is completed, you will be transferred to a recovery room. Your blood pressure, oxygen level and heart rate will continue to be monitored. The length of time in the recovery room may be two or more hours, depending on the type of anesthesia you received.

When you are awake and your vital signs are in normal range, you will be transferred to your room, if staying overnight. If staying in the hospital, your blood pressure, pulse and breathing rate will continue to be monitored at regular intervals. If you are having outpatient surgery, you may be transferred to an outpatient recovery room and monitored for several more hours before being discharged. Your family members will be able to join you during this time.

After you wake up from surgery, you may have a slight headache or nausea from the residual anesthesia. This is not unusual and is often caused by the long period of time without food or caffeine. A nurse will administer pain or nausea medication, if needed, and offer you something to drink.

You may notice that your throat feels sore when swallowing. The soreness is caused by the tube that was inserted to keep your airways open during surgery. Soreness in the back or shoulder area is another common post-surgical problem because of the position you were placed in during surgery. This soreness will last for several days.

Surgical Dressing and Drain Bulbs

Most patients have a surgical gauze dressing on their chest and may have one or more surgical drain bulbs. Drain bulbs are used to drain lymphatic fluid from the surgical site. Some types of surgery may not require a drain. At first, the drainage will be bright red from blood, but it will gradually change to a light straw color over the next few days. If, at any time, you notice that your bandage feels wet or you see bright red blood coming through your bandage, notify your physician. Drains usually remain in place when you return home and are removed at a later time.

Discomfort After Surgery

Most women are surprised at the small amount of pain they experience after breast cancer surgery. Pain medication is placed on order for the hospital nurses to administer if you are hospitalized. You must request the pain medication from the nurse when needed. If you are going home on the day of surgery, you will be given a prescription for pain medication. When you begin to feel uncomfortable, take pain medication as prescribed. Do not wait until pain is severe because severe pain can increase other post-operative symptoms, such as nausea. Your goal is to take what you need to be as comfortable as possible. Remember, there are no rewards for suffering unnecessarily.

The pain experienced after breast surgery has been described as a generalized discomfort in the breast area, accompanied by numbness or tingling in the arm. Some women have reported sensations from the nipple or feeling pain in the removed breast that felt like a heaviness. Doctors call this "phantom pain" because even though the breast is gone, the brain perceives the sensation of pain from the remaining nerves. Some of the nerves on the chest wall may be irritated or cut during the surgical procedure, which can cause a feeling of numbness across the chest. Most women state that the greatest surgical discomfort was under the arm where the lymph nodes were removed. This pain often radiates down the arm, and you may feel as if needles or pins are pricking you. These pricking sensations will improve over the coming months. The arm may also feel numb, which is not unusual. Incisional pain is usually gone in a week to ten days, and the arm sensations will improve as arm mobility is restored. For additional information, refer to the *Surgical Discharge Questions* on page 269.

Seat Belt Use After Surgery

On the car ride home after surgery, place your travel pillow between the seat belt and your surgical incision. The pressure of a seat belt during sudden stops can cause pain and potential injury to the mastectomy or lumpectomy area. Continue using the pillow for several weeks when wearing a seat belt.

Personal Hygiene After Surgery

Most women return home with some type of dressing covering their incision. If you have a gauze dressing, it is important to keep it dry. If the dressing becomes wet, it will need to be changed. Damp dressings that remain over the incision can cause a local infection. Follow your physician's recommendations for bathing and shampooing your hair. Do not use deodorant under the surgical arm for the first several weeks, or until your incision heals. You may wipe the area with an alcohol pad if you feel a need to cleanse the area. Do not allow the alcohol to run into the surgical incision, because it will sting.

Post-Surgical Arm Care:

- Use the hand on the side of your surgery to feed yourself, comb your hair and wash your face if surgery was on your dominant side. These activities will help reduce the soreness.
- Keep your surgical arm propped up on a pillow above the level of your heart when lying down to prevent fluid accumulation. Fluid accumulation increases swelling and pain in the arm.
- Place a small pillow between your surgical arm and your body to keep the arm from pressing tightly against the body. This position also promotes drainage and reduces swelling.
- Do not lift anything over 1 – 2 pounds or begin exercising until your physician gives you permission.
- Get in and out of your bed on the side opposite your surgery.
- Elevate your arm above the level of your heart for 45 minutes twice daily for the first six weeks.

Your Surgical Incision

A lumpectomy will leave an incision on the breast and another under the arm if lymph nodes were removed. Mastectomy will leave a single scar. Your surgical incision(s) may be closed with sutures, staples or skin glue with Steri-Strips™.

Your first dressing change will occur before you leave the hospital unless you have outpatient surgery—in which case, it will occur when you return to the physician's office. Some women report it was difficult to view the incision for the first time, but afterward they were glad they did. Viewing the incision may also be difficult for your partner. Many women felt that viewing the incision together the first time was helpful for their future adjustment. Postponing the viewing does not make it easier for either of you.

It is important that you observe the incision area carefully to learn what is normal for the scar area. This will help as you monitor the incision for changes after you return home. Since it is difficult to change a dressing on your own chest, it will be helpful if a family member is present during the instructions to help you understand and be able to assist you with dressing changes and managing drains. If your incision(s) is closed with skin glue, home dressing changes are usually not required. If dressing changes are needed, ask your nurse for dressing supplies to take home with you when you are discharged.

Surgical Dressing Care

If you have a surgical dressing, the goal is to keep it clean and dry. A wet dressing creates an environment for bacteria to breed and may cause an infection. If your dressing becomes damp, follow your physician's instructions for changing it. If you have sutures or staples, they will be removed in the surgeon's office five to ten days after surgery. If you have skin glue and Steri-Strips™, the strips will be allowed to fall off naturally.

When changing your dressing, observe the old bandage for signs of drainage. Normal drainage is a blood-tinged, watery discharge. Discharge that is thick and yellowish to greenish in color may be a sign of infection. Often, this type of discharge will have a foul odor. If you notice this occurring, notify your healthcare provider.

Dressing Change Instructions:

- Gather all dressing supplies: disposable bag, dressing, tape, scissors, alcohol wipes or gauze pads.
- Wash your hands.
- Pre-cut tape into strips to apply to the new dressing.
- Remove the old dressing and record the color, any odor and the amount of drainage on the dressing.
- Place the removed dressing in the disposable bag. Wash your hands.
- Observe the incision as you wipe off any blood or tape residue with an alcohol wipe. Always begin by wiping near the incision, and wipe away from the incision. Do not wipe back over the incision.
- Place a clean dressing on the area and tape it into place.
- Dispose of the bag containing the old dressing and alcohol wipes. Wash your hands.

Carefully monitor your incision site. An increase in tenderness, warmth, redness, swelling or signs of discharge anywhere along the incision may indicate a potential infection. Call your physician's office and ask for instructions.

Drain Bulbs

During surgery, the lymphatic system vessels are cut, causing the microscopic lymph vessels to empty fluid into the surgical area. To keep this fluid from accumulating and causing pain, drain bulbs are placed to drain the fluid. Clear tubing with an attached bulb is anchored to the surgical site during surgery to allow the fluid to drain. A plug on the bulb allows collected fluid to be emptied.

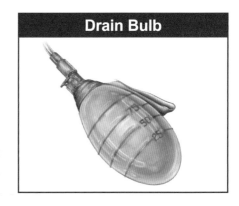

Drain Bulb

The fluid that accumulates in the drain bulb is a mixture of blood cells and lymphatic fluid. The drainage will be dark red at first because of the large amount of blood cells in the area. It will gradually begin to change to a pink-tinged color and finally to a light straw color. The amount of drainage varies, and there is no way to predict how much drainage a woman will accumulate. Some women have a large amount, while others have a minimal amount. Gradually, these small vessels seal themselves off, and the fluid stops accumulating. The time this takes varies among women. Neither body size nor age seems to determine the amount; however, the amount of drainage during the first 24 hours often predicts the future accumulation volume.

Physicians remove drains when the amount of drainage is between 20 to 50 ccs (0.5 to 1.5 ounces; 4 to 10 teaspoons) per drain, per 24 hours. Women with little drainage may have their drains removed the first week. Others may need to keep their drains longer. If the drains are removed too soon, the fluid can accumulate under the skin, forming a seroma (collection of fluid), and become painful if it puts pressure on the surgical site. Neither the amount of fluid produced, nor the length of time you require drains, has anything to do with your cancer. It is only related to the amount of fluid your lymphatic system produces.

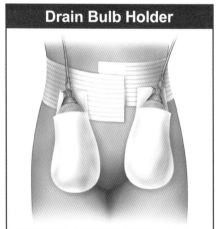

Drain Bulb Holder

It is important not to allow bulb drains to hang loosely or allow drains to drop away from your body. Always secure them to your clothing, and empty them before they become heavy. For this reason, a drain bulb holder or a post-surgical camisole with drain bulb pockets is helpful. Pressure from a heavy drain can pull on your incision site and cause pain and scar formation at the drain insertion site. The scar will heal, but it will be thick and have an uneven appearance.

Emptying and Recording Drainage

Empty drains before they become heavy or over half-filled with fluid. On the first day, your drains may require emptying every several hours. Later, twice a day should be sufficient. If you have more than one drain, place a piece of tape on each one and mark them with a number (drain 1 and drain 2). When you empty a drain, record the drainage amount on your record sheet, indicating which drain bulb was emptied.

Instructions for Emptying Drain Bulbs:

- Gather supplies: a *Drain Bulb Record* (located on page 271), a pen and a measuring cup.
- Remove the plug in one drain bulb and empty the drainage into a measuring cup.
- Squeeze the air out of the empty bulb. Keep the bulb squeezed as flat as possible as you replug the drain. This compression of the bulb encourages the flow of fluid from the surgical site into the bulb.
- Wipe any spilled drainage on the outside of the bulb with a damp, soapy cloth or an alcohol wipe.
- Secure the bulb by pinning it to your clothing or placing it into a surgical drain bulb holder or camisole pocket. Do not allow the bulb to hang freely.
- Measure the drainage that is in the cup.
- Observe the color of the drainage. If you notice that the fluid has changed color, becoming a darker red, or if fresh blood reappears after the color had changed to a light pink, contact your physician's office and inform them of the change.
- Empty the drainage into the toilet, and flush. Do not save the drainage.
- Wash your hands with soap and water.
- Record drainage on your record sheet, documenting the time and the amount emptied.
- If you have a second drain, repeat the process.
- Take the written drain record to the surgeon on your return visit. An accurate record will assist the physician in determining when to remove your drain(s).

Potential Post-Surgical Problems

Fluid Leakage at Drain Site

Occasionally, a small amount of fluid will leak from the insertion site of the drain tubing. This is not alarming. However, you should remove the damp dressing and apply a clean one. Change the dressing as often as needed to prevent irritation of the skin. If large amounts of fluid begin leaking from the site, call your physician and ask for instructions.

Clogged Drains

Bulb drains may clog due to a small blood clot in the tubing. This is not an unusual occurrence. If you notice that there is no fluid in the drain bulb, check the tubing for a possible blockage caused by a clot.

Instructions for Opening a Clogged Drain:

- Wash your hands with soap and water.
- Look for a small clot in the tubing. If one is seen, gently squeeze the tubing over the clot.
- After breaking up the clot, place your fingers on the tubing near the insertion site on your chest and squeeze downward toward the drainage bulb (the entire length of tubing). Do not pull on the tubing. Repeat the process several times.
- Monitor the drain bulb for fluid accumulation. If no drainage accumulates after several hours, notify your physician for further instructions.

Drain Bulb Site Infection

It is very rare for infections to occur at the bulb drain sites. However, if you notice that the insertion site begins to have increased redness, discharge of pus (yellowish or greenish) or has a foul odor, notify your physician of these changes.

Seromas

Before or after your drains are removed, you may notice a lump in an area under the skin, near the incision site on the chest or in the underarm area. This soft, spongy lump that feels like a water balloon is caused by fluid accumulation and is called a seroma. If a seroma continues to increase in size and puts pressure on your incision, it can become painful. This fluid accumulation has nothing to do with your cancer. It is related only to lymphatic fluid accumulation in the area.

Seromas are the most common complication after surgery. Painful seromas may require the withdrawal (aspiration) of the fluid by the surgeon, using a small needle connected to an empty syringe. This procedure is performed in the physician's office. Withdrawal of the fluid is relatively painless, and relieves the pain. However, as with any invasive procedure, the potential for infection increases after aspiration. You will need to monitor the area and report any redness, swelling or pain to your physician. The fluid may continue to accumulate after aspiration and require additional aspirations. Although it is very rare, some patients require surgical opening of the area if fluid continues to accumulate.

Drain Removal

Drains are removed by the surgeon or an assistant during an office visit. During drain removal, a tugging feeling with a moderate amount of pain lasting for a few seconds is felt. A small bandage is placed over the drain removal site. This site will need to be monitored for infection for the next several days.

Recovering at Home

Recovery from breast cancer surgery usually requires two to three weeks. Discomfort in the incisional area(s) will improve daily, usually resolving within ten days. In five to six weeks, most women report that they are able to resume their normal activities. Remember, we all heal differently. Listen to the cues from your body, rest when needed and resume your normal activities when your energy returns.

Your incision will change color as it heals; this is normal. The surgical scar will be red and raised for several months following surgery. The redness is caused by the additional blood flow in the area to promote healing. The redness and thickness of the scar will subside over the next one to two years, and the area will become less obvious and very faint in color.

Plan to begin your arm exercise program to restore your normal range of motion in the surgical arm as soon as the physician gives you permission. Report any problems you have when performing the exercises to your physician. Refer to *Surgical Arm Exercises* beginning on page 279 for illustrated exercise samples.

It is important that you keep your post-surgery, follow-up appointments. You will be monitored for proper healing and for the return of full range of motion in your surgical arm.

Uncommon Post-Surgical Problems

Most women have very few problems after breast surgery. However, there are some uncommon surgical procedure problems that you may need to be aware of. These problems have nothing to do with the cancer and are only due to the surgery.

Phlebitis

Occasionally, some women will have very little pain after their surgery only to experience increased pain that begins days after surgery. The pain may radiate down the arm, usually to the elbow, but sometimes to the wrist. This occurs when the basilic vein in the arm becomes inflamed after surgery. This inflammation, called phlebitis, is not serious, but it causes pain that can be relieved with an analgesic such as aspirin or ibuprofen. Phlebitis will resolve in several days to a week. This pain may limit your ability to perform your arm exercises. Inform your physician if you experience phlebitis.

Breast Sensations

During the surgical healing process, it is common to experience a variety of sensations. The brain interprets the signals from the remaining nerves on the chest wall and may cause some patients to experience a sensation of pins and needles, itching, pressure or extreme skin sensitivity to clothing or touch.

If you experience these sensations after mastectomy and they become bothersome, inform your physician. Ice packs are usually helpful, but check with your physician before using them. Physical therapists are trained to treat these symptoms with a procedure called desensitization. Desensitization decreases the sensations from the nerve endings remaining in the area. The therapist can instruct you on how to perform the procedure at home and, if needed, it can become part of your daily exercise routine. Massage of the area may also be recommended. If the sensation does not decrease, medications may be prescribed by your physician. This is a time-limited problem that usually resolves as healing progresses.

Frozen Shoulder

Failure to restore your range of motion after the physician has given you permission to begin exercises can result in a condition called frozen shoulder. This condition causes pain and the inability to move the shoulder freely. Frozen shoulder is directly related to the lack of arm movement. Any complication that can keep you from performing your arm exercises should be brought to the surgeon's attention. Restoring full range of motion is accomplished by gradually increasing arm movements and performing surgical arm exercises such as the ones beginning on page 279.

Shoulder Bursitis

After breast surgery, some patients experience pain that radiates to the chest area and, less frequently, to the shoulder. This pain may be caused by shoulder bursitis. The bursa is a sac of lubricating fluid located in the shoulder. The sac becomes inflamed due to lying flat with the arm extended during breast surgery. Anti-inflammatory medications can help reduce pain. If pain is severe, cortisone injections into the bursa area may be required.

"I had never had such a serious surgery (bilateral mastectomies with immediate implant reconstruction), so I didn't know what to expect. At first, I questioned why I was so tired when all I was doing was resting on the couch. My sister, a nurse, explained that the fatigue was VERY normal. Being under anesthesia for seven hours takes a great toll on the body. My body needed time to heal. This was hard for me to accept, as I was always so vibrant and full of energy. But I learned that I had to be patient with my body. Week by week, my energy increased, and eventually my 'old self' came back."

—Lisa DelGuidice

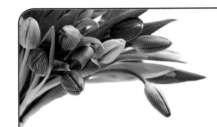

Remember...

- *Surgery for breast cancer is usually not very physically painful, but it may be very emotionally painful.*

- *Ask your healthcare team for what you need to make this time as easy as possible for you—additional information or instructions, pain medication, access to a chaplain, etc. You are employing them to meet your needs.*

- *Tell your support partner, family or friends how they can be helpful during this time. Be honest.*

- *Do not hesitate to call your physician if any problems arise when you return home.*

- *Use your surgical recovery time to rekindle your emotions and energy. Rest when needed. Be good to yourself. Think about any changes you would like to make in your life. At no other time in life will people give you as much permission to make changes.*

Additional Information

Tear-out Worksheets
Drain Bulb Record - page 271
Surgical Discharge Questions - page 269
Surgical Arm Exercises - page 279

Your Pathology Report

"I was serious about wanting to know about breast cancer. I wanted to be a part of my treatments. I wanted to know what was being done and why. The secrets to my individual tumor lay in my final pathology report."

—**Harriett Barrineau**

The preliminary pathology report you received after your biopsy contained a lot of information about your cancer. A second, final pathology report will be prepared after your breast cancer surgery. This report will give additional information about your cancer and the status of cancer in your lymph nodes, if any were removed. These two pathology reports will be combined with your personal history, family history and other testing to determine which course of treatment is best for your individual case. The most common treatments after surgery are chemotherapy, targeted therapy, radiation therapy and hormonal therapy. Your treatment may consist of one or more types of treatment. For a few women, no further treatment may be needed after breast cancer surgery, only close surveillance by the physician. A brief explanation of each type of treatment will be discussed in later chapters. Because of the wide variety of treatment plans, your physician will provide you with specific information regarding your planned treatment.

Your Pathology Report

Treatment decisions will be based on your pathology reports. Because your pathology report contains information vital to treatment decisions, it is helpful to understand the major factors that determine how a physician makes treatment recommendations. However, some patients do not want to know these details. If you are a patient who does not want to know every detail, or if you feel overwhelmed with information at this time, feel free to skip this chapter. If at some point in the future you have questions about your pathology report or treatment recommendations, you can refer back to this chapter.

After your tumor is removed from your breast, it will be sent to a pathology laboratory where it will be carefully processed. A pathologist, a physician who specializes in diagnosing diseases from tissue samples, will analyze

"I asked for and kept copies of my pathology reports. Over the years, I have found this to be helpful."
—**Anna Cluxton**

"My doctors explained and then gave me my report. I looked over it, but I wasn't really interested in what was on that piece of paper. There was nothing there that was going to change my circumstances in life one bit. I was more interested in what we were going to do to take care of it."
—**Earnestine Brown**

your tissues. The pathologist will look at the tumor with the naked eye and record what is observed. The tumor will be cut into very small slices and studied under a microscope. From these observations, critical interpretations will be made; and a pathology report will be prepared and sent to your physician. If additional treatment is needed after surgery, the pathology report will be used as a guide for your physicians to develop a treatment plan for your cancer.

In the future, if additional studies are needed or if research unfolds new tissue diagnostic tests, your samples will be available at the pathology lab.

Characteristics of Cancer Cells

Normal ducts and lobules are lined with one or more layers of cells in an orderly pattern. When normal cells become cancerous, they change their appearance. They may remain in the area where they started or they may grow through the wall.

Cancer Will Be Reported As:

- **In Situ Cancer**: Cancer cells are contained within the duct or lobule where they originated. The cancer cells have not grown through the walls and invaded surrounding tissues. Cancer is non-invasive. This type of cancer has a good prognosis.

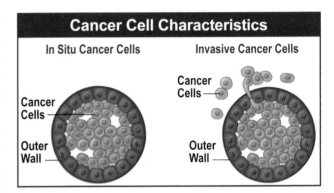

- **Invasive (Infiltrating) Cancer**: Cancer cells have grown through the wall of the duct or lobule and are growing into surrounding tissues. Microinvasive means that only a small amount of cells have grown through the duct or lobular walls.

Types of Breast Cancer

The most common types of breast cancer are listed below. There are also various other rare types of breast cancer and combinations of the following types. The percentage of occurrence shown below is approximate.

- Invasive (infiltrating) ductal (52%)
- Ductal carcinoma in situ (20%)
- Invasive lobular (10%)
- Medullary (6%)
- Inflammatory breast cancer (5%)
- Mucinous or Colloid (3%)
- Lobular carcinoma in situ (2%)
- Tubular (2%)
- Paget disease with intraductal (1%)
- Paget disease with invasive ductal (1%)

Remaining Cancers, Occurring in 1% or Less:

- Cribiform
- Papillary
- Micropapillary
- Adenoid Cystic
- Secretory
- Mixed Ductal and Lobular
- Other Cancers

Tumor Characteristics

Tumor Shape

The shape of the tumor is reported as round, spherical or having irregular contours (edges), such as stellate or spiculated.

Tumor Size

Tumor size is measured at the widest diameter and is reported in millimeters (mm) or centimeters (cm).

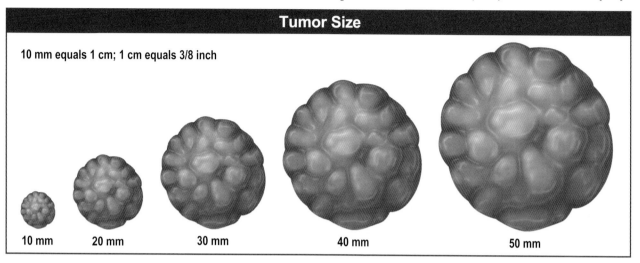

Tumor Size

10 mm equals 1 cm; 1 cm equals 3/8 inch

10 mm   20 mm   30 mm   40 mm   50 mm

Margins

Margins report the shortest distance between a tumor edge and the surgical edge of the tissue removed during surgery.

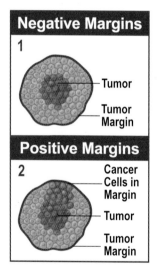

Negative Margins

1 — Tumor / Tumor Margin

Positive Margins

2 — Cancer Cells in Margin / Tumor / Tumor Margin

Pathology Margins May Be Described As:

- **Negative, Clear, Clean or Uninvolved:** There was no evidence of cancer cells in the margins *(illustration 1)*
- **Positive, Involved or Residual Cancer:** Cancer was found in the margins and will probably require more surgery *(illustration 2)*
- **Close:** Cancer cells are close to margins and may require more surgery
- **Indeterminate:** Pathologist could not determine margin status

Lymph Node Status

If your surgery included lymph node removal, the report will state the area from which they were removed, the number of nodes removed and how many nodes tested positive for cancer cells. Nodes are reported as:

- **Lymph Node Negative:** No cancer was found in the lymph nodes
- **Lymph Node Positive:** Cancer was present in the lymph nodes

Nuclear Grade

Nuclear grade reports the size and shape of the nucleus in tumor cells and considers the percentage of tumor cells that are in the process of dividing or growing.

- **Grade 1:** Grow and spread at a slower rate
- **Grade 2:** Grow and spread at a medium rate
- **Grade 3:** Grow and spread at a rapid rate

Cancer Receptors

One of the major pathology studies performed on your tumor will test for receptors on the cancer cell surface. Receptors are like little chairs with different shapes that sit on the surface of all cells, including breast cancer cells. When blood passes a cell, different elements in the blood may be a perfect match in size and shape to fit into the chairs. When an element in the blood fits a cell chair, it sends a signal to the cell to grow. Receptors that influence breast cancer growth include estrogen, progesterone and HER2. These receptors are evaluated during the pathology studies of your tumor.

Prognostic Tests

A variety of marker tests may be performed to look at specific characteristics of the tumor cells, including:

- **Cell Proliferation Rate:** Determines the cancer cells' growth rate and can be evaluated during pathology by:
  - **S-phase Fraction Test:** Identifies the number of cells in the "synthesis phase" (the period right before a cell divides). Counts below 6 percent are considered low; counts of 6 to 10 percent are considered intermediate; counts over 10 percent are considered high.
  - **Ki-67:** A proliferation study that measures a protein in a cell that increases prior to dividing. Study results below 10 percent are considered low; counts of 10 to 20 percent are considered borderline; counts over 20 percent are considered high.

- **Hormone Receptor Assay Test:** Measures the quantity of estrogen (ER) and progesterone (PR) receptors in the tumor cell nuclei. It tells the physician whether the tumor growth was stimulated by female hormones and is very important in determining the type of treatment after surgery. If a tumor is ER or PR positive, it means it was stimulated by estrogen or progesterone hormones.
  - **Tumors May Be:**
    - » ER positive (+) PR positive (+)
    - » ER positive (+) PR negative (-)
    - » ER negative (-) PR positive (+)
    - » ER negative (-) PR negative (-)

- **HER2/neu:** A protein on the cell surface that stimulates cell growth. It is evaluated to determine if it is over-expressed or amplified. Approximately 25 percent of patients have elevated HER2 levels. Elevation of HER2 indicates a more aggressive cancer. For women with HER2 elevation, a targeted therapy, called Herceptin®, targets the HER2/neu receptor and is an appropriate treatment choice.

- **Blood Vessel or Lymphatic Invasion:** Determined by microscopic examination of the tumor. No blood vessel or lymphatic invasion offers a better prognosis. *Note: Lymphatic invasion is different than lymph node involvement.*

- **Multigene Testing:** May be ordered from outside labs for Stage 1 or Stage 2 cancers. Multigene tests may include OncoType DX® or MammaPrint®. These tests analyze a large group of genes that are known to affect cancer aggressiveness. Test results

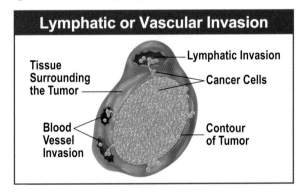

help predict the potential for cancer to spread to other parts of the body or to recur. This information helps physicians determine which patients will benefit from chemotherapy. If ordered, these test results may not be included in the final pathology report, but will be sent to your physician.

Triple Negative Breast Cancer

The term "triple negative" breast cancer describes a woman's cancer that is estrogen negative, progesterone negative and HER2 negative. Many drugs used in cancer treatment target one of these three receptor sites, thus a triple negative breast cancer diagnosis limits the use of some medications. Triple negative women, however, are typically responsive to general chemotherapy drugs that are not specifically targeted at ER/PR or HER2 receptor sites.

Tumor Grading Systems

Tumor grading systems have been developed to evaluate different components of a tumor for levels of potential aggressiveness. Tumor grades are used as a guide for treatment planning. Your pathology report may indicate that one of the following systems was used to grade your tumor.

Ductal Carcinoma In Situ Grading System

Patients diagnosed with ductal carcinoma in situ may have their tumor evaluated with a tumor grading system to determine the most appropriate treatment. A common grading system, The Van Nuys Prognostic Index, evaluates the size, nuclear grade, tumor margins and age as an indicator of tumor aggressiveness.

A score of 1 – 3 is given to each parameter, and the total score is calculated. Final scores may range from 4 – 12. The lower the score, the less aggressive the tumor. Higher scores indicate the need for more aggressive surgery. Physicians use the grading system score to indicate the need for radiation therapy after lumpectomy or for the need for mastectomy for better disease control.

Invasive Carcinoma Grading System

Patients diagnosed with invasive carcinoma tumors may be evaluated with a grading system to determine the most appropriate treatment. A common grading system, The Nottingham Scale (also called the Elston-Ellis modification of the Scarff-Bloom-Richardson grading system), evaluates three tumor characteristics:

- **Tubular Formation:** How much of the tumor is arranged as tubules
- **Nuclear Grade:** Size, shape and color of the nucleus in the tumor cells
- **Mitotic Rate:** How fast the tumor cells are growing and dividing

Each tumor characteristic is given a score of 1, 2 or 3. The score of each characteristic is added to produce a final grade. The final grade may range from 3 – 9. A lower score indicates a less aggressive tumor. A higher score indicates a more aggressive tumor and a need to consider more aggressive treatment.

Final Pathology Report

The final pathology report is sent to your physician which provides a description of the characteristics of your cancer after surgery. The report describes the extent of cancer spread and the biological characteristics of your cancer (biomarkers). The pathology report is your cancer's fingerprint, unique only to you, and contains the vital information needed to stage your cancer and plan further treatment.

Cancer Staging

Staging places your cancer in a category according to the extent of spread in the body. Staging is determined by three components: **TNM** (**T**=tumor; **N**=nodes; **M**=metastasis).The T and N information is found in the written pathology report. The metastasis (M) information is derived from any diagnostic test that finds cancer has spread to distant parts of your body.

Breast cancer stages range from Stage 0 to Stage 4. A Stage 0 cancer is the earliest form of breast cancer, and Stage 4 is the most advanced. Grouping in stage numbers allows physicians to communicate more effectively and accurately because they understand the characteristics needed to compose each stage number. A physician can know, just by hearing the stage number, the major components of your cancer. It is like understanding grades in school. We immediately know the difference between a child that is in the first grade and one that is in the fourth grade.

Understanding the TNM Components of Staging

To accurately define the extent of spread, additional letters or numbers are added after the T, N and M. These letters or numbers further define the extent of the cancer.

Tumor (T) Components

- **TX:** Primary tumor cannot be assessed
- **T0:** No evidence of a primary tumor
- **Tis (DCIS):** Ductal carcinoma in situ
- **Tis (Paget):** Paget Disease not associated with invasive carcinoma and/or carcinoma in situ
- **T1:** Tumor 20 mm or less in greatest dimension

- **T2:** Tumor more than 20 mm but not more than 50 mm in greatest dimension
- **T3:** Tumor more than 50 mm in greatest dimension
- **T4:** Tumor of any size with direct extension to the chest wall and/or to the skin

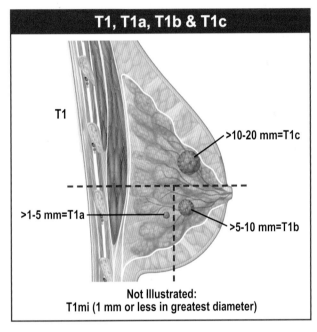

T1, T1a, T1b & T1c

T1

>10-20 mm=T1c

>1-5 mm=T1a

>5-10 mm=T1b

Not Illustrated:
T1mi (1 mm or less in greatest diameter)

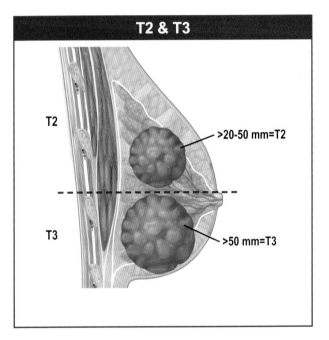

T2 & T3

T2

>20-50 mm=T2

T3

>50 mm=T3

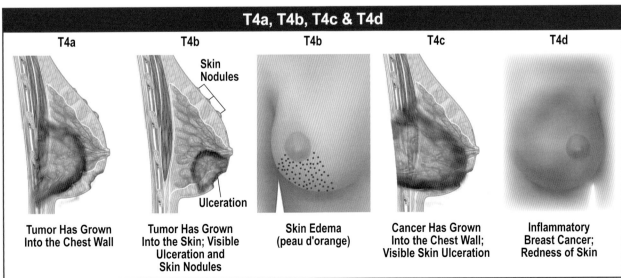

T4a, T4b, T4c & T4d

| T4a | T4b | T4b | T4c | T4d |

Skin Nodules

Ulceration

| Tumor Has Grown Into the Chest Wall | Tumor Has Grown Into the Skin; Visible Ulceration and Skin Nodules | Skin Edema (peau d'orange) | Cancer Has Grown Into the Chest Wall; Visible Skin Ulceration | Inflammatory Breast Cancer; Redness of Skin |

Node (N) Components

- **NX:** Regional lymph nodes cannot be assessed
- **N0:** No regional lymph node involvement
- **N0(i+):** Isolated tumor cell clusters (ITC)
- **N1mi:** Micrometastasis (<2 mm)
- **N1 – 3:** Involvement of regional lymph nodes (number or extent of spread)

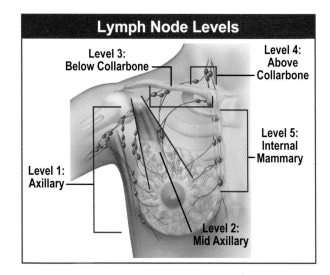

Lymph Node Levels

Level 3: Below Collarbone

Level 4: Above Collarbone

Level 5: Internal Mammary

Level 1: Axillary

Level 2: Mid Axillary

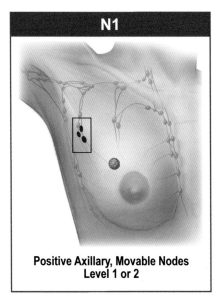

N1

Positive Axillary, Movable Nodes
Level 1 or 2

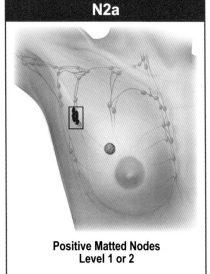

N2a

Positive Matted Nodes
Level 1 or 2

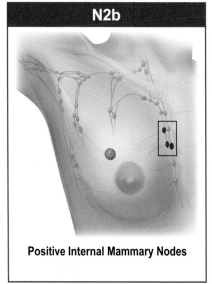

N2b

Positive Internal Mammary Nodes

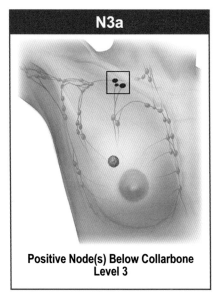

N3a

Positive Node(s) Below Collarbone
Level 3

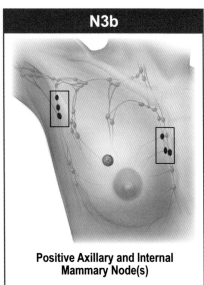

N3b

Positive Axillary and Internal
Mammary Node(s)

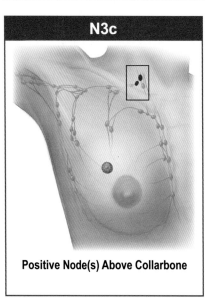

N3c

Positive Node(s) Above Collarbone

Metastasis (M) Components

- **MX:** Distant spread cannot be evaluated
- **M0:** No evidence of distant metastasis (cancer has not spread)
- **M0(i+):** Microscopic evidence of tumor cells in the blood, bone marrow or lymph nodes
- **M1:** Distant metastasis (cancer has spread to distant parts of the body)

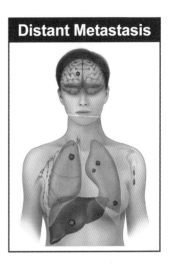

Distant Metastasis

Systemic Treatment Determining Factors

To determine treatment, the TNM stage is supplemented with additional information from your pathology report that describes the biology of your cancer (biomarkers). Biomarkers describe the unique details of how your cancer behaves in your body. These biomarkers include estrogen and progesterone (ER/PR) receptor status, HER2 receptor status, tumor grade and proliferation rate (Ki-67; how fast the tumor was growing). These biomarkers, combined with TNM staging, provide the data needed for an oncologist to determine the most appropriate type of systemic chemotherapy drugs or medications.

Multigene Testing

For some patients, additional information about the biology of their tumor through multigene testing (Oncotype Dx ®, Mammaprint®, EndoPredict®, PAM 50®, and Breast Cancer Index®) may be helpful for making final treatment decisions. Multigene testing provides an expanded genomic profile of a cancerous tumor that predicts potential for recurrence as well as predicting sensitivity to certain chemotherapy drugs. Currently, these genomic tests are designed for patients with T1 or T2 tumors who are ER/PR positive, HER2 negative and lymph node negative. Testing results provide a potential recurrence score for a patient. Knowing the level of potential recurrence may allow some patients to avoid treatment and for others to get the most appropriate drug protocol for their cancer.

New Prognostic Staging for Breast Cancer

In 2018, new staging guidelines went into effect for breast cancer that expands the previous TNM staging to include all factors known about a patient's breast cancer. Staging now includes any multigene testing results, if performed, along with tumor grade, proliferation rate, estrogen and progesterone receptor status and HER2 status. Staging based on these factors is called **Clinical Prognostic Staging**.

Note: It is **not** essential for you to understand staging information. It is included in this book to guide you if you have questions about your cancer stage. Some patients prefer to leave this to their physicians. You may want to ask a member of your healthcare team to help you identify your cancer stage in the following graphics.

Stage 0

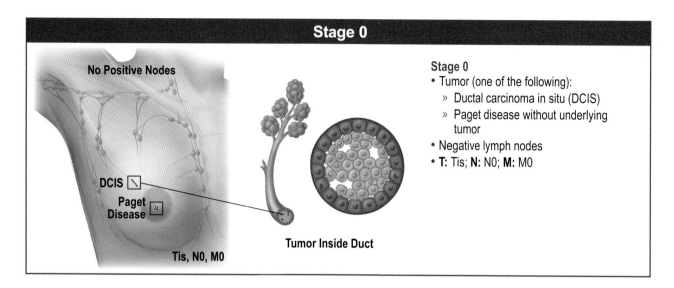

No Positive Nodes

DCIS

Paget
Disease

Tumor Inside Duct

Tis, N0, M0

Stage 0
- Tumor (one of the following):
  - » Ductal carcinoma in situ (DCIS)
  - » Paget disease without underlying tumor
- Negative lymph nodes
- **T:** Tis; **N:** N0; **M:** M0

Stage 1A

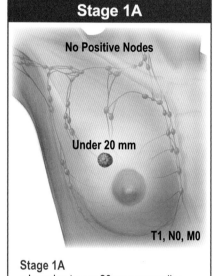

No Positive Nodes

Under 20 mm

T1, N0, M0

Stage 1A
- Invasive tumor 20 mm or smaller
- No positive lymph nodes
- **T:** T1; **N:** N0; **M:** M0

Isolated tumor cells and clusters less than 0.2 mm are conisdered "negative", N0(i+).

Stage 1B

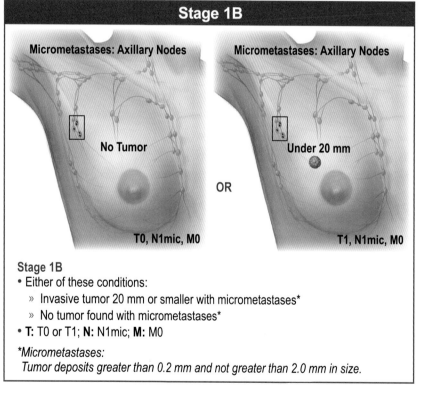

Micrometastases: Axillary Nodes

Micrometastases: Axillary Nodes

No Tumor

Under 20 mm

OR

T0, N1mic, M0

T1, N1mic, M0

Stage 1B
- Either of these conditions:
  - » Invasive tumor 20 mm or smaller with micrometastases*
  - » No tumor found with micrometastases*
- **T:** T0 or T1; **N:** N1mic; **M:** M0

Micrometastases:
Tumor deposits greater than 0.2 mm and not greater than 2.0 mm in size.

CHAPTER 10

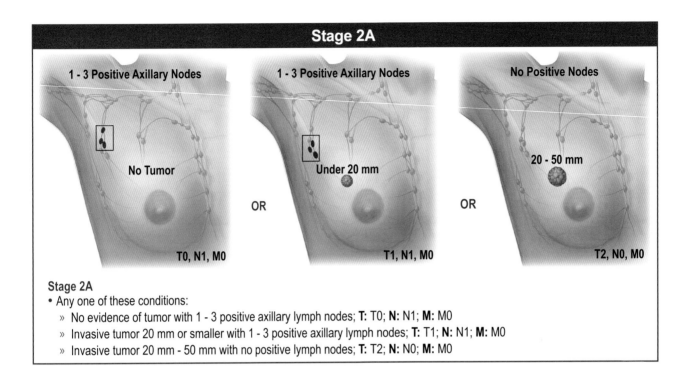

Stage 2A

Stage 2A
- Any one of these conditions:
  - » No evidence of tumor with 1 - 3 positive axillary lymph nodes; **T:** T0; **N:** N1; **M:** M0
  - » Invasive tumor 20 mm or smaller with 1 - 3 positive axillary lymph nodes; **T:** T1; **N:** N1; **M:** M0
  - » Invasive tumor 20 mm - 50 mm with no positive lymph nodes; **T:** T2; **N:** N0; **M:** M0

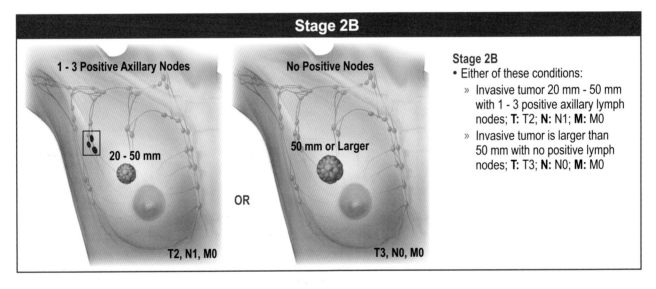

Stage 2B

Stage 2B
- Either of these conditions:
  - » Invasive tumor 20 mm - 50 mm with 1 - 3 positive axillary lymph nodes; **T:** T2; **N:** N1; **M:** M0
  - » Invasive tumor is larger than 50 mm with no positive lymph nodes; **T:** T3; **N:** N0; **M:** M0

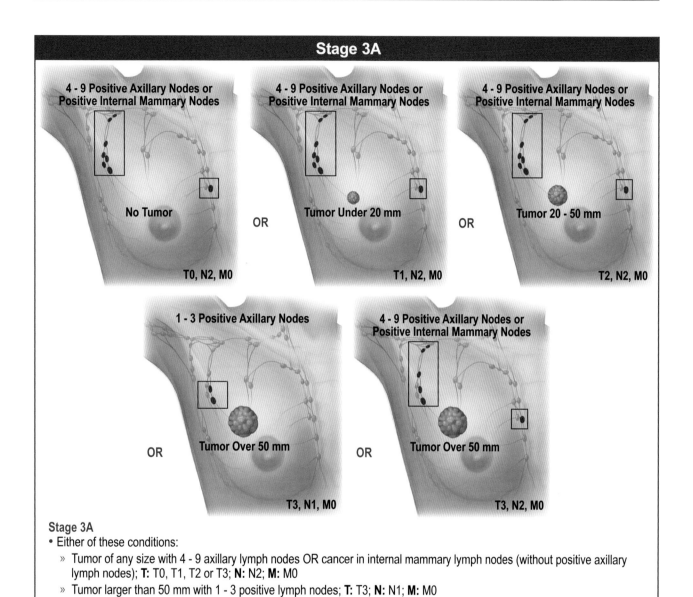

Stage 3A

4 - 9 Positive Axillary Nodes or
Positive Internal Mammary Nodes

No Tumor

T0, N2, M0

OR

4 - 9 Positive Axillary Nodes or
Positive Internal Mammary Nodes

Tumor Under 20 mm

T1, N2, M0

OR

4 - 9 Positive Axillary Nodes or
Positive Internal Mammary Nodes

Tumor 20 - 50 mm

T2, N2, M0

1 - 3 Positive Axillary Nodes

Tumor Over 50 mm

T3, N1, M0

OR

4 - 9 Positive Axillary Nodes or
Positive Internal Mammary Nodes

Tumor Over 50 mm

T3, N2, M0

OR

Stage 3A
• Either of these conditions:
  » Tumor of any size with 4 - 9 axillary lymph nodes OR cancer in internal mammary lymph nodes (without positive axillary lymph nodes); **T:** T0, T1, T2 or T3; **N:** N2; **M:** M0
  » Tumor larger than 50 mm with 1 - 3 positive lymph nodes; **T:** T3; **N:** N1; **M:** M0

Stage 3B

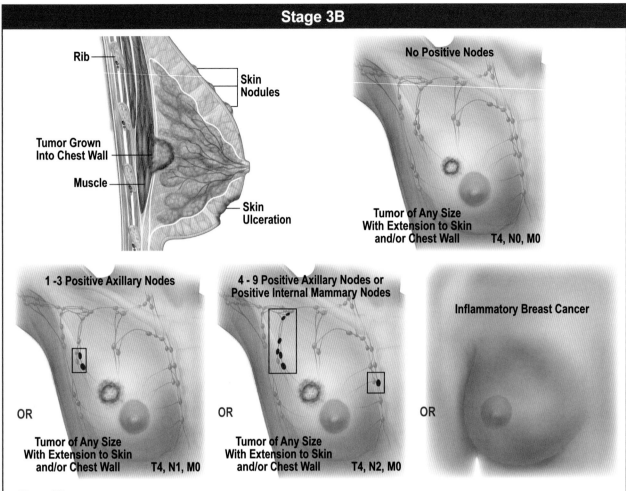

Rib

Skin Nodules

Tumor Grown Into Chest Wall

Muscle

Skin Ulceration

No Positive Nodes

Tumor of Any Size With Extension to Skin and/or Chest Wall   T4, N0, M0

1 -3 Positive Axillary Nodes

OR

Tumor of Any Size With Extension to Skin and/or Chest Wall   T4, N1, M0

4 - 9 Positive Axillary Nodes or Positive Internal Mammary Nodes

OR

Tumor of Any Size With Extension to Skin and/or Chest Wall   T4, N2, M0

Inflammatory Breast Cancer

OR

Stage 3B

- Invasive tumor, any size, that has not spread to other body parts, but has spread to the chest wall **OR** caused skin swelling **OR** ulceration of the breast with **one** of the following:
  - » No positive lymph nodes
  - » 1 – 3 positive axillary lymph nodes
  - » 4 – 9 positive axillary lymph nodes
  - » Positive internal mammary nodes
- Inflammatory breast cancer
- **T:** T4; **N:** N0, N1, N2; **M:** M0

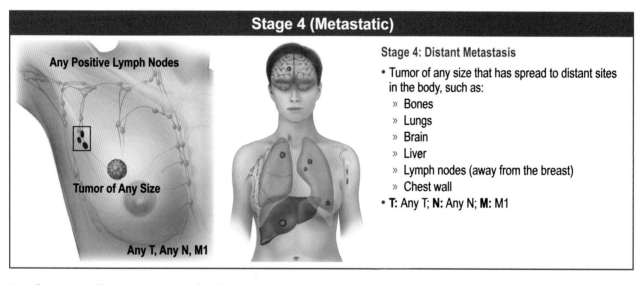

Stage 3C

10 or More Positive Axillary Nodes or Positive Infraclavicular Nodes or Positive Supraclavicular Nodes or Positive Internal Mammary Nodes

Tumor of Any Size

Any T, Any N, M0

Stage 3C
- Invasive tumor of any size/type that has not spread to distant parts of the body, but has spread to at least **one** of the following:
  - » 10 or more axillary lymph nodes
  - » Supraclavicular (above collarbone) lymph nodes
  - » Infraclavicular (below collarbone) lymph nodes
  - » Internal mammary lymph nodes
- **T:** Any T; **N:** N3; **M:** M0

Stage 4 (Metastatic)

Any Positive Lymph Nodes

Tumor of Any Size

Any T, Any N, M1

Stage 4: Distant Metastasis
- Tumor of any size that has spread to distant sites in the body, such as:
  - » Bones
  - » Lungs
  - » Brain
  - » Liver
  - » Lymph nodes (away from the breast)
  - » Chest wall
- **T:** Any T; **N:** Any N; **M:** M1

Understanding Your Pathology Report

To help you understand your pathology report, there are two worksheets located at the back of this book. The worksheets are designed to help you receive the amount of information you prefer about the biology of your cancer. The first worksheet, *Pathology Report Questions*, contains general questions to ask your surgeon or oncologist (page 277). The second worksheet, *Essential Pathology Report Information,* is designed to be filled in by your physician, identifying the major components of your pathology report that influence treatment decisions (page 278).

Review the two worksheets and determine which of the two meets your information needs. A vital part of recovery is receiving the amount of information that you feel is helpful.

Additional Information

Tear-out Worksheets

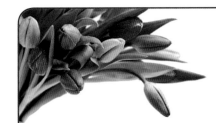

Remember...

- *Your final pathology report serves as the foundation for future treatment decisions. It contains the unique fingerprints of your breast cancer and is a guide to help your physician make the most effective treatment recommendations.*

- *Pathology reports are complicated to read and understand. As a patient, it is not necessary to understand all of the information contained in the report. The main components a patient needs to know about her cancer are hormone receptor status, HER2 receptor status, lymph node status and stage of cancer.*

- *Acquire an understanding of the treatment options. This will allow you to communicate with your healthcare team and become an active participant in decisions. Understanding will serve to alleviate many unfounded fears and restore a sense of control to your life.*

- *Employ the best of all medicines—your attitude. The most productive approach that you can bring, and one that the physician cannot provide, is a positive, cooperative attitude. Determination, combined with optimism, creates a healing environment that only you can provide.*

CHAPTER 11

Chemotherapy Treatments

"My doctor told me, 'If you can't remember everything you want to ask me about, write it down.' That's what I did. I had so many questions, and he would sit down there and answer every last one of them."

—Earnestine Brown

You have had your surgery, received your final pathology report and your cancer has been staged. The next step will be determining the need for additional treatment of your breast cancer. For a few women, it will be observation only. However, the majority of women receive some type of additional treatment—radiation therapy, chemotherapy, targeted therapy and/or hormonal therapy. These treatments are called adjuvant (additional) therapy. Adjuvant therapy is given to prevent a recurrence of cancer by killing or controlling any undetected cancer cells that may remain in your body after surgery. Adjuvant therapy may be local or systemic and is given to prevent a cancer recurrence.

Local Therapy (Specific Area):
- **Radiation Therapy:** Targets cancer cells only in the area that receives radiation treatment. The breast or nearby lymph nodes may be radiated to kill any remaining local microscopic cells.

Systemic Therapy (Throughout the Body):
- **Chemotherapy:** Travels in the blood to reach all distant areas of the body to kill any remaining microscopic cells. Most often given through an I.V.
- **Hormonal Therapy:** Travels to all parts of the body to block hormone receptors on the breast and control the growth of hormone positive breast cells. Most often given orally.
- **Targeted Monoclonal Antibody Therapy:** Travels to all parts of the body to target specific abnormalities within cancer cells. Most often given by I.V.

Your physicians will study your pathology report and tell you which treatment or combination of treatments are the most advisable for your type and stage of cancer.

"I kept a binder notebook with all of my reports and labs, along with a calendar of my appointments. I asked ahead what kind of treatments they predicted would be prescribed so I could look them up. I read everything I could about the type of treatment that was being recommended. I wanted to be prepared to ask the appropriate questions before treatments were given. This gave me a sense of being involved in my treatment decisions."
—Anna Cluxton

91

Your First Oncologist Visit

It is very important to carry a list of all medications you take to your first oncology appointment. Along with prescription drugs, include all nonprescription medicines, such as cold or sinus medications, aspirin, antacids, laxatives, vitamins and herbs. Many drugs can alter the response of the treatment. Your oncologist will determine if you can continue each medication. Check with your oncologist before starting any new medication (prescription or over-the-counter) or herbal preparation during chemotherapy.

During your first appointment, your oncologist will review your pathology report and any other tests, perform a thorough physical exam and then prescribe a treatment plan according to:

- Cancer cell type
- Size of tumor
- In situ or invasive cancer
- Lymph node involvement
- Tumor grade: how much cells have changed from original cells and cell growth rate
- Estrogen and progesterone hormone receptor status
- HER2 status
- Your menopausal state
- Evidence of cancer in other parts of the body
- Your personal and family medical history

Remember, there is more than one kind of breast cancer, and different types of cancers may require different treatments. Do not compare your treatment with another patient's treatment because you will probably be comparing two completely different cancers. It is also important to remember that the information you get from Internet sites, newspapers, magazines, radio or television may not be applicable to your cancer or may be experimental treatments that have not been tested extensively. Rely on your physician to make sure you are receiving accurate information that is relevant to your cancer diagnosis.

Clinical Trials

During your discussion about your breast cancer treatment plan, your physician may ask if you would consider participating in a clinical trial. Clinical trials are investigational studies that research the effectiveness of treatments for patients. Participating in a clinical trial may include receiving a new drug or a new combination of drugs, comparing two different drugs or evaluating new drug dosages. The goal of a clinical trial is to determine if a new treatment works, if it is safe or if it is more effective.

Participating in a clinical trial does not prevent you from getting any additional medical care you may need. If asked to participate, your physician will explain the clinical trial in detail. For additional information, refer to *Appendix C: Understanding Clinical Trials* on page 213.

Genomic Testing

Genomic testing (also called multigene testing) is designed to study the genes in a tumor which predict your potential for recurrence over the next 10 years. Early stage breast cancer patients who meet specific criteria are candidates for testing. If your doctor recommends testing, a pathology slide of your tumor, removed during surgery, is shipped to a specialized lab. You do not have to undergo any additional procedures. *(Do not confuse genomic testing with genetic testing, which is performed on saliva or blood to determine the presence of a gene mutation for hereditary breast cancer.)* Oncotype DX® is presently the most widely ordered genomic test. Other genomic tests include MammaPrint® and Breast Cancer Index®.

Genomic Testing Report

Test results are returned to your physician with a prediction for recurrence potential. Oncotype DX® reports a Recurrence Score® from 0 to 100. The score corresponds to the potential for breast cancer recurrence within a period of 10 years from the time of diagnosis.

Women with lower Recurrence Scores have a lower risk that their cancer will return. It is important to note that a lower score does not mean that there is no chance that a woman's cancer will return. Women with a higher score have a greater chance that their breast cancer will return; however, a higher score does not mean that a woman's breast cancer will definitely return. The test analyzes a wide range of genes and serves as a prediction for recurrence, not an absolute fact.

Stage 0 patients with a low Recurrence Score may be less likely to benefit from radiation therapy. Stage I and II patients with a low Recurrence Score may be less likely to benefit from chemotherapy. A high Recurrence Score indicates that chemotherapy benefits are greater than the risks of side effects. Knowing the genomic profile of a cancer allows your physician to tailor a treatment plan for you and your cancer. If you have early stage breast cancer, ask your physician if you are a potential candidate for genomic testing.

Chemotherapy

Chemotherapy is a compound of two words that mean "chemical" and "treatment." We have all experienced treatment with chemicals, such as antibiotics and cold medicines, for other illnesses. The word chemotherapy usually refers to treatment of cancer with drugs. Chemotherapy is systemic treatment that travels to all parts of the body through the bloodstream. A combination of several drugs may be used to fight your cancer. The drugs selected will have different side effects and work in different ways to kill or control the growth of any cancer cells that may be left in your body. Most often, people think of the drugs that cause hair loss and nausea when they think of chemotherapy; however, anti-hormonal drugs that alter the hormonal environment of the body and cause few side effects are also included in this category. The goals of chemotherapy drugs include:

- Destroy cancer cells in other parts of the body
- Stop cancer spread to other parts of the body
- Slow cancer growth
- Relieve symptoms of advanced cancer

Hormonal Therapy

Hormonal therapy may be recommended by your oncologist. This type of therapy is prescribed after surgery for women if their pathology report reveals that their tumor growth was dependent on the female hormones estrogen or progesterone. Tumors that have a significant number of estrogen receptors (ER) are considered "ER positive," and tumors that have a high number of progesterone receptors (PR) are considered "PR positive." The receptor status of the tumor determines which treatments will best control your cancer. The use of hormonal drugs often depends upon whether you are premenopausal (having your monthly menstrual periods) or post-menopausal (not having your monthly menstrual periods). Patients who have estrogen receptor positive (ER+) and/or progesterone receptor positive (PR+) cancers are often given hormonal therapies as part of treatment. It is currently recommended that hormonal therapy be given for 5 – 10 years. Hormonal therapies include:

- **Tamoxifen Citrate (Nolvadex®):** This is the most commonly used hormonal drug. While doctors don't know exactly how tamoxifen works, they acknowledge that it blocks the effects of estrogen on breast cancer cells. It does not kill, but it may control, any remaining cancer cells that have been left in the body after surgery. It does not cause the same side effects as chemotherapy. There is no hair loss or fatigue. The most frequently reported side effects are hot flashes (80 percent on tamoxifen and 68 percent on placebo) and vaginal discharge (55 percent on tamoxifen and 35 percent on placebo). Tamoxifen is given by pill once or twice a day.

- **Aromatase Inhibitors:** A newer class of hormonal drugs called aromatase inhibitors, Aromasin® (exemestane), Femara® (letrozole), and Arimidex® (anastrozole), may be prescribed for women who are naturally, or chemically, post-menopausal. In post-menopausal women, the enzyme aromatase can convert androgens (male hormones) found in body fat and muscle into estrogen. Aromatase inhibitors block or prevent the enzymes from converting these androgens into estrogen. Your physician will tell you if your cancer treatment will include an aromatase inhibitor.

Targeted Therapy

A targeted therapy (biological response modifier) is a drug that binds with certain proteins on a tumor to prevent their growth. For women whose tumors test positive for over-expression of HER2 receptors, Herceptin® (trastuzumab) or Pertuzumab (Perjeta®) may be used. These drugs attach to the HER2 protein found on the cancer cell to prevent the cell from growing or dividing. Your pathology report will show if your tumor is HER2 positive. Herceptin® or Perjeta® are only indicated in treatment when a tumor tests positive for over-expression of HER2.

Chemotherapy Drugs		
Chemotherapy Class of Drugs	**Drug Action**	**Drug Names**
Anthracyclines *(antibiotic-based)*	Alters the structure of cellular DNA	**Adriamycin®** (doxorubicin) **Ellence®** (epirubicin) **Doxil®** (doxorubicin HCl liposome)
Taxanes	Prevents cancer cells from dividing	**Abraxane®** (plasma bound paclitaxel) **Taxol®** (paclitaxel) **Taxotere®** (docetaxel)
Alkylating Agent	Interferes with cellular metabolism and growth	**Cytoxan®** (cyclophosphamide)
Antimetabolites	Interferes with cancer cell division	**Gemzar®** (gemcitabine) **Methotrexate®** **5-FU®** (5 fluorouracil) **Xeloda®** (capecitabine)
Miscellaneous Anti-Neoplastic	Interferes with microtubule assembly	**Navelbine®** (vinorelbine tartrate)
Platinum Analog	Binds with DNA	**Paraplatin®** (carboplatin)
Hormonal and Biological Response Modifier Drugs		
Breast Cancer Class of Drugs	**Drug Action**	**Drug Names**
SERMs *(Selective Estrogen-Receptor Modulators)*	Drug binds to estrogen receptors in breast, controlling cancer growth	**Nolvadex®** (tamoxifen) **Fareston®** (toremifene)
Aromatase Inhibitors	Reduces estrogen production by blocking enzyme aromatase	**Aromasin®** (exemestane) **Femara®** (letrozole) **Arimidex®** (anastrazole)
Targeted Therapy *(Biological Response Modifier)*	Drug binds with certain estrogen proteins on breast cancer cells, preventing growth in HER2 positive women	**Tykerb®** (lapatinib) **Herceptin®** (trastuzumab) **Kadcyla®** (ado-trastuzumab emtansine) **Perjeta®** (pertuzumab) **Afinitor®** (everolimus)
Miscellaneous Hormonal	Used for breast cancers that are estrogen dependent	**Zoladex®** (goserelin acetate) **Faslodex®** (fulvestrant) **Lupron®** (leuprolide)

How Chemotherapy Drugs Work

Chemotherapy drugs work by killing cells that are dividing in your body, unlike the hormonal and targeted therapy drugs, which prevent or slow growth. Cancer cells are constantly dividing until something disrupts this cycle, which is the role of chemotherapy. Even when the surgeon has removed all evidence of your tumor, you may receive adjuvant chemotherapy. This is because there is a possibility that some cells may have broken away from the original site and moved through the lymphatic or blood vessels to other parts of your body, where they cannot be detected; this is called micrometastasis (the cells are too small to be detected). Adjuvant chemotherapy helps to destroy these cells and is effective in all parts of the body except the brain.

Don't listen to anyone else and their stories about the side effects of chemotherapy. Instead, ask your nurse for the names of the drugs prescribed for you and the side effects of those particular drugs. There are approximately 15 different types of breast cancer, and there are many drugs being used to treat cancer. Therefore, it would be difficult to get accurate information from anyone but the medical professionals involved with your cancer treatment.

Chemotherapy Scheduling

Chemotherapy is given in cycles. Your oncologist will let you know the planned schedule for your chemotherapy administration. Each treatment cycle is followed by a period of rest to allow your body time to recover from the side effects of the drugs. Your schedule may be altered during treatment, depending on how your body responds to the drugs. Determining if your body has recovered enough to receive another treatment is done by drawing your blood to see if your blood counts have returned to a safe range.

Traditionally, most breast cancer patients receive their treatments every three weeks. The three-week period allows the side effects of lowered blood counts to naturally return to a safe level that allows for another treatment. Some patients may have their treatments scheduled every two weeks instead of every three weeks, called dose-dense chemotherapy. This allows the same amount of medication to be delivered in a shortened time frame. This shortened schedule may not allow the white blood cells enough time to return to a range that is safe for more chemotherapy to be given. To address this issue, a medication called a "growth factor" is given as an injection to stimulate the production of necessary white blood cells. In a dose-dense schedule, Neupogen® (filgrastim), Neulasta® (pegfilgrastim) or Leukine® (sargramostim) may be needed to support the more rapid return of white blood cells to a normal range.

Neoadjuvant Chemotherapy

Chemotherapy treatments usually begin after surgery; however, some types of breast cancer require chemotherapy to be given before surgery, which is called neoadjuvant chemotherapy. Neoadjuvant chemotherapy may be given to shrink a large tumor to a size that allows for breast conservation in a woman with smaller breasts. It is also given for triple negative breast cancer, inflammatory breast cancer or advanced stage tumors.

How Chemotherapy Is Administered

Most chemotherapy for breast cancer is given intravenously (I.V.). Chemotherapy may be administered in a doctor's office, a hospital or a clinic.

If your veins are hard to locate or if you are to receive certain types of chemotherapy drugs, your physician may request the insertion of a special catheter for I.V. administrations. This is commonly called a vascular access device. A vascular access device prevents repeated needle sticks to arm veins and prevents potential damage to the small veins in the arm from chemotherapy drugs. A vascular access catheter can also be used for blood draws.

Two Basic Types of Venous Access Devices:

- **Intravenous Port:** (Also called a vascular access device, life-port or port-a-cath) This is the most commonly used device. The port is surgically placed under the skin through a small incision in the chest, opposite the surgical breast. The port consists of an injection hub (smaller than a quarter) and a catheter. The catheter is threaded into a large vein in the area near the heart. The injection hub has a hollow space inside that is sealed by a soft silicone covering. The silicone portion of the injection hub is accessed by a needle when needed for I.V. treatments. When treatment is complete, the needle is removed. Because the port is completely under the skin, you are able to bathe and swim without restrictions. The port can remain in place for an extended period of time, if needed. A minor surgical procedure is required to remove the port.

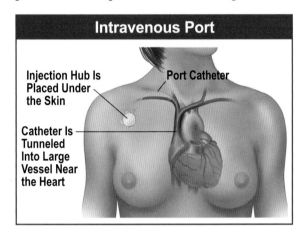

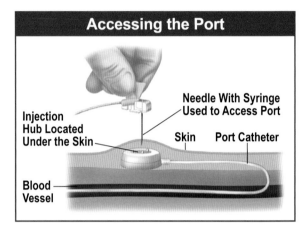

- **PICC Line:** (peripherally inserted central catheter) A catheter is inserted into a vein in the arm and threaded up to a large vein in the chest near the heart. A PICC line does not require surgery to insert. The needle insertion site is located outside the skin and requires dressing changes. The insertion site cannot get wet. A PICC line can remain in place for several months and does not require a surgical procedure to remove it.

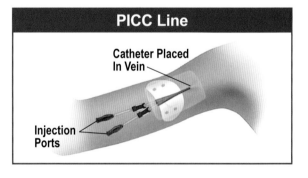

Understanding Chemotherapy Nadir

Nadir is the time in your treatment when chemotherapy drugs that impact blood counts cause blood values to fall to their lowest level. Different drugs impact different blood components. Your physician will tell you about the expected side effects of the drugs you are taking and when the nadir is expected. During this time, you will feel most fatigued if red blood cells are impacted. You will be most susceptible to acquiring an infection or virus if white blood cells are lowered. You will have the highest potential for spontaneous bleeding if platelets are decreased. Usually the nadir is midway between scheduled treatments. Blood values are allowed to come back to near normal before your next treatment is given.

Chemotherapy Side Effects

Because chemotherapy kills rapidly dividing cells, it not only kills cancer cells, but it also damages healthy cells in the body that may be dividing at the time of drug administration. The most common cells affected are in the bone marrow (causing lower blood counts), digestive tract, reproductive system and hair follicles. The good news is that most of the side effects are short-term and will go away when cancer treatment is completed. Ask your doctor to tell you about the expected side effects of your treatment.

Nausea and Vomiting

Nausea, a common side effect, is a wave-like feeling of distress, causing an uneasy feeling in the stomach or in the back of the throat, which signals the potential for vomiting. Dry heaves (no stomach contents are released) or vomiting may or may not accompany nausea. People with a history of motion sickness or pregnancy morning sickness are more prone to experience these problems during chemotherapy treatment.

Medications for Nausea and Vomiting

Before chemotherapy is administered, you will be given medication to prevent nausea and vomiting. You will also be given a prescription to relieve nausea at home. After returning home, plan to take the medication with a small amount of fluid at the first sign of nausea. It may take at least 30 minutes for the medication to begin to work. After the nausea passes, try small amounts of fluid before eating a meal.

Recognizing the symptoms that occur prior to nausea is helpful. The center in the brain that controls vomiting is closely related to the respiratory and heart functions. These organs may have signs that can serve as cues to take action to prevent a vomiting episode. Symptoms preceding vomiting include an increase in oral secretions, an uneasy feeling in your stomach, an increase in your heart rate and increased skin warmth. These are signs to take your nausea medication immediately. After taking your medication, lie down in a cool, well-ventilated environment, if possible. Place a cool, damp cloth on your head or neck. Take a series of long, deep breaths and hold each breath for five seconds before slowly exhaling.

If you do vomit, rinse your mouth with cool water and wipe your face with a cool, damp cloth. After taking medication, try to remain quiet and still. Sip on ice chips or take small sips of fluid before trying to drink a large amount. If vomiting is frequent, it is best to avoid solid food for four to eight hours past the last vomiting episode. It is extremely important that you are able to continue to drink to remain hydrated.

Preventing or Reducing Nausea and Vomiting:

- Select room temperature or cold foods; warm or hot foods have odors that often stimulate vomiting.
- Select bland foods for your diet, such as mashed or baked potatoes, applesauce, yogurt, cottage cheese, sherbet, crackers or toast. Highly seasoned food often aggravates nausea.
- Sip clear, cool liquids to reduce nausea. Apple juice, cranberry juice, lemonade, broths, Gatorade®, ginger ale, tea, colas and gelatins are usually well-tolerated in small amounts.
- Try sour foods such as lemons, pickles, hard candy or lemon sherbet; rinse your mouth with lemon juice and water if your mouth is not sore from chemotherapy.
- Avoid fried, greasy, highly salted, spicy foods and foods with strong odors.
- Avoid smelling strong odors such as perfume, cleaning chemicals or food cooking.
- Avoid being around other people who are vomiting.
- Eat light meals often, rather than large, heavy meals.
- Try to relieve nausea or vomiting with the same foods or beverages that you used in the past when you were sick with the flu or during pregnancy; often these foods will give effective relief.
- Maintain regular bowel movements. Constipation and bowel obstruction can be contributing causes of nausea. Many drugs used during cancer treatment contribute to constipation.
- Narcotic pain medications often cause nausea, vomiting and constipation.

Persistent nausea and vomiting can lead to fluid and electrolyte imbalances, which causes dehydration and fatigue. While nausea and vomiting are expected side effects of treatment, they need to be addressed and treated by your healthcare provider to maintain the highest quality of life possible during your treatment. If you are unable to keep clear fluids down for four to five hours, call your doctor.

Fatigue

Fatigue is a major complaint of patients undergoing chemotherapy treatment. After each treatment, fatigue will be the greatest when your blood counts are at their lowest level. Your energy will gradually increase as your blood counts increase, with your energy reaching its highest level several days before your next scheduled treatment. The degree of fatigue you can expect is related to the type of drugs you receive. Ask your physician or nurse what level of fatigue you can expect.

Fatigue has a cumulative effect, increasing as treatment progresses. Plan to get additional rest by taking naps or sleeping later. Reduce as many tasks of daily living as possible during your highest levels of fatigue. Take the initiative to divide household responsibilities among family members, or consider hiring help during this time. Since you will be the least fatigued the week before your next treatment, plan activities requiring more energy during this time.

It is recommended that you stay as physically active as possible during treatment, while being careful not to overdo it. Moderate exercise, such as a walking program, has been shown to increase energy and reduce fatigue. Exercise also reduces other side effects of chemotherapy. The key is to balance exercise and rest.

Be sure your meals are nutritionally adequate; good nutrition is required to build new cells to replace those that chemotherapy destroys. You may be too tired to prepare nutritionally balanced meals and may need help in this area. Some patients find it helpful to prepare and freeze meals prior to their next treatment, while their energy is at its highest level. Diet and exercise are fully discussed in *Chapter 20*.

Diarrhea

Chemotherapy destroys the rapidly dividing cells that line the intestines, which often results in diarrhea. The degree and duration of diarrhea depend on the drug, the length of time it is given and the amount given. Persistent diarrhea can cause electrolyte imbalances that have the potential to become serious. Management of diarrhea is essential.

Diarrhea Management Tips:
- Take an over-the-counter antidiarrheal medication as directed. Continue taking the medication for 12 hours after your last loose stool.
- Eat foods high in potassium, such as baked potatoes and bananas.
- Drink extra fluids such as bouillon, grape juice, Gatorade® and weak, warm tea.
- Avoid carbonated beverages.
- Eat small, frequent meals.
- Avoid milk products; buttermilk and yogurt are permitted.
- Keep the rectal area clean and dry by washing with soap and water; dry well and apply a protective ointment (such as Desitin® Cream or zinc oxide) to prevent tissue breakdown.
- If diarrhea lasts more than 24 hours, call your healthcare provider and report the number of diarrhea stools in the past 24 hours along with any medication you have taken.

Constipation

Some chemotherapy drugs or narcotic medications may cause the colon to become less active, which results in constipation.

Constipation Management Tips:

- Eat foods high in fiber, such as fresh raw fruits and vegetables, whole grain cereals, breads and pastas, dried beans and peas, nuts, corn, popcorn, raisins, dates and prunes. These foods absorb water and keep the stool soft.
- Drink extra fluids, especially water; 3,000 ccs. of fluid a day is recommended (3,000 ccs = 12 cups).
- Avoid cheese and refined products made with white flour.
- Increase physical activity; physical activity promotes the movement of stool through the intestines.
- Drink a warm fluid early in the morning to stimulate the colon.
- Take a cellulose, bulk-producing product, such as Miralax® or Metamucil®, to increase your fiber.
- Establish a time for elimination that is regular and not rushed.
- If constipation occurs and the above methods do not give results, consult your physician about a mild laxative or a stool softener to prevent constipation. If you do not have a bowel movement in 72 hours, consult your physician again.

Stomach Irritation

Chemotherapy irritates cells in the gastrointestinal system of your body. The main complaints of gastritis (stomach irritation) include a burning, gnawing sensation in the stomach or abdominal pain with cramps. These conditions are temporary and are relieved when treatment is over. Factors that increase the potential for irritation include: excessive stomach acid caused by stress; alcohol; excessive caffeine; smoking; eating fatty, acidic or spicy foods that are not easily digested; aspirin; non-steroidal anti-inflammatory medications (Motrin®, Advil®, etc.); cortisone, and some antibiotics.

Stomach Irritation Management Tips:

- Take non-prescription antacids on a regular basis, according to directions on the bottle, until symptoms improve.
- Do not take aspirin or ibuprofen for pain; instead take acetaminophen (Tylenol®).
- Try a liquid diet to allow the stomach to rest. Resume a normal diet slowly, by beginning with bland foods.
- Eat a bland diet until symptoms improve—no spicy, hot, acidic or fatty foods.
- Eat a small amount of bland food frequently. Avoid large meals.
- Stop smoking. Do not drink alcohol while experiencing stomach irritation.
- Take any medication that irritates your stomach with food.
- Inform your healthcare provider if symptoms do not improve. Medications may be ordered to reduce or block the secretion of stomach acid, which may include:
  - **Acid Reducers:** famotidine (Prevacid®), nizatidine (Axid®), ranitidine (Zantac®) or cimetidine (Tagamet®). Recent studies show cimetidine may interact with some chemotherapy drugs.
  - **Acid Blockers:** omeprazole (Prilosec®), lansopraxole (Prevacid®), esomeprazole (Nexium®), pantoprozole (Protonix®) or rabeprazole (Aciphex®).

Notify Healthcare Provider If:

- Pain is severe and persists after several days of antacids and diet modification.
- Vomit looks like coffee grounds or bowel movements appear dark and tarry because of bleeding.
- Prescribed medications cannot be taken because of abdominal pain or vomiting.
- Prescribed medications for stomach irritation do not bring pain relief within a week.

Mouth Irritation (Stomatitis)

Stomatitis is a condition that refers to an inflammation of the lining of the mouth and throat, causing discomfort or pain. Stomatitis causes your mouth and throat to hurt or burn when you eat or drink. Mouth sores or ulcers may occur. Usually, a sore mouth from chemotherapy administration will improve, and cells will repair themselves within a week, if additional chemotherapy is not given during that time.

Mouth Irritation Management Tips:

- Cleanse your mouth thoroughly after every meal; brush your teeth with a very soft toothbrush, being careful not to injure your gums; soak your toothbrush in hot water to soften the bristles and prevent irritation to gums; use a non-irritating toothpaste or baking soda.
- Rinse your mouth with water to remove food particles if you cannot brush after a meal.
- Prepare a mouthwash solution of 1 tablespoon baking soda in 2 cups water, or ½ teaspoon salt and 1 teaspoon baking soda in 4 cups water. Avoid commercial mouthwashes containing alcohol. Alcohol-free mouthwashes (such as Biotene®) can promote healing and prevent infection by stimulating the body's own immune system in the mouth and saliva.
- Keep your lips moist with lip balm, Vaseline®, K-Y Jelly® or Aquaphor®.
- Avoid tobacco and alcohol.
- Avoid very hot or very cold foods; avoid foods that are spicy, acidic or have a coarse, irritating texture.
- Floss between teeth, but avoid any contact with gums. Stop flossing if it causes pain.
- Apply Orabase®, an over-the-counter oral protective paste, to irritated areas to relieve discomfort.
- Apply Vitamin E oil to the irritated areas. Puncture a Vitamin E capsule and apply with a cotton swab.
- Ask your physician for a prescription for a topical analgesic to deaden the area at mealtime if pain is preventing you from eating or drinking. Swish and swallow or spit it out to temporarily relieve pain.
- Notify your healthcare provider if white or yellowish patches develop on your tongue, inside your cheeks or in your throat and do not come off after rinsing your mouth with salt water. This is a sign of thrush, a fungal infection that requires a prescription medication.
- Notify your healthcare provider if your mouth irritation continues after trying the tips listed above.

Chemo Brain

Some chemotherapy patients complain that their treatments cause changes in their ability to concentrate. They struggle to find the right words, and their short-term memory seems unreliable. Some people refer to this as chemo brain. Recently, the phenomenon patients have been reporting for years has been validated by research.

Many factors can contribute to the fuzzy thinking women experience during chemotherapy treatment. One of the major causes is the decrease in female hormones caused by chemotherapy. Other conditions that can contribute to fuzzy thinking are stress, anemia, fatigue, anxiety, depression, side effects of anesthesia and medications. Some doctors recommend taking B-Complex vitamins to combat chemo brain, but be sure to consult your healthcare team to get their best advice for you.

If you find that your thinking feels fuzzier than usual, use a calendar to keep track of dates and appointments. Make lists, and leave yourself notes. Participate in thinking exercises that encourage your brain to try new pathways. Consider playing memory games, working crossword puzzles or doing other activities that require concentration. Keep a family calendar with everyone's schedule—several online sites offer free calendar programs that can make this easier. Most of all, remember that your symptoms will gradually improve when your treatments are complete.

Nerve Damage (Peripheral Neuropathy)

Several chemotherapy drugs that treat breast cancer have the potential to cause damage to peripheral nerves in the body, called peripheral neuropathy. The symptoms of early nerve damage are numbness, pain, burning, tingling sensations and weakness in the hands or feet. One of the first peripheral neuropathy signs you may notice is that you have difficulty buttoning a button.

The most common drugs that cause peripheral neuropathy are the taxanes (docetaxel and paclitaxel). If you are receiving a taxane drug and begin to experience any of the above symptoms, no matter how minor, report it to your doctor or nurse immediately. Reporting these symptoms early can prevent future and lasting damage to your peripheral nerves.

Hot Flashes

Hot flashes are not a disease, even though they may feel that way. Hot flashes are sensations of increased body temperature, which are caused by a lack of estrogen. A hot flash usually begins in one region of the body and spreads throughout the body quickly. A sudden wave of warmth in the face, neck and chest occurs and usually lasts between a minute and several minutes. Hot flashes can also be associated with nausea, dizziness, headache, irregular heartbeat pattern and sweating. Researchers attribute hot flashes to irregular expansion and contraction of the small blood vessels of the skin, which produce perspiration and blushing. The sensation from a hot flash is unexpected and can be very bothersome. Most chemotherapy drugs, including anti-hormonal drugs such as tamoxifen, cause hot flashes.

Most women notice that their hot flashes tend to occur during certain times of the day. The best management technique is to control body temperature and the immediate environment.

Hot Flash Management Tips:

- Notice a time or pattern for your hot flashes. Anticipating hot flashes can give you a sense of control.
- Dress in light, layered clothing so that outer garments can be removed during a hot flash. Avoid turtleneck sweaters. Wear slip-on shoes that can be quickly removed so that you can place your feet on the cold floor.
- Avoid hot environments or activities that can increase body temperature, such as hot baths, saunas and sunbathing.
- Drink cold liquids; avoid hot drinks. When a hot flash starts, try drinking cold water to reduce the sensation and to keep yourself hydrated.
- Sleep in a cool room. Use cotton sheets and bed coverings that can be quickly removed. Select cotton pajamas or nightgowns to absorb perspiration. Sleeping naked is another helpful option.
- Use an electric fan to keep cool.
- Avoid highly seasoned foods, alcohol and drinks with large amounts of caffeine (coffee, tea, sodas).
- Avoid stressful situations that can stimulate you emotionally.
- Learn mental visualization techniques that can reduce the intensity of the hot flash sensations.

Medications for Hot Flashes

If your hot flashes are interfering with your quality of life and are not managed with the above suggestions, talk to your doctor. Several of the selective serotonin reuptake inhibitor medications (SSRIs) have been proven effective in reducing hot flashes. If you are taking tamoxifen, recent clinical studies show that these medications do not interfere with its effectiveness: citalopram (Celexa®), escitalopram (Lexapro®), venlavaxine (Effexor®) and fluvoxamine (Luvox®).

Hair Loss

Hair loss (alopecia) is visible evidence of your battle with cancer, and it may be more difficult to deal with than your breast surgery. Hair loss can further compound your struggle with body image changes caused by surgery and further diminish your sense of femininity. Hair loss, most often, can be an emotionally draining experience.

In EduCare Focus Groups, women who had been given chemotherapy and lost their hair were asked which was more emotionally painful—their surgical experience or the loss of their hair. The answer was, overwhelmingly, hair loss—74 percent said hair loss was more difficult; only 26 percent said that their surgery was more difficult emotionally.

When you lose your hair, people may try to offer you consolation and support by pointing out how insignificant hair loss is compared to battling a life-threatening disease. As well-meaning as this is, most can say this because they have never lost their hair. If you have a hard time dealing with your hair loss, don't feel alone; most women feel the same way. During this time, it is helpful to remind yourself that hair loss is the visible proof that chemotherapy is killing cells—both good and bad. Losing your hair is evidence that cancer cells are also dying.

Facts About Hair Loss

Chemotherapy causes temporary alopecia that varies from hair thinning to complete baldness, depending on the type of drugs given, the length of time they are given and the dosage given. Taking multiple drugs increases the risk of hair loss. Chemotherapy drugs damage growing hair cells, causing the hair follicles to produce weak, brittle hair that either breaks off at the scalp surface or falls out. Most hair loss occurs within 7 – 21 days after the administration of drugs and is usually preceded by scalp tingling.

Some drugs cause hair thinning. The degree of hair thinning is an individual response and varies among women being given the same treatment. Total alopecia drugs may cause hair to fall out in clumps over several days, or the hair may all fall out in one day while shampooing. For this reason, many women who are expecting total hair loss choose to shave their heads to take charge of when and how they will lose their hair.

Some drugs may also cause hair loss in other sites such as the eyebrows, eyelashes, pubic hair and facial hair. This hair loss ranges from thinning to total loss. Because these hair follicles have a slower growth rate they usually suffer less damage.

Chemotherapy Drugs and Hair Loss:

- 5-Fluorouracil (5-FU®): Minimal hair loss
- Cyclophosphamide (Cytoxan®): 3 – 6 weeks; partial to total hair loss
- Doxorubicin (Adriamycin®): 7 – 21 days; 90% average loss
- Epirubicin (Ellence®): 7 – 21 days; total hair loss

- Methotrexate: 3 – 4 weeks; 33% average loss
- Taxol® and Taxotere®: 7 – 21 days; total hair loss (Taxol® given weekly causes hair thinning)

Ask your healthcare provider about the amount of hair loss and when you can expect it to occur.

Preparing for Hair Loss

A decision that each woman must make for herself, after losing her hair, is whether to cover her head or not. Women respond differently when dealing with the loss of their hair. Some women prefer not to wear a wig or cover their head during treatment. Instead, they are very comfortable with their appearance and find that their visible hair loss becomes an opportunity to share information with other women about early breast cancer detection. However, the majority of women prefer to cover their heads.

If you plan to cover your head, it is recommended that you purchase head-covering items before you begin losing your hair. Today, there are many options available, and many can be found on the Internet. The American Cancer Society offers an online store that sells a variety of hair loss products, wigs, human hair accents, turbans, hats and scarves, at a very reasonable price.

Plan to purchase a turban, sleep cap or hair net to wear at home to control loose hairs as they fall out at night. Cotton items tend to stay on the smooth scalp better than synthetic ones. During the day you can select a hat, turban, scarf or wig.

Wigs are available in natural or synthetic hair and come in all colors and lengths. It is helpful to try on wigs to determine which type you prefer. Select a wig prior to losing your hair, when your natural hair color and style can be closely matched. Consider buying more than one wig to allow time to have one cleaned and styled. Synthetic wigs require less frequent styling. Some insurance companies cover most, or all, of the cost of a wig and require a prescription for reimbursement. Wigs are a tax deductible medical expense.

Hair Thinning Management Tips Before Treatment Begins:

- Consider getting a short, easily managed haircut that will minimize the appearance of hair thinning. Save a lock of your hair in case you decide to purchase a wig after you lose your hair.
- Plan to shop for a wig. Some women prefer to purchase a wig before hair thins; others prefer to wait until after they see how much hair they will lose.
- Talk to your hairdresser. Ask if a perm prior to treatment would help add volume to your hair and conceal hair thinning. A perm helps reduce stress from styling tools.
- Ask about coloring your hair a lighter shade so that hair thinning will not show the scalp as easily.
- Wear a hair net, turban or sleep cap at night to keep fallen hair off bed linens when hair loss begins.
- Use a satin pillowcase to reduce hair tangling while sleeping.

Hair Thinning Management Tips During Treatment:

- Plan to use a protein-based shampoo and follow with a conditioning rinse.
- Plan to shampoo less often; every three to five days.
- Avoid excessive hair combing and brushing.
- Dry hair on a low temperature setting, or allow it to dry naturally.
- Minimize the use of hot styling tools; avoid use of hair clips, barrettes and elastic ponytail holders.
- Use hair spray sparingly.

Total Hair Loss Management Tips Before Treatment Begins:

- Prepare your family. Explain to young children that hair loss does not hurt and that your hair will grow back when treatment is over.

- Consider getting your hair cut short. Some women experience scalp tingling just prior to their hair falling out. Short hair eases this symptom.

- Consider shaving your head just prior to hair loss. This puts you in charge of your hair loss.

- Purchase hair nets, sleep caps, turbans, scarves, hats or, if you decide, a wig.
  - Do a web search to locate local wig retailers, online ordering companies and local specialty boutiques for cancer patients.
  - Purchase head coverings online at the American Cancer Society: www.tlcdirect.org.
  - Consider purchasing hair accents—pieces of human hair that you wear as bangs under turbans or hats. Baseball hats made with bangs, ponytail or hair attached are also available.

- Investigate having a wig, bangs or ponytail made from your own hair if it is long enough.

- Provide your stylist a photo of yourself taken on a good hair day as a guide to style your wig.

- Wear your new wig occasionally before you have hair loss to help with the adjustment.

Total Hair Loss Management Tips During Treatment:

- Keep your head covered during cold weather to prevent body heat loss. Sleep with a turban if your bedroom is cool.

- Keep your scalp moisturized to prevent dryness. Coconut oil is a good, all-natural moisturizer.

- Apply sunscreen to your scalp if it is exposed to sunlight.

Hair Regrowth

Hair regrowth starts during treatment or shortly after treatments are completed. When your hair grows back, it may have a different texture and slightly different color. Very often, the hair has a wavy pattern or is curly and darker. Most women like the texture and manageability of their new hair. However, the new hair growth is also fragile and is prone to breaking off. Continue to treat your new hair growth with the tips offered in this chapter for thinning hair. Avoid hair dye and perms for several months. It is also helpful to keep your hair short and easy to style until the hair becomes healthy and strong. Minoxidil (Rogaine®) is a drug approved for restoring hair loss in both women and men and is used by some patients to promote hair regrowth after chemotherapy.

Hair Loss Perspective

To deal with hair loss, it is essential to remind yourself that hair loss is evidence that chemotherapy is working to kill cancer cells. Undergoing hair loss for a short period of time is the price of obtaining a cancer-free future. During this time, it may be helpful to reach out to another cancer patient who has experienced hair loss and share your feelings. She will understand how you feel.

Skin and Nail Care

Chemotherapy causes the skin to undergo changes, becoming drier and more sensitive. You may find that you are sensitive to chemicals or products you have used for years. You will also be more sensitive to sun exposure. After treatment is over, your skin will gradually return to normal.

Skin Care Management Tips During Chemotherapy:

- Use a mild cleanser designed for sensitive skin: Dove®; Cetaphil Gentle Skin®; CeraVe® or Keri®.

- Do not scrub your skin; use a soft washcloth and warm water; avoid hot water and steam facials; pat your skin dry, do not rub.
- Use a facial moisturizer free of irritating chemicals:
  - Dry skin: Eucerin® (recommended by Skin Cancer Foundation because of SPF 30 sun protection)
  - Oily skin: Cetaphil®, SPF 15 protection
  - Acne prone skin: apply toner on the t-zone of face; moisturize with Cetaphil®
- Apply sunscreen with a minimum of SPF 30. Zinc or titanium oxide sunscreens scatter ultraviolet light and are less likely to be irritating to sensitive skin.
- Protect your skin from sunburn by wearing a hat and long-sleeved clothing. Polyester is better than cotton or linen at blocking harmful rays. UV-protective clothing, available at sporting goods stores, is specifically designed to block the sun.
- Keep your lips moist by applying a lip balm, Vaseline®, Aquaphor®, coconut oil or almond oil frequently.

Irritated Hands and Feet Management:

- Avoid putting your hands or feet in hot water.
- Soak your hands and feet in cool water to reduce discomfort.
- Keep hands and feet moisturized by applying lotions during the day. At night, apply Aquaphor® or Vaseline® and cover with gloves and socks overnight.
- Avoid any type of friction to the palms of your hands or the soles of your feet. Wear well-fitting shoes with cotton socks. Avoid wearing sandals.

Makeup Tips During Chemotherapy:

- Correct temporary complexion color changes caused by chemotherapy by applying a color-correcting concealer before your foundation. (Yellow for blue/purple undertone such as dark circles; pink for gray undertone; purple for yellow undertone; green for redness or blotchy discoloration.)
- Select a foundation closest to the color of your skin. Mineral makeup is less likely to irritate sensitive or dry skin. Moisturizing foundation provides a dewy, softer appearance for dry skin. Select a cream-based blush and eye shadow.
- Try a bronzing powder or lotion instead of foundation to help maintain a healthy glow.
- Select a moisturizing lipstick instead of a drier, matte lipstick.
- Wash your hands before applying makeup to the face with your fingers.
- Enhance thinning eyebrows by using an eyebrow brush dipped into a very small amount of powdered eyeshadow in a shade closest to your eyebrows. Apply to brows sparingly and then brush brows into shape to remove excess powder.
- Recreate eyebrows lost during chemo by purchasing an eyebrow stencil that provides a pattern to fill in brow using an eyebrow pencil. Available at www.tlcdirect.org.
- Consider false eyelashes, if lashes have thinned.
- Remove makeup with a gentle cleanser such as Cetaphil Gentle Skin Cleanser®.
- Keep all makeup brushes clean by washing in alcohol; do not share makeup; discard mascara after several months; do not use lipstick or mascara testers at makeup counters because of possible bacterial contamination.

Nails Care Tips During Chemotherapy:

- Do not cut cuticles during a manicure.

- Avoid artificial nails from a salon because of the electric files and strong chemicals.

- Treat dry, cracked or peeling nails by placing a small amount of olive oil in a dish and heating it in a microwave for 30 seconds. Soak your nails and cuticles for five minutes. Push your cuticles back with the pad of your finger. Massage remaining oil into the skin. Repeat three times a week.

- Buff your nails before applying non-formaldehyde nail polish to reduce potential ridges.

- Wrap your hands and feet in a warm washcloth or soak in warm water for five minutes; apply natural oil (olive or coconut), Vaseline® or a moisturizer. After treatment, put on gloves and socks to help the oil absorb. Leave them on overnight for maximum effectiveness.

- Apply one drop of tea tree oil under the nails daily before bedtime for prevention or treatment of an active fungal infection.

- Soak hands, then feet, in a mixture of one half cup white vinegar to one gallon of warm water for 5 - 10 minutes a day to reduce a fungal infection. Begin as soon as you notice nail changes.

- Apply Vicks Vapor Rub® to your feet and cover with socks overnight to treat toenail fungus. This will also moisturize your feet.

Learning Grooming Techniques From the Experts

The American Cancer Society offers a program called "Look Good, Feel Better." These sessions, led by licensed professionals, provide makeup techniques specifically for cancer patients and are held at most large cancer centers. They also provide information on ways to wear hats, scarves and head coverings to enhance your appearance during cancer treatment. By learning techniques from professionals, you can better deal with the grooming changes chemotherapy brings. If the program is not available in your area, their website, www.lookgoodfeelbetter.org, has videos for self-paced learning to enhance your personal appearance during cancer treatment. Call your cancer center to see if this free program is offered.

Report to Your Doctor

During chemotherapy, your blood cell counts will be lowered. If your white blood cells are affected, you will be at higher risk for infection. If your platelet count is lowered, you will be at higher risk for bleeding. If your red blood cells are lowered, you will have increased fatigue. Be sure to track your symptoms and side effects so that you can report them to your doctor during your next visit. To help you track your symptoms, refer to the *Health Symptoms Record* on page 291.

Symptoms to Report Immediately:

- Fever greater than 100.5° F

- Shaking chills with or without fever

- Sore throat; mouth sores; swallowing problems because of pain

- Cough with sputum (saliva mixed with mucus) production

- Pain or burning when urinating; sudden increase in urinary frequency; inability to control urine

- Discharge or redness around any wound, incision or sore

- Clear blisters on the skin

- Bleeding from any site that is not controlled after 20 minutes of pressure to the area

- Vomit that has a coffee ground appearance; dark tea-colored urine; blood-tinged sputum

- Racing or irregular heartbeat

- Fainting or sudden onset of dizziness
- Severe headache
- Shortness of breath; difficulty catching your breath; chest pain
- Sudden vision changes
- Sudden onset of severe pain in any area of the body
- Nausea not controlled in 24 hours with medication
- Diarrhea not controlled in 24 hours with medication

Ask your physician if there are any other symptoms specific to your care that you should report.

Treatment Response Terminology

At the completion of chemotherapy, your oncologist will report and document how your cancer responded to treatment. Terms used to describe your response to treatment include:

- **Remission, Cancer Free or Disease Free:** No signs of cancer can be found based on your symptoms, physical exam, radiology scans, X-rays or lab tests. This does not mean you will never have recurrence, but it does mean that with the current diagnostic studies, no evidence of cancer was found and that treatment was successful.

- **Incomplete Remission or Residual Disease:** Your cancer has been reduced after treatment, but there are still some signs of cancer based either on physical exam, radiology scans, X-rays or lab tests. Your healthcare team may recommend additional treatment or observation to see if the disease remains stable and does not progress.

- **Disease Progression:** Scans, X-rays or lab tests show that your disease did not respond to treatment but continued to increase, indicating the need for a different drug or treatment.

Dealing With the Stress of Chemotherapy

Going through chemotherapy often stresses your coping skills and causes you to wonder if all of the side effects are worth it. Indeed, this is not an easy time. The old saying, *"You can't control the waves of the ocean, but you can learn to ride them"* applies to getting through treatment. During treatment, try to mentally reframe the side effects experienced as time-limited and the price you are paying for your cancer-free future. During chemotherapy, pause and remember that:

- These unwanted symptoms are time-limited, like during pregnancy. They will come to an end.
- Hair loss is proof that you are killing cancer cells that may be hiding in your body and could return to harm you.
- Fatigue is like the yellow light on your car dashboard that serves as a warning of potential future problems if it is ignored. Fatigue warns you that your body needs rest. Just as you don't ignore the flashing yellow light in your car, don't ignore your body's fatigue. Instead, honor it and physically rest. While resting your body, also replenish your spirit with music or inspirational reading.

Keep your eye on the goal of chemotherapy—a cancer-free tomorrow.

Treatment Success Evaluation

Absolute Risk Reduction or Relative Risk Reduction

One of the challenges in making treatment decisions is understanding how a treatment will increase longterm outcomes in survivorship. Often this is a great source of confusion. When percentages are used to describe a benefit of a treatment or drug, it can cause confusion because there are two ways that percentages can describe the outcome. Both ways are truthful, but the percentage is derived in two very different ways. Therefore, it is essential to understand these two terms, **absolute risk reduction** and **relative risk reduction**, and their implications on your decisions.

Study Example: New drug to prevent breast cancer is given to two groups of 10 women each. One group is given a new drug and the other is given a placebo (dummy pill). At the end of five years, the findings are: 1 woman has breast cancer in the new drug group and 2 women in the placebo group have breast cancer.

The same data from the study could be reported as either:

1. *"New drug reduces breast cancer by 50 percent."*
2. *"New drug results in a 10 percent drop in breast cancer."*

Both are accurate. How can this be? The first is reported using relative risk reduction percentages, and the second is reported using absolute risk reduction percentages. This distinction is very important to understand if you are a patient making a decision about your healthcare. Let's look at how these figures are derived.

Study with two groups of ten women each.
Women in the first group get a new drug.
Women in the second group get a placebo (dummy pill).

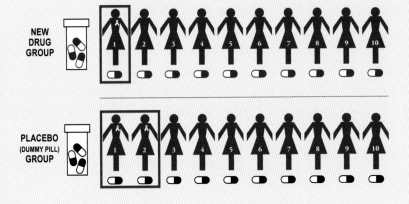

NEW DRUG GROUP

PLACEBO (DUMMY PILL) GROUP

At End of Study
- New Drug Group:
  - 1 diagnosis (10%)
- Placebo Group:
  - 2 diagnoses (20%)

Treatment Success Evaluation

Two Ways to Report the Outcome of the Study:

1. Absolute Risk Reduction: 20% – 10% = 10%
- *"The new treatment reduces breast cancer diagnoses by 10%."*

  OR

- *"After treatment, 1 woman in 10 was diagnosed instead of 2 in 10."*

2. Relative Risk Reduction: One diagnosis in the New Treatment Group is half as many as the two diagnoses in the Placebo Group, and that equals 50%.
- *"After treatment, only half as many women got breast cancer."*

  OR

- *"New treatment reduces breast cancer diagnoses by 50%."*

The media often reports **Relative Risk Reduction**. Both of the above statements are true, but **absolute risk reduction** allows you to make better choices. Be sure to always ask your doctor for your **absolute risk reduction**.

Not knowing if your healthcare provider is quoting you **absolute risk reduction** figures or **relative risk reduction** figures can be very misleading and confusing. If percentages are used, ask if these are **absolute risk reduction** figures or **relative risk reduction** figures. It is best to always know the absolute benefit from a drug or treatment in order to make an informed decision. Simply ask, *"What is the actual number of women out of 100 that benefited from taking the drug/treatment?"*

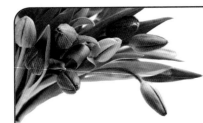

Remember...

- *Chemotherapy has significantly contributed to an increase in breast cancer survival.*

- *Surgery removes the cancerous tumor, and radiation therapy destroys any local cancer cells that may have been left after surgery. Chemotherapy is treatment that travels throughout your body to kill or control any microscopic cells that may have escaped the local area of the breast via the blood or lymphatic systems. The goal is to prevent these escaped cells from starting new tumor sites in other areas of the body.*

- *Chemotherapy decisions are not cookie-cutter. Your treatment plan is designed by your oncologist based on the unique features of your pathology report and any additional studies performed. Chemotherapy recommendations are based on national guidelines showing the most effective treatment known to prevent recurrence and increase survival.*

- *Chemotherapy has some undesirable side effects that vary according to the drug. However, most side effects resolve after treatment is completed.*

- *During treatment, be proactive and ask your treatment team how to manage any side effects of treatment.*

Additional Information

Tear-out Worksheets

Appendix

Radiation Therapy

Radiation therapy involves delivering X-rays to the breast area to destroy microscopic cancer cells. Radiation treatment is designed and administered under the care of a radiation oncologist—a physician who specializes in using radiation to treat diseases. Cancer cells so small they can't be seen with the human eye may remain in the body after surgery. The goal of radiation therapy is to destroy any remaining cancer cells in the surgical area to prevent future recurrence. Radiation destroys these microscopic cancer cells by making them unable to divide and multiply. When these cells die, the body naturally eliminates them. Healthy tissue is able to repair itself in a way that cancer cells cannot.

Lumpectomy patients usually have radiation therapy to the breast for three to six weeks. Mastectomy patients may also receive radiation therapy if their pathology report shows certain characteristics, such as a large tumor, positive lymph nodes or a tumor close to the chest wall. Your radiation oncologist will review your pathology report and write a prescription for the dose of radiation and the exact area to be treated. If you require chemotherapy, radiation usually starts about four weeks after your last chemo treatment is given. If you do **not** require chemotherapy, radiation usually starts about three to six weeks after surgery, or when the breast has healed.

When Radiation Therapy Is Not a Treatment Option:
- You had previous radiation to the chest area on the same side
- You are pregnant (may be an option if you can safely deliver the baby within six weeks and then receive radiation therapy)
- You have connective tissue disease such as scleroderma
- You cannot commit to the daily radiation therapy schedule
- You cannot lie on your back with your arm positioned above your shoulder for about 15 minutes (if receiving external beam radiation)

"I actually looked forward to my treatments every day, because I knew I was taking care of what I needed to do. Each day was a day that was behind me until I got through my thirty-three treatments."
—Earnestine Brown

Radiation Therapy Types

There are two methods to deliver radiation therapy for breast cancer—external and internal. External beam radiation is the most common type. Internal breast radiation, also called brachytherapy or partial breast radiation, is a newer method being used after lumpectomy. Internal breast radiation is being compared to whole breast external radiation in clinical trials.

External Beam Radiation

External beam radiation therapy is delivered by a machine called a linear accelerator that produces high-energy X-rays. Treatments are given daily, Monday through Friday, for up to six weeks. **Accelerated whole breast radiation** administers a higher dose of radiation in a shorter period of time and reduces treatment time to three weeks.

External Radiation Therapy Preparation

Before treatment begins, you will be scheduled for an appointment to map out the area to be treated. This visit will involve having X-rays and/or a CT scan to precisely identify the area to receive the therapy. When the area is identified, your therapist will make tiny marks, the size of a freckle, to outline the treatment area. The marks can be made with permanent ink (tattoo) or non-permanent ink. Your therapist will tell you which type you will receive. If permanent ink is used, you will feel a small pinch, like an insect bite, when the marks are being created with a needle and a drop of ink.

Receiving External Radiation Treatment

During external radiation therapy, you will lie on your back on a table with your arm above your head. The radiation device that delivers your treatment will be overhead. The therapist will use the marks on your chest to properly align the machine over the planned area of treatment. You will be alone in the room during the treatment, but a two-way communication system allows you and your technologist to talk. The therapist views your procedure on a screen from outside the room. Each treatment usually takes only 10 – 15 minutes in the treatment room but requires that you allow approximately 30 minutes for each visit. During the course of treatment, you will see your radiation oncologist weekly.

Internal Radiation: Accelerated Partial Breast Irradiation (APBI)

Accelerated partial breast irradiation (APBI) is a localized radiation treatment commonly called brachytherapy. It involves the insertion of radioactive seeds to kill breast cancer cells that may remain after lumpectomy surgery. Specialized catheters to deliver treatment are inserted into the cavity where the tumor was removed. Treatment starts one to four weeks after a lumpectomy.

APBI Patient Criteria Includes:

- 50 years of age or older
- Tumor measuring 3 cm or less
- Negative tumor margins
- Negative lymph nodes

APBI Advantages:

- Shorter treatment time than external beam radiation. Five to seven days versus three to six weeks.
- Radiation dose is concentrated on the tissues surrounding the lumpectomy cavity, which is the most likely site for local recurrence. Treatment spares the heart and lungs from unnecessary radiation.

Current APBI Devices:

- **SAVI™ (Strut Assisted Volume Implant):** A catheter is inserted into the lumpectomy site and is then expanded like a tiny umbrella to snugly fit the tumor cavity. A machine delivers radiation seeds through the catheter twice a day, six hours apart, for five days. The catheter is then removed.

- **Mammosite®:** A balloon-like device is inserted into the lumpectomy cavity at the time of surgery and is then inflated with saline water. The Mammosite® has four catheters through which a machine connected to a computer delivers the radioactive seeds for treatment twice a day, for five days. The catheter is then removed.

- **Contura™ MLB:** A balloon-like device with five catheters through which the radiation seeds travel. Contura® has vacuum ports on either end of the balloon to remove air or fluid between the balloon and breast tissue to ensure a snug fit. A machine connected to a computer delivers treatment twice a day, six hours apart, for five days. The catheter is then removed.

Newer APBI Methods:

- **3D-Conformal Radiotherapy:** This method uses a specialized machine to target radiation to the tumor area, which allows more of the healthy breast to be spared. Treatments are given twice a day for five days.

- **Intraoperative Radiation Therapy (IORT):** This method delivers a single, large dose of radiation to the tumor area while you are still in the operating room after lumpectomy surgery. IORT requires special equipment and is not widely available. This method is still in clinical trials.

Undergoing Radiation Therapy

During radiation therapy, it is suggested that you wear loose-fitting, cotton clothing, without a bra, to prevent irritation to the radiated tissues. Breakdown of the tissues can result in discomfort and delay of treatment. The ideal garment to wear is a cotton camisole. Some camisoles are designed with mastectomy pockets to hold a prosthesis or a lightweight fiber-fill insert, which allows you to maintain your body image during treatment. Before radiation therapy starts, it is helpful to purchase at least two soft cotton camisoles. These camisoles are available at the American Cancer Society's online store (www.tlcdirect. org). Insurance may reimburse the cost.

Radiation therapy does not make you radioactive, nor does it make you a danger to your family. Throughout radiation therapy, your therapist and radiation oncologist will monitor side effects from treatment. The side effects from radiation are usually mild and well tolerated. However, it is common for side effects to increase for one to three weeks after treatment is completed.

Potential Radiation Side Effects:

- Skin redness similar to a sunburn, which causes sensitivity and itching during treatment
- Tanning of the radiated area after redness subsides
- Breast swelling that is mild to moderate; potential for arm swelling
- Fatigue (mild) that begins during the third or fourth week; gradually improves after treatment ends
- Sore throat may occur during therapy
- Blisters and breaks in the skin, called wet desquamation, may occur and require that you stop radiation for a short period of time (more common after a mastectomy)
- Cough occurring six weeks to several months after treatment (uncommon)

- Increased risk for future arm lymphedema if underarm lymph node area is radiated
- Increased risk for future breast lymphedema

Skin Care During Radiation Therapy:

- Avoid extremely hot water when bathing; use only mild soaps (Tone®, Dove®, Basis® or baby soap) on the area being treated; avoid scrubbing or vigorous wiping with a washcloth or towel.
- Avoid extremes of hot or cold to the skin: no heating pads, ice packs, hot-water bottles, sun lamps, tanning beds or sunbathing.
- Avoid shaving under your arm with a razor blade to avoid nicking the skin; use an electric razor.
- Avoid underarm deodorant, powder, perfumes, lotions or other scented or alcohol-containing skin preparations on the treated area during therapy.
- Ask your nurse if you may apply pure aloe vera gel or Lubriderm® lotion to dry or peeling skin.
- Report any painful areas or blisters that occur. Ask if you can apply cool compresses moistened with water or saline (salt) water to blisters that burst. If the area is being rubbed by clothing, ask about applying a sterile dressing such as Op-Site® or Tegaderm® (available in a pharmacy) while it heals. Expose the covered area to air for 10 – 15 minutes two or three times per day. Moist desquamation usually heals within one to two weeks after treatment ends. Occasionally, the removal of the damaged tissue (debridement) is performed to speed healing to the area.
- Wait until two weeks after treatment to wear your regular bras or prosthesis. If you have a breakdown of the skin, you will need to wait until you are completely healed.
- Avoid sun exposure to the treated area.

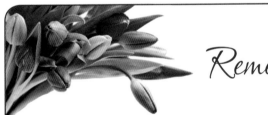

Remember...

- *Radiation therapy is used to destroy any microscopic cancer cells located in the area that is radiated.*
- *Radiation treatments are painless.*
- *Radiation therapy does not make you radioactive. You are not a danger to those around you.*
- *Ask your healthcare provider about how to best care for the radiated area.*

Additional Information

Tear-out Worksheet

Radiation Oncologist Questions - page 275

CHAPTER 13

Complementary and Alternative Medicine

In the treatment of cancer, there are proven and unproven treatments. The doctors, nurses and other healthcare providers involved in your cancer care are practicing conventional, Western, mainstream or biomedicine, which is backed by research.

After a diagnosis of cancer, you will hear about treatments for cancer from many sources—friends, family and the media. Some of the information will sound very appealing, especially when you are faced with choosing between treatments that have unpleasant side effects and those that do not. It is true that chemotherapy and radiation therapy have some unpleasant side effects; however, these treatments have proven results. They have been found to be effective in fighting your type of cancer. The treatments recommended by your physicians have many years of scientific study and clinical trials supporting their effectiveness. Many of the alternative therapies have never been the subjects of scientific studies, and their effectiveness has not been proven. Some healthcare organizations, including hospitals, cancer clinics and physicians, however, are engaged in clinical trials to test the effectiveness of some alternative therapies. Choosing to forego conventional therapy and replace it with an alternative treatment alone calls for a critical, thorough and wise investigation.

Cancer Treatment Terms
Various terms are associated with healthcare therapies. As a patient, it is important to understand what the terms mean, which approaches are considered safe and where you can find accurate information about various types of treatments.

Standard Medical or Clinical Treatments
Medical or clinical treatments are those that have been clinically tested for years, following a strict set of guidelines, and have been found to be safe and effective. The results of such studies have been published in medical journals and peer reviewed by other doctors and/or scientists in the field.

"I did a lot of meditating and I did a lot of praying."
—Earnestine Brown

"I explored and used a number of complementary therapies for both physical and emotional issues. I wanted to give myself every opportunity to be happy inside and out."
—Lisa DelGuidice

The Food and Drug Administration (FDA) grants approval for the treatments or procedures to be used in mainstream medicine.

Investigational Treatments

Investigational treatments or research treatments or therapies are studied in a clinical trial. Clinical trials are research-based projects that determine if a new treatment is effective and safe and, if applicable, the optimal dose for treatment. Before a drug, device or other treatment can be widely used to treat patients, it is studied and tested. If a clinical trial proves the effectiveness of the treatment or drug, the FDA may approve it for regular use by healthcare providers. Only then does the treatment become part of the standard, recommended collection of proven methods used to treat or diagnose disease in human beings.

Complementary Therapies

Complementary therapies are used along with your medical treatment and are often encouraged by physicians. Complementary therapies and activities that may enhance your recovery include:

- Nutrition
- Biofeedback
- Aromatherapy
- Hypnotherapy
- Herbal therapy
- Healing energy
- Art and music therapy
- Massage therapy
- Journaling
- Chiropractic therapy
- Counseling
- T'ai chi
- Psychotherapy
- Exercise
- Spiritual practices
- Reflexology
- Prayer
- Yoga
- Meditation
- Acupuncture

Integrative Therapy

Integrative therapy is a term that refers to the combination of both evidence-based (mainstream) medicine and complementary therapies.

Alternative Therapies or Quackery

Alternative therapy refers to a treatment that is used in place of conventional medical therapies and may be promoted as a cure. Most often, alternative treatments have never been scientifically tested according to US standards. They may have been tested and been found to be ineffective. Choosing alternative therapies instead of traditional medical treatments may cause a patient to put her health at risk.

Quackery refers to treatments, drugs or devices that claim to prevent, diagnose or cure diseases, but are known to be false or have no proven scientific evidence. These methods are most often based on a few patient testimonials or so-called doctor recommendations as evidence for their effectiveness and safety. Often, the treatment is claimed to be effective for multiple diseases as well as cancer. The elderly or chronically ill are often targets of quackery therapies.

These practitioners play on the emotional vulnerability of cancer patients by offering miracle cures. If an alternative therapy has caught your attention, it is highly recommended that you ask key questions about the therapy.

Alternative Therapy Questions:

- How much scientific evidence from clinical studies on humans has been published that proves the effectiveness of this treatment for my type of cancer?
- Are the testimonials from reputable healthcare professionals or are they only anecdotal reports?
- Are the claims validated with clinical data such as X-rays or laboratory tests that prove effectiveness?

- Is the person promoting the therapy benefiting financially?
- Do the promoters claim that if the product fails, it is because of a patient's lack of faith?
- What will the treatment cost? Will insurance cover it?
- Can I continue my regular treatments and try the alternative therapy at the same time?

Making the Right Choices

After a cancer diagnosis, you deserve every opportunity to restore your health to optimal levels. Choosing appropriate treatments is the foundation for your recovery. Many people find that it is helpful to combine complementary therapies with the treatment recommended by their healthcare providers, but they feel reluctant to share this decision with their physician. However, it is important to tell your healthcare providers about any treatments, therapies, drugs, vitamins or herbal products you are considering. There are many therapies you can safely use along with standard medical treatment to relieve symptoms, reduce side effects, ease pain and enjoy your life more. However, there are also some therapies that could interfere with the effectiveness of traditional treatment and even cause harmful side effects. Recovery is a partnership between you and your physician. You must communicate to receive the best care possible.

Internet as a Source of Information

The Internet is an easily accessible source of helpful information. Be careful, though, because the Internet can also be a source of misinformation.

Guidelines for Using the Internet:

- Select websites created by major medical centers, universities, government agencies and well-known advocacy groups like the American Cancer Society, Susan G. Komen for the Cure or Young Survival Coalition. You will find that they offer clinically proven advice for the treatment of cancer.
- Look for a board of qualified professionals who review information before it's published. What expertise do they have?
- Avoid commercial sites or personal testimonials that push a single point-of-view or sell miracle cures.
- Avoid sites that don't clearly distinguish between scientific evidence and advertisements.
- Ask your healthcare team about treatment advice that conflicts with their recommendations.
- Beware of scams and healthcare frauds. Many individuals or companies make their alternative treatments sound very persuasive. Remember, if it sounds too good to be true, it probably is.

FDA Clues To Identify Fraudulent Websites:

- Red-flag words: satisfaction guaranteed, miracle cure or new discovery.
- Pseudomedical jargon terms such as purify, detoxify and energize.
- Cure-all claims suggesting the product treats a wide range of symptoms and cures or prevents a number of diseases. No single product can do all of this.
- Anecdotal evidence. Testimonials are no substitute for solid scientific documentation. If the product is scientifically sound, it's actually to the manufacturer's advantage—and ultimately yours—to promote the scientific evidence.
- False accusations. The manufacturer of the product accuses the government or medical profession of suppressing important information about their product's benefits. Neither the government nor any medical profession has a reason to withhold information that could help people.

Reputable Internet Sources:

- Alternative and Complementary Medicine:
  - American Cancer Society: www.cancer.org
  - CancerGuide by Steve Dunn: www.cancerguide.org
  - National Cancer Institute: www.nci.nih.gov
  - National Center for Complementary and Alternative Medicine (NCCAM): www.nccam.nih.gov

- Herbal and Food Supplements:
  - American Botanical Council: www.herbalgram.org
  - Office of Dietary Supplements (ODS), NIH: www.ods.od.nih.gov
  - U.S. Food and Drug Administration (FDA): www.cfsan.fda.gov

- Research on Alternative/Unproven Methods:
  - National Council Against Health Fraud: www.ncahf.org

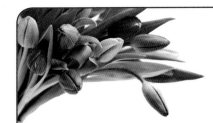

Remember...

- *Cancer treatment is not easy to undergo, yet standard medical treatments are proven to be safe and effective in increasing survival.*

- *Alternative therapies are often promoted as a cure. These claims are not based on proven clinical evidence but, rather, on a few patient testimonials. Often, the person promoting the treatment will financially benefit from the promoted treatment.*

- *Keep your healthcare team informed of any additional supplements you take during treatment because some supplements can block the effectiveness of the chemotherapy.*

- *Complementary therapies such as massage and yoga can enhance your recovery and are often recommended during treatment. Ask your physician for additional information.*

CHAPTER 14

Prosthesis Selection

Restoring your body image after breast surgery is an important part of your recovery. If you do not choose reconstruction, selecting and wearing a breast prosthesis is an alternative option. A breast prosthesis is a form molded into the shape of a breast and worn inside a bra. Choosing a prosthesis eliminates the need for a series of additional surgeries required for breast reconstruction. Many women decide that a prosthesis best suits their needs for restoring their body image.

Prosthesis Selection
Breast prostheses come in various types of material, shapes and colors, offering every woman a solution to restore her body image. A prosthesis fitter is trained to assess your chest wall, your non-surgical breast and your lifestyle, in order to recommend a form that will best restore your body image, both cosmetically and functionally.

A prosthesis is also available for patients who have had lumpectomy surgery that removed a large amount of breast tissue, which has caused their breasts to be mismatched in size. This prosthesis has a hollow back that fits over the lumpectomy breast to supplement existing breast tissues. This form is lightweight and fits into a regular bra.

If you have a mastectomy, you will need two types of prostheses. The first one is temporary to wear while your surgical incision is healing. The second one is permanent and will be worn when your incision has healed, or at the completion of radiation therapy.

Temporary Prosthesis
A temporary breast prosthesis is a fiber-filled form that can be adjusted to match the size of your remaining breast by adding or removing fiberfill. This lightweight form will fit into a bra and is an ideal option for women who desire to maintain their body image after surgery. It is also a good choice for wearing under night clothes.

It is suggested that you purchase a temporary prosthesis before surgery. You can purchase your temporary prosthesis at a local boutique or online

"The day I was fitted with my prosthesis was a major step in my road to recovery. For the first time in weeks, I began to feel that life just might return to normal again."
—Harriett Barrineau

since they do not require a fitting by a professional. The American Cancer Society has an online shop, www.tlcdirect.com, that has a wide variety of mastectomy and post-surgical products. You may also want to consider purchasing a mastectomy camisole designed to hold the temporary prosthesis. Some camisoles also have pockets to hold your surgical drains after breast surgery.

Permanent Prosthesis

When your incision has completely healed, or you have completed radiation therapy, it is time to select a prosthesis to balance the weight of your remaining breast. A weighted prosthesis prevents posture shift, which can eventually lead to back pain. Double mastectomy patients have the option of continuing to wear the lighter weight prostheses since they do not have to balance breast weight.

A permanent prosthesis requires a professional fitting. Make an appointment with a prosthesis fitter, allowing 1 to 2 hours for the fitting. Wear a tight sweater or a man's t-shirt to show the contour of the prosthesis when it is on your chest. Take someone with you who will provide honest feedback on how the prosthesis looks. Ask the professional fitter which prosthesis she recommends for you. Many women choose to purchase both a weighted prosthesis and a lightweight prosthesis to allow them to choose between the two according to their activity.

Types of Permanent Prostheses Available

Prostheses are made from foam, silicone or a combination of materials and come in a variety of shapes—teardrop, asymmetrical or triangle. Each type has advantages and disadvantages.

Foam Prosthesis:

- Less expensive option
- Lighter weight than a silicone prosthesis
- Not waterproof

Silicone Prosthesis:

- Feels and looks more natural than a foam prosthesis
- Molds to chest wall to provide a secure fit over uneven or concave surgical sites
- Weighs more than foam; larger-breasted women may find that a silicone prosthesis is too heavy and puts a strain on their shoulders
- Feels warmer than foam; silicone causes perspiration in hot weather or during exercise
- Available in models that adhere to the chest wall with adhesive strips (higher in cost); prosthesis stays in place for five days and does not require a special bra
  - It is recommended you try the adhesive strips to test for adhesive sensitivity before purchasing.
- Available in models with or without a nipple and areola
- Available in a variety of shades, as well as colorless to blend with any skin color
- Completely waterproof; but it is not recommended to wear in a hot tub

Micro-Bead Prosthesis:

- Made of thousands of tiny plastic beads inside a hypo-allergenic fabric covering
- Waterproof and molds to the body
- Looks and feels natural
- Lighter weight than a foam prosthesis by 80%
- Good selection to wear in swimsuits, night clothes and leisure wear

- Can be worn by bilateral mastectomy patients anytime
- May not be recommended for long-term use by single mastectomy patients

Combination Prosthesis:

- Three-layer construction of silicone gel, polyurethane beads and a hypo-allergenic fabric that wicks away perspiration
- Lighter weight than silicone prosthesis by 50%
- Soft and natural-looking
- May not be recommended for long-term use by single mastectomy patients

Bra With Built-In Prosthesis:

- Bra has a permanently sewn-in lightweight form made of soft plastic beads that mold naturally to the body
- Prosthesis is washable
- Form is customized to match your size with either left, right or bilateral placement
- May not be recommended for long-term use by single mastectomy patients

Prosthesis Fitter Questions:

- How do I clean my prosthesis?
- Can I get my prosthesis wet?
  - If so, how long will it take to dry?
- Will pool or hot tub chemicals damage the prosthesis?
- Does perspiration damage the prosthesis?
- Can I wear my regular bras with this prosthesis if they are altered?
- Is there an exchange policy if I decide the prosthesis does not meet my needs?
- How much will my insurance provider pay on my prosthesis?
- How many bras will my insurance cover each year?
- How many mastectomy camisoles will my insurance cover each year?
- How often will my insurance pay for the replacement of my prosthesis?

Altering Clothes for Prostheses

You can alter many of your clothes to accommodate a prosthesis. Swimsuits, sportswear and night clothes are examples. Your prosthesis fitter can give you instructions on how to sew a pocket into your clothing and recommend the most appropriate prosthesis to use.

Prostheses Cost

Prices for a prosthesis vary according to the type you choose. A temporary fiber-filled prosthesis, which is adjustable by removing filling, is approximately $12. Lightweight, microbead forms are usually under $75. A foam prosthesis is usually less than $100. A silicone prosthesis ranges from $165 to $300. Custom-made models and models that adhere to the chest are more expensive. Mastectomy bra prices range between $36 – $65.

Prosthesis and Bra Reimbursement

Most professional prosthesis shops will assist you in understanding the amount covered by your insurance and help you fill out your claim for reimbursement.

Medicare, Medicaid and private insurers cover the cost of a prosthesis after breast cancer surgery. Ask your physician for a prescription so that you can get reimbursed by your insurer. Most insurers will also cover the cost of camisoles designed to hold a prosthesis after surgery. If your weight changes (increases or decreases), your prosthesis or bras may no longer fit correctly. Ask your doctor to write a letter documenting the weight change and send it to your insurance provider asking them to allow you to purchase new ones.

Current Medicare Replacement Guidelines:
- Foam form replacement: Every 6 months
- Silicone form replacement: Every 2 years
- Bras: 4 – 6 each year or as medically necessary for weight loss or gain
- Camisoles: As many as medically necessary, but not more than 3 per month

When You Cannot Afford a Prosthesis

If you cannot afford a prosthesis, some local American Cancer Society units or cancer centers have loan closets that can help you. Some women who have undergone delayed reconstruction donate their prosthesis to a loan closet to be given to other women. Call your local cancer center to ask if anyone in your area provides this service or if there are any organizations that provide financial support for patients who cannot afford a prosthesis.

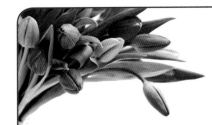

Remember...

- *Plan to shop for a prosthesis when you have time to carefully evaluate which breast form best suits your need. Make an appointment with a specialized prosthesis fitter.*

- *Take someone with you who will be supportive and honest in helping you evaluate how it looks. Take a t-shirt or tight sweater to try on over the new form to see how it looks under your clothing.*

- *Do not try to save a few dollars on a prosthesis you do not like or feel uncomfortable wearing. Restoring your body image is a very important part of recovery.*

Chapter 15

Monitoring Your Emotional Recovery

"My one-year diagnosis anniversary date blindsided me a little bit. My mother sent a huge bouquet of pink roses to work, and I broke down crying. But I still reflect back upon the entire thing as a gift of change. Going to a support group, even if there were no other young women in the group, was incredibly helpful. I found an online 'virtual' support group with discussion boards. Later, I joined the organization as a volunteer. Getting involved in breast cancer advocacy work has helped me with the need to give back and continue the fight."

—Anna Cluxton

"I actually started taking care of ME after my diagnosis—the way you're supposed to. I had to realize that there are only 24 hours in a day and not 99 like I thought there were before."

—Earnestine Brown

The unexpected diagnosis of breast cancer can serve as a threat to your self-esteem, body image, sexuality, social life and career. That's a lot of unexpected threats and changes to deal with after diagnosis. During this time, you may experience many confusing emotions—things you may have never felt—as these threats are individually worked into your life. After receiving a cancer diagnosis, the biggest surprise for many women was the struggle they had emotionally—they thought dealing with treatment would be their biggest challenge, but they found that the hardest part was dealing with their fluctuating emotions.

The problem they had dealing with their anxiety and depression threw them a curve ball. One patient shared about her emotional struggles:

I have always been so strong and able to handle anything that came my way ... until now, and now I feel as if I am falling apart many days. My doctor assures me I am doing great and have a good prognosis. I know that this should make me happy, and I should be grateful, but somehow I can't feel that way. I feel so alone in my struggle to make sense of this. What is happening to me?

"My physical recovery went well. At first, it seemed, so was my mental and emotional state. After three or four months, things began to change. I knew people still cared, but the initial interest and concern began to wane. I was still surrounded by so much love, yet I was feeling totally alone."

—Harriett Barrineau

If you have had difficulty with your emotional recovery, you are not alone. Somehow the emotional struggle is seldom talked about. It may not be discussed by your healthcare team because they are trained to treat your cancer, and that is their main focus. You may have to approach the topic with them to receive the same good treatment for your emotional struggles as you do for your cancer.

This chapter will share insights to help you understand the normal emotional challenges you may or may not face, what you can do about them and when you should seek help from a professional.

Major Emotional Challenges

Anxiety and depression are the major emotional challenges patients deal with. Anxiety is a signal that you are under too much stress, and it is defined as the time spent fighting the problem. Depression, on the other hand, signals that you have stopped struggling with a problem, have given in to it and have given up the fight. It is helpful to understand how the symptoms of anxiety and depression differ and when you should seek professional help for either.

Anxiety

Anxiety occurs throughout life when someone is faced with a new challenge and feels frightened or threatened by it. A breast cancer diagnosis is certainly one of these times. High anxiety is expected during the diagnostic period, immediately after a diagnosis and anytime a new stressor (an event that is frightening and perceived to be a threat) happens.

Signs and Symptoms of Anxiety:

- Nervousness and shaking inside; lips quiver; hands shake; speech is rapid
- Racing heart; tightness in chest; choking sensation; palpitations (heart skips a beat)
- Rapid breathing; lightheadedness
- Tingling or numbness in arms, hands, legs and feet
- Pacing, can't sit still; lack of concentration and short-term memory about events; confusion
- Constant worry; intrusive thoughts; sense of dread
- Difficulty falling asleep and staying asleep; restless, unsatisfying sleep

Anxiety symptoms are real and indicate that you are dealing with something that is frightening to you. Anxiety can rob you of your ability to make decisions, cause you to be fatigued and irritable and, if experienced for a long period of time without relief, can impede your recovery. Anxiety may be a short-term problem that resolves itself and only reappears when a new challenge arises, or it can be long-term. When a person experiences anxiety on a daily basis, week after week, it is considered chronic anxiety.

Depression

Depression occurs when you give in to a situation—life is just too hard, so you withdraw. It often follows an extended period of anxiety. Depression symptoms manifest themselves differently than anxiety. Depression varies in degree of severity from a short period of feeling down and blue to a debilitating depression that continues day after day. It is essential to understand the difference between a normal reaction of feeling depressed for a short period of time and prolonged clinical depression, which needs intervention by health professionals.

Reactive Depression

After a breast cancer diagnosis, most women suffer from an expected short-term depression called a reactive depression. A cancer diagnosis is a real loss that has to be incorporated into your life. Scattered throughout the months after your surgery and during treatment, sometimes for unknown reasons, you may find yourself feeling blue, down or depressed. If the feeling lasts for several days and then you begin to feel better, this is a normal reaction (reactive depression) after a loss in your life.

Common Times for Reactive Depression:

- **Check-Ups:** Depression may occur around the time of a return visit to your physician for a check-up after breast cancer. We refer to this normal reactive depression as check-up anxiety. Most women are anxious the week or days surrounding their check-up, worrying if anything new will be found. If the exam is negative, the blue mood lifts.

- **Treatment Conclusion:** Many women feel depressed at the conclusion of all of their cancer treatments. This depression is referred to as post-treatment depression and is very common.

- **Anniversary Dates:** Dates of diagnosis, surgery or treatments can cause an anniversary date reaction. These dates may bring back vivid memories and the feelings you experienced during the original event. It is normal for these dates to create a sad reminder of the experience, but anticipating and planning for them can significantly reduce the emotional strain.

It can be helpful if you anticipate these common times for experiencing reactive depression and plan to accommodate for your blue feelings. When check-ups are due, share your anxiety and concerns with someone. On anniversary dates, plan a time away from your routine duties and do something special with friends. At the conclusion of treatment, set new goals and do things you have always wanted to do.

Depression That Needs Intervention: Clinical Depression

For some women, incorporating the changes a cancer diagnosis brings becomes a problem. Their depressed feelings and tears do not cease; they continue for extended periods of time during or long after surgery and treatments are completed. These periods may occur often or remain as a constant companion. This is a sign of **clinical depression** that needs intervention by a professional. Clinical depression is a serious condition with real symptoms that affect the mind, body and relationships. Symptoms are prolonged, severe and will increasingly incapacitate your ability to return to normal functioning.

The first step in distinguishing the difference between feeling blue and clinical depression is to know the warning signs of clinical depression and to feel comfortable about seeking appropriate help. Feeling blue means a person may feel sad but can still enjoy and look forward to parts of life, such as a family gathering, a movie or seeing a friend. Depression, on the other hand, steals all joy from a person's life.

Clinical Depression Is Often Manifested By:

- Continuous (week after week) feelings of sadness during or after surgery and treatment
- Social withdrawal from friends or family
- Feelings of worthlessness
- Excessive feelings of guilt
- Excessive fear of the future
- Slowness in physical movement or speech
- Constant jitters or nervousness with no apparent reason
- Low energy level; feeling tired all of the time
- Inability to make decisions
- Negative thinking; constant anger or mistrust
- Persistent aches, pains or digestive disorders that do not respond to treatment

- Obsessions about health and cancer

- General disinterest in food, or eating excessively

- Disinterest in work or day-to-day activities (things which used to interest you)

- Disinterest in intimacy or sex

- Insomnia (inability to sleep, waking early or being unable to go to sleep)

- Hypersomnia (sleeping too much, wanting to sleep all of the time)

- Suicidal thoughts (If you have suicidal thoughts and feel that death would be an easy choice, please call your physician or nurse immediately.)

If you find that you are experiencing several of these symptoms (some experts say five) for a period of two weeks or longer during or after treatment completion, you should talk to your physician. Breast cancer patients who take chemotherapy also have to deal with hormonal fluctuations caused by treatment, which greatly increases the potential for mood changes and other side effects that increase stress and contribute to the potential for depression. It is essential to understand that seeking help for your depression is not a sign of weakness; instead, it is a sign of strength.

Is It Anxiety or Depression or Both?

Sometimes it is difficult to determine if you are suffering from anxiety, depression or a combination of both. A quick assessment may help you determine which you are experiencing. Answer the questions below by marking a yes or no for each question to help determine whether your struggle is with anxiety, depression or both.

Anxiety or Depression Assessment

Set I

1. Do you feel nervous or edgy most of the day for no reason? . . . . Yes   No
2. Do you sometimes panic when something happens? . . . . Yes   No
3. Do you often feel scared, as if something bad is going to happen? . . . . Yes   No
4. Are you sometimes too nervous to do anything? . . . . Yes   No
5. Do you constantly feel stressed out? . . . . Yes   No

                                                        Totals ___   ___

Set II

1. Do you no longer feel confident in yourself to handle problems? . . . . Yes   No
2. Do you feel hopeless about what is happening in your life? . . . . Yes   No
3. Do you feel helpless about what is happening in your life? . . . . Yes   No
4. Do you feel worthless as a person? . . . . Yes   No
5. Do you sometimes think life is not worth living? . . . . Yes   No

                                                        Totals ___   ___

Assessment Score

Total up the yes and no answers to each set of questions. Generally, if you answered yes to more of the questions in Set I, you are experiencing anxiety. If you answered yes to more of the questions in Set II, you are likely experiencing depression. If you answered yes to more than three in each set, you may be suffering from both anxiety and depression. Discuss this questionnaire with your physician or someone on your healthcare team.

Treatments for Depression and Anxiety

The good news is that there are treatments available for anxiety and clinical depression. Both are treated through learning new personal coping skills, seeking professional counseling and drug therapy.

Counseling

In some cases, counseling—talking to a professional—may be all that is needed. Counseling identifies weaknesses in coping skills and works to strengthen them. Often, talking to an understanding person accomplishes a lot for a depressed or anxious person. Counseling, often called "talk therapy" or psychotherapy, allows a person to talk about past and present experiences, relationships, feelings, thoughts and behaviors that may be contributing to the problem. The counselor's aim is to identify major causes of stress and then help you determine the best approach to solve your problems. Ask your nurse or physician for local counseling resources. Most often, counseling after breast cancer is short-term.

Drug Therapy for Anxiety and Depression

Medication may be needed to assist the therapeutic process and requires a prescription from a medical physician or an advanced care practitioner. Some people feel there is a social stigma to taking anti-anxiety or antidepressant medications. However, taking medications for anxiety or depression is no different than taking medication for diabetes. Both conditions are uninvited and attack the body, and both can be successfully managed with medication. Denying yourself medication to help with your acute anxiety or depressed mood is like denying yourself insulin to treat diabetes.

Anti-Anxiety Medication

Anti-anxiety drugs (benzodiazepines) are used to calm your nervousness or agitation and they begin to work immediately. Many women diagnosed with acute anxiety find that taking an anti-anxiety drug allows them to regain their composure, to concentrate on treatment decisions and to sleep much better. When taken correctly, symptoms of anxiety are reduced within 30 to 90 minutes. If you are experiencing a high level of anxiety after your diagnosis, do not hesitate to ask your physician for help. This will allow you to get the rest you need and to make decisions in a more timely, informed manner.

Medications for Anxiety
■ Alprazolam (Xanax®)
■ Lorazepam (Ativan®)
■ Chlordiazepoxide (Librium®)
■ Clonazepam (Klonopin®)
■ Diazepam (Valium®)

Your doctor will usually prescribe these medications only for a short time to help you get through a particularly rough period of anxiety. Long-term anxiety is better controlled with other medications. Anti-anxiety drugs for acute anxiety may be prescribed on a regular schedule or to be taken as needed during periods of high anxiety. Don't drive while taking these drugs; they cause drowsiness. Remember, your healthcare team does not know what you are experiencing or need unless you tell them.

Antidepressant Medications

Antidepressants are often prescribed to stabilize your mood. They will take approximately two to three weeks to become effective. There are numerous categories of antidepressants to treat depression. Both the drugs and the dosages must be carefully matched with a patient's symptoms and overall health.

Antidepressant medications are not a one-size-fits-all approach. Physicians consider numerous factors. For example, if you are experiencing depression accompanied by fatigue, the selective serotonin reuptake inhibitors (SSRIs) will help with the fatigue, and some will reduce hot flashes. The SSRIs are the most commonly prescribed group of antidepressants. If you are experiencing anxiety with your depression and are not able to fall asleep or stay asleep, another type of antidepressant may be a better choice because of its sedating effect. Wellbutrin® is another antidepressant for patients who do not have anxiety with their depression. Wellbutrin® has no sexual dysfunction associated with use. Some antidepressants may interfere with tamoxifen. Preferred drugs for patients taking tamoxifen include: Wellbutrin®, Cymbalta®, Effexor® and Lexapro®.

It is important to understand that not all antidepressant medications are effective in all people. It may take several attempts before your physician finds the most effective medication for your needs. Since it takes time for antidepressant medication to build up in your body before you feel the full effects, it is important to contact your physician when you first recognize symptoms of depression.

Medications for Depression

- Bupropion (Wellbutrin®)
- Citalopram (Celexa®)
- Desvenlafaxine (Pristiq®)
- Duloxetine (Cymbalta®)
- Escitalopram (Lexapro®)
- Fluoxetine (Prozac®, Prozac Weekly®)
- Fluvoxamine (Luvox®)
- Paroxetine (Paxil®, Paxil CR®, Pexeva®)
- Sertraline (Zoloft®)
- Venlafaxine (Effexor®, Effexor XR®)

Antidepressants are usually prescribed for an extended period of time and are withdrawn gradually when you and your physician feel you are ready. They need to be taken as prescribed, without skipping doses or stopping when symptoms are controlled. Anti-anxiety medication and an antidepressant may initially be prescribed at the same time. When the antidepressant begins to take effect, the anti-anxiety drug is reduced, discontinued or used only when needed. Talk to your healthcare team about getting the help you need to regain control of your emotions and improve your quality of life.

Self-Care for Anxiety and Depression

If you are reading this and are in the acute phase of anxiety or have moved to depression, talk to your physician about the appropriate medication to restore you to a state where you can function. You can then tackle adding the self-care tips discussed below. If your anxiety or depression is mild, allow yourself to experience the benefits of self-care for stress. The following suggestions do not require a prescription and do not cost anything—only your determination to implement the proven methods of stress control.

Controlling Stress With Self Care

Stress control begins with identifying exactly what you are afraid of and taking steps to do what you can to make it less threatening. Dr. Herbert Benson of Harvard Medical School, recognized as the world's leading expert on elicitation of the relaxation response, advises patients to use the following formula: **stop**, **breathe**, **reflect** and **choose**.

- **Stop:** Recognize you are at the beginning of a stress response.
- **Breathe:** Take several deep breaths and let them out slowly. This slows down the body's physical response and allows you to think more clearly.
- **Reflect:** Ask yourself:
  - What am I afraid of that is causing these feelings?
  - What about this event or thought is upsetting or distressing me?
  - Am I jumping to conclusions about what happened or may happen?
  - Is this a present reality or a future worry?
  - If a present reality:
    - » What can I do to change it?
    - » What information can I gather?
    - » With whom can I talk to understand what I need to do?
  - What is the worst thing that can happen? If that happens, can I handle it?

- **Choose:** Take the steps of action you identified—you may still feel fearful, but addressing your fears is the way to make them manageable. Make a deliberate decision not to think about them so anxiously—remember, 90 percent of what we worry about never happens.

Stress Control by Self-Talk

An important part of recovery is self-talk, or what your mind is saying to you. It is helpful to choose some encouraging phrases to say repeatedly to yourself when you begin to be fearful or worried. Sometimes self-talk is the quickest and easiest way to calm your nerves.

Calming Self-Talk Phrases Include:

- *"I can handle this."*
- *"I am doing the best I can."*
- *"I've done hard things before; I can do them again."*
- *"I don't have to be perfect; I'd rather be happy."*
- *"Let it go; it's not worth it."*
- *"This, too, will pass."*
- *"My health is more important than my need to be right."*
- *"I have so much to be thankful for."*

Using the stop, breathe, reflect and choose formula and repeating positive self-talk phrases allows you to reduce your stress when an event occurs. Chronic stress can also be reduced by using methods that elicit the relaxation response to calm the body. These techniques include deep breathing, meditation or imagery (focused thinking about something positive), praying or repetitive prayers, repetitive exercise, progressive muscle relaxation and yoga.

The Relaxation Response

Dr. Benson identified the relaxation response (deep breathing and repetitive phrases) as a means to manage stress when you are dealing with things you cannot control. The relaxation response has been clinically proven to reduce heart rate and blood pressure, thus relaxing the entire body and counteracting the harmful effects of chronic stress.

Learning To Elicit the Relaxation Response

To learn any new skill requires practice and perseverance. Most people have difficulty relaxing their bodies and need a way to free themselves from the stress of their environment to enter into a state of relaxation. Relaxing begins with a conscious effort.

How To Elicit the Relaxation Response:

- Find a quiet room away from interruptions, and sit up straight in a chair.
- Place your hands comfortably in your lap. Relax your muscles.
- Close your eyes.
- Select a focus word, phrase or prayer that gives you a sense of peace, love and safety. Some suggestions are:
  - **General:** One; Peace; Calm; Relax; Let go; Let it be; Love; My time
  - **Christian:** Come, Lord; Lord, have mercy; Our Father, who art in heaven; Lord Jesus Christ, have mercy on me; Hail Mary; The Lord is my Shepherd
  - **Jewish:** Sh'ma Yisroel (Hear, o Israel); Shalom (Peace); Hashem (The Name)

- **Eastern:** Om (the universal sound); Shantih (Peace)
- **Aramaic:** Maranatha (Come, Lord); Abba (Father)
- **Islamic:** Allah

■ Breathe slowly and naturally, and, as you do, silently repeat the phrase or word you have selected as you exhale.

■ Continue inhaling and repeating your phrase while exhaling. Do this for approximately 20 minutes.

■ When your mind wanders to another thought, refuse to entertain it and gently bring your thoughts back to your breathing and repetitive phrase.

■ Open your eyes and gradually reorient yourself to your surroundings.

As you practice the relaxation techniques, you may find it is difficult to keep your mind focused. Admittedly, it is hard, but don't get discouraged. Fortunately, there are a number of ways to focus your mind. Mindful breathing is one of the keys. As you practice, take a few deep breaths to help turn your attention inward, and then allow your breathing to follow its own natural rhythm. During relaxation you may feel sensations such as a tingling, a sense of floating, drifting or dropping. This indicates that your body is relaxing. It is suggested that the relaxation response be practiced twice a day to provide maximum benefit from stress.

Mini Relaxation Responses

You may find yourself in a stressful situation such as a diagnostic test or an I.V. stick when you cannot leave or escape to a quiet place. Simply concentrate on breathing and repeating your phrase either silently or quietly with your eyes open, if necessary. Taking a deep breath increases the oxygen to the brain and clears the thinking. Focusing on a word or phrase during concentrated breathing interrupts the anxiety produced by the stressful situation. Many patients have said this technique has been invaluable and comforting when confronting a stressful event such as receiving chemotherapy or radiation, having an I.V. stick, enduring a diagnostic test or undergoing a new procedure. Keep your body in a more relaxed state by practicing the mini relaxation response anytime, anywhere.

Visualization Relaxation

Another relaxation technique is to replace the repetitive phrase with a mental picture of a scene that brings a sense of peace and safety—a garden, park, seashore, etc. As you breathe slowly, mentally feel and explore the beauty of this favorite place in your mind—smell the fragrances, feel the warmth of the sun and hear the familiar sounds.

Additional Chronic Stress Busters

One of the major ways to control chronic stress is to start a program of regular exercise. You may not feel like you have the energy to do anything, but any effort to increase your daily movement will bring positive benefits. Set goals for yourself to gradually increase your daily activity. Exercise has proven to be one of the best ways to reduce stress and improve your mood. Exercise promotes the release of endorphins, chemicals in your body that naturally increase mood and decrease pain. Massage and sexual activity have also been proven to increase the release of your natural endorphins.

Another way to control chronic stress is to watch what you eat. A nutritious diet and adequate hydration (water intake) promote a better mood and increase energy. Mayo Clinic psychiatrist, Daniel K. Hall-Flavin, M.D., reported that some people with depression have low blood levels of eicosapentaenoic acid (EPA), a fatty acid found in fish oil. These omega-3 fatty acids have been shown to play an important role in brain function as well as normal growth and development. A good way to get more omega-3 fatty acids, including EPA, is to simply eat more fish. Try salmon, mackerel and tuna. Other dietary sources of omega-3 fatty acids include flaxseed, canola oil, soybeans, pumpkin seeds and walnuts. Increase your intake of these foods.

Conquering Anxiety and Depression

No one can avoid daily events which cause anxiety. We are usually able to manage these everyday stressors until a crisis comes. During a crisis, we have to deal with so many threatening unknowns that we become overwhelmed with stress and experience acute anxiety. Acute anxiety is a natural response to something we find frightening. Depression often comes after acute anxiety has exhausted our ability to cope. The underlying cause of acute anxiety and depression is fear. Worry is our mental effort to manage our fears during a crisis. Every negative, worrisome thought we have releases a cascade of stress hormones that negatively affects our physical health and lowers our ability to fight infections. Ignoring worry has physical health consequences. Taking steps to learn how to deal with our fears and reduce worry is a step towards creating better health. This is a hard change for many people to make because they feel that paying attention by worrying is necessary.

One patient shared her advice to other women going through treatment:

> When the news is good, I don't allow myself to get too high, and when it is bad, I don't allow myself to get too low because I know that things will constantly change. My job is to manage my emotions; the doctor's is to manage my cancer. You've got to get off of that emotional roller coaster; it will destroy you.

We can't change what happens to us, but we can change many of our responses. We can change what we think about the event. We can get support and help to understand what we can do. We can manage stress by incorporating physical activity and eating a nutritious diet. Then, if we don't find relief, there are medications for anxiety and depression. Remember, it's hard enough to fight breast cancer physically. You do not have to tough it out emotionally, dealing with anxiety or depression that robs you of your ability to function. Reaching out for help is a sign of strength—not weakness. If you need help, don't hesitate to call your healthcare team.

Understanding The Stress Response

On the following pages is a complete explanation of the stress response that occurs after a threatening event in a person's life, such as a cancer diagnosis. The response to an event impacts a person's mind and behavior, which results in physical symptoms in the body. Understanding this process will help you to identify how you are responding to a new threatening stressor and will provide you with insight on how to prevent any negative effects by interrupting the process. Tips on how to keep a stressful event from negatively impacting your mental and physical health are also discussed.

The Stress Response

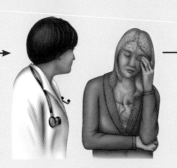

1
The Event
Perceived in Mind as a Threat or Danger

Examples:
- Cancer Diagnosis
- Surgery
- Death in Family
- Chemotherapy
- Radiation Therapy
- Car Accident

2
Brain's Perception
Sets off Physical and Emotional Responses

4
Evaluation of Event or Stressors
Making Choices to "Fight" or "Flight" (Flee)

Determined By:
- Previous Life Experiences
- Personal Belief System
- How One Sees Self as Able to Handle Stressor (Physically and Emotionally)
- Problem-solving Skills
- Communication Skills
- Available Resources and Support (People, Information, Etc.)

3
Automatic Response

Physical Responses:
- Blood Pressure Increases
- Heart Rate Increases
- Breathing Rate Increases
- Muscles Tense
- Eyes Dilate
- Digestive System Slows
- Bladder Relaxes
- Saliva Increases

Emotional Responses:
- Panic
- Fear
- Anxiety/ Nervousness
- Tension

5
Mental Outlook Decision

5A
Mental Outlook: "Fight" or Optimism
- Take Problem on as a Challenge
- Commit to Solve the Problem
- Take Control of Problem by Learning Options
- Develop Support System

Physical Responses:
- Stronger Immune System
- Sleep Soundly
- Increased Energy

Emotional Responses:
- Calm
- Patient
- Relaxed
- Self-confident
- Even-tempered
- Hopeful
- Assertive

5B
Mental Outlook: "Flight" or Pessimism
- View Self as a Victim
- View Situation as Hopeless
- Negative Thoughts About Situation
- Irrational Beliefs About Situation
- Unable to Make Decisions or Communicate

Physical Responses:
- Headaches
- Weakened Immune System
- Sleep Disturbances
- Appetite Changes
- Stomach Disorders
- High Blood Pressure
- Heart Disease
- Chronic Pain

Emotional Responses:
- Emotional Withdrawal
- Persistent Anxiety
- Long-term: Major or Clinical Depression

6
Exhaustion State: Clinical Depression
If a person remains in this state for weeks or longer, the stress can lead to harmful physical and emotional damage to the body.

The Stress Response

Understanding The Stress Response During Cancer

The word stress is defined by Webster's dictionary as *"a state of mental tension and worry caused by problems in your life; something that causes strong feelings of worry or anxiety caused by adverse or very demanding circumstances."* Stress can come from interactions between people or an environmental situation that a person perceives as threatening to their well-being.

Stress is a normal response to a new or unknown situation. When faced with a stressor, our bodies automatically release a flood of stress hormones throughout the body that cause physical and mental changes. This flood of hormones can prepare us to jump out of the way of a speeding car in a split second to save our life. However, the same flood of hormones that can save our life can become health-threatening if the stress is not reduced. In psychology, this physiological process is known as the stress response.

The Stress Response

The Stress Response, also called the General Adaptation Syndrome, was first identified in the early 1900s by Hans Selye. It is a basic description of the role of stress, the way people respond to stress in their environment and how, if not relieved, stress can negatively impact one's health. No one can avoid stress; it is a part of life. However, we can learn to control and change some of the things that cause stress. This skill is especially important after a cancer diagnosis because cancer brings many stressors that need to be handled effectively so that the negative effects of stress will not slow your recovery.

One of the secrets to reducing the harmful effects of stress in your life is to understand the stress process and learn how you can intentionally interrupt it.

Where Does Stress Begin?

The process begins when a new event—stressor—is perceived by a person as a threat to their well-being. The stressor can be a real or an imagined threat. No matter whether the stressor is real or imagined, the first and natural response of humans is to respond with a stress reaction called the **fight or flight** (flee or run away) reaction. This reaction makes people feel they are in danger and have to do something to protect themselves or others. The brain sends signals to the body to secrete high levels of stress hormones. High levels of anxiety caused by the event and the release of the hormones prepare the body to remove itself from danger.

If we hear a siren as we are crossing the road, we tense and run quickly to get out of its way—it's a natural instinct for self-preservation. It can also happen when an event, such as a loud noise, awakens us at night—we do not know whether it is threatening or not, until it is evaluated. This fear experience may also occur when we remember a time in our lives when a tragic event happened—simply thinking about it brings back feelings of stress and anxiety.

The Stress Response

This stress reaction, although normal, can turn into complete physical and emotional exhaustion (depression) if it lasts too long. The secret to stopping this downward spiral is to use all available tools to manage your reactions to stress. A diagnosis of breast cancer is a real threat. It makes sense that your anxiety will be acute until you find how to regain your control and make the problem manageable—assemble your treatment and support team, get information, etc. The best advice is to take advantage of all the support available from your treatment team and then add a program of self-care. You will find that even though your reality doesn't change, taking active steps will drastically change your thinking. With the change in thinking comes a big reduction in stress, and with reduction in stress comes an improvement in mood and increased energy. In this section, we will examine the stress response and help you learn how you can manage the impact of stress on your life.

Dealing With the Fight or Flight (Flee) Response

When an unexpected event happens and is perceived as a threat, we naturally respond with a heightened sense of awareness. The shock can either give us a healthy surge of emotions and energy that prepares us to move from danger, or it can cause us to become completely overwhelmed with fear. This is called the fight or flight (flee) response. A number of changes occur throughout the body as we prepare to fight or flee from this unexpected event. Sometimes the fight or flight response occurs when we merely remember or think about something that is frightening.

After years of working as a Nurse Navigator, I realized how this stress response model was evident in patients. Understanding the main principles of stress could help them identify what was happening to them and how they could manage their response. The diagram on page 132 illustrates the stress process. The following numbers correspond with the diagram.

1. **The Event: A Cancer Diagnosis**
   A cancer diagnosis comes with little warning and is naturally perceived as a threat. It sets off the stress response spiral. Other events during cancer treatment, such as surgery, chemotherapy, radiation therapy and diagnostic tests, can also cause high levels of stress.

2. **Brain's Perception**
   The event is interpreted in the mind as unknown or threatening and is viewed as dangerous. This is an initial and automatic response.

3. **Body's Automatic Reaction**
   The brain releases a cascade of stress hormones, mainly cortisol and adrenaline, to prepare the body to take action. These stress hormones can cause changes in every body system, preparing the person to fight or flee.

The Stress Response

Physical Responses include tensed muscles, increased blood pressure, racing heart, rapid and shallow breathing, dilated eyes, slowed digestion, relaxed bladder, increased saliva and numerous other changes.

Emotional Responses include panic, fear, anxiety, nervousness and tension.

4. **Evaluation of Event or Stressors**

After the initial stress happens and the body panics, an evaluation of what to do occurs. Does this event really require you to take action? Do you fight or flee the stressor? You'll probably decide whether to fight or flee based on your past preparation for coping, including:

- Previous life experiences (*"Is this something I know how to deal with?"*)
- Personal belief system (*"Is it the right thing to do in this situation?"*)
- How capable you feel of handling the stress physically and emotionally (*"Can I face this and not be destroyed emotionally or physically?"*)
- Problem-solving skills (*"Do I know what to do?"*)
- Communication skills (*"Can I ask for help and feel that someone will respond?"*)
- Available resources, support and people (*"Do I have enough information about the stressor to understand what to do? Do I have someone to help me with this problem?"*)

5. **Mental Outlook Decision**

Depending on how you evaluate your ability to deal with the stressor, you'll either respond by saying, (5A) *"I will fight this"* (an optimistic response) or (5B) *"I can't do this—I will try to flee"* (a pessimistic response).

5A. **Mental Outlook:**
Fight or Optimism

"I am going to do all I can." This leads to seeing the event as a problem to be solved. It becomes a challenge, and you make a commitment to take control of the situation and learn what can be done to change things. Part of this decision is reaching out to find the information you need and getting help from others to fight this new battle.

When the stressor is viewed as a challenge and a problem to be solved, the emotional and physical reactions change. Emotionally, you will notice reduced nervousness and a sense of calm because you believe that you are capable of dealing with the stressor. You will probably feel more assertive as you ask questions and begin your quest for information about what you can do. As you change your perception from victim to challenger, you reduce the stress hormones in your body. With reduced stress hormones, you'll sleep better, experience increased energy and boost your immune system. *"I will fight this!"* is the decision.

The Stress Response

5B. Mental Outlook:
Flight (Give In) or Pessimism

The other option is to give in. The stressor seems to be too overwhelming to deal with. You might not view yourself as having the skills needed to fight the stressor. The decision (most often subconsciously) is to surrender to the stressor—*"I give in."* You might view yourself as a victim of the stressor and see your future as hopeless. Negative, frightening thoughts that may be irrational cause you to be unable to communicate your fears, make decisions about what could be done or ask for help. These thoughts are frightening and cause emotional withdrawal from people and activities. *"My situation is hopeless and it is useless to fight; I will give in,"* is the decision. You withdraw.

Giving in keeps the body under stress and allows the stress hormones to continue to be secreted. This chronic anxiety may manifest itself with symptoms such as constant fatigue, high blood pressure, heart disease, chronic back or generalized muscle pain, chronic headaches, sleep disturbances, appetite changes and stomach and bowel disorders. The prolonged presence of stress hormones weakens the immune system, and you may notice an increase in infections, colds and viruses.

6. Exhaustion State: Clinical Depression

If the state of hopelessness with its host of symptoms is maintained for longer than a few weeks, it will lead to a condition psychologists call a state of exhaustion or clinical depression. Clinical depression is a condition that should be considered serious and needs treatment, like any other malfunction in the body.

Stress Buster Skills

Now that you understand how the stress response works, you can learn to recognize it when it begins and take steps to manage or reduce your stress. We can never prevent events that threaten us from entering into our lives. We can, though, learn what we can do that will reduce their impact on our health.

"While we cannot direct the winds that enter our lives, we can adjust our sails."

—*Author Unknown*

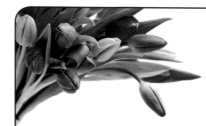

Remember...

- *Breast cancer comes as an unexpected event in a woman's life and brings with it many emotional stressors.*

- *The biggest surprise for many women is the struggle they have emotionally—they thought dealing with treatment would be their biggest challenge, but they found the hardest part was dealing with their emotions.*

- *Anxiety is the initial response to a new stressor and is expected. However, if anxiety remains high for an extended period of time, it negatively affects your physical health.*

- *Depression may occur after a period of acute, unresolved anxiety. Depression signals that a person has exhausted one's coping skills and feels overwhelmed, helpless and hopeless.*

- *Depression is not a sign of weakness. It is a sign that you are human and that you have been overwhelmed by a situation and simply need help dealing with it.*

- *Common to both anxiety and depression is worry. Worry is the mental struggle to deal with a situation.*

- *Ninety percent of what people worry about never happens. Constant worry leads to increased anxiety and potential for depression.*

- *Each negative thought we have has serious health consequences. Each thought releases a cascade of stress hormones into the body that lowers our immunity.*

- *Learning to control stress and the worry it brings is a conscious decision. It requires taking action to acquire skills to deal with stress.*

- *Keeping your family and friends involved in your life while undergoing treatment is a great buffer to stress. Ask for their help when needed.*

- *Learn self-care skills to interrupt and deal with anxiety. Practice the relaxation response to calm your mind and relax your body when under stressful situations.*

- *Seeking help for anxiety and depression is as important as seeking treatment for your cancer. Reach out to your physician, or seek the help of a counselor.*

Thoughts To Ponder...

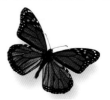

When we feel fear or stress, our hormones tell the cells in our bodies to either fight or flee. When we feel joy or love, our hormones tell our bodies to spend time repairing broken cells, digesting foods and healing infections. Our bodies are either fighting/fleeing or healing, not both.

So, in order to turn on the body's healing mode, we must first turn off the fight or flight mode. One powerful way to do this is to release suppressed emotions from the past (anger, bitterness, resentment, unforgiveness). As soon as we are out of the fight or flight mode, the body naturally begins to repair cells and heal itself.

However, we can turn up that healing—much like turning up the volume on a stereo—by purposefully trying to feel positive emotions such as love, joy and happiness. That's because positive emotions are like rocket fuel for the immune system.

Whenever we feel the emotions of love, joy or happiness, the glands in our brains release a surge of healing hormones into our blood streams, including serotonin, relaxin, oxytocin, dopamine and endorphins. These hormones instantly communicate with all the cells in our bodies telling them to do things such as lower blood pressure, heart rate and cortisol (the stress hormone); improve blood circulation; deepen our breathing and bring oxygen to our cells; digest our food more slowly, which helps the body absorb more nutrients; increase white and red blood cell activity, which helps the immune system fight cancer; clear out any infections; scan our body and remove cancer cells.

—**Kelly Turner, Ph.D.**
Radical Remission: Surviving Cancer Against All Odds

Worry takes our past negative experiences and projects them into the future. This becomes self-torture and does not prevent anything from happening. We have to say "no" to our negative, defeating thoughts or we will spend our time in a mental prison built from our own thoughts.

—**Judy Kneece**

Worry is like a rocking chair: it gives you something to do but never gets you anywhere.

—**Erma Bombeck**

I learned to never worry alone. When anxiety grabs my mind, it is self-perpetuating. Worrisome thoughts reproduce faster than rabbits. To stop this spiral of worry, I simply talk to a friend about my worry. Their simple act of reassurance becomes a tool to cast out my fear because peace and fear are both contagious.

—**John Ortberg, Jr.**

CHAPTER 16

Sexuality After Breast Cancer

"Resuming sexual relations with my husband after surgery was not easy for me. I was not comfortable with my own sexuality and wasn't sure what I wanted or expected from my husband. Fortunately, he was more comfortable with this than I was. He very tenderly and lovingly helped me come to terms with this part of our recovery."

—Harriett Barrineau

Breast cancer has changed many things in your life. One of the potential changes you may experience is a problem restoring your normal sexual functioning. Surgery, chemotherapy and hormonal therapy, while they are ridding your body of the devastating threats of cancer, all have side effects that may negatively affect sexual functioning. In this chapter, we will discuss these potential side effects and what you can do to alleviate or reduce their impact on your sexuality.

Focus Group Research
In an effort to determine the impact of cancer treatment on breast cancer patients' sexuality, EduCare conducted research by holding focus groups of breast cancer survivors. The groups were convened in 11 different hospitals nationwide and consisted of women who had taken chemotherapy. The goal was to define the impact surgery and chemotherapy had on their sexual functioning and quality of life. The focus groups investigated the physical and sexual changes experienced and the impact these changes had on the relationship with their sexual partner.

A total of 126 survivors attended and responded to 143 questions using handheld computer pads that allowed all answers to be anonymous. Each woman was free to express her true feelings without anyone knowing how she answered. The computer analyzed the data entered at each site and then combined the 11 sites for the final analysis. Throughout this chapter, findings from the research will be shared to help you better understand what other breast cancer patients have experienced.

Surgical Side Effects on Sexuality
Breast cancer surgery alters or removes one or both breasts, which physically changes your body image. The most important factor in determining whether surgery will impact your sexuality is what you or

"We had to learn to navigate my new body. It was important for us to resume the intimate part of our life as it was the one thing we, and we alone, shared. Also, after the tremendous assault on my body, we looked upon the tenderness together as healing."

—Anna Cluxton

your partner think about your new body image. Breasts add pleasure to the sexual relationship but are not essential for sexual pleasure to occur. It is not the loss or change in a breast that impacts the sexual relationship, but the way you and your partner accept the change. Facing the change in your body image together and openly communicating are the first steps to keeping surgery from impacting your sexual relationship. I encourage you to talk to your partner if you have fears and concerns that your new body image may have an impact on your sexuality. Having this conversation early will help both of you.

One of the hardest, but most important, steps is viewing your incision and the changed or missing breast. This is difficult, but it is an essential step to recovery. Your partner shares your pain and loss and, when allowed to join you in viewing the incision, will be better able to respond to your needs. Not allowing your partner to participate in seeing your new body image and share in your loss can potentially build a wall of separation that can affect future sexual intimacy.

To avoid this separation, it is helpful to plan to view the surgical incision as early as possible after surgery. The first dressing change is a good opportunity; however, some women find that they prefer a time more emotionally suitable for them. The goal is to allow your sexual partner to view your new body image. This is an important step to restoring normal intimacy. Delaying this step may make it even more difficult in the future.

Surgical Scars
Partners' viewing of scar:
■ 75% replied that it was within days after surgery
■ 6% reported that their partner had never seen their scar. These women still dress and undress behind closed doors or in the dark.
Perception of partners' response when viewing the scar:
■ 80% reported their partners were accepting and supportive
■ 15% reported a neutral response
■ 5% reported a negative response

Resuming Physical Intimacy After Surgery

If no complications arise, your surgical incision should heal in about four weeks. However, you may resume your sexual relationship as soon as both of you feel ready. The surgical scar area will naturally be sore and sensitive, but you can lead your partner in how to prevent pain by altering positions to avoid pressure on the area.

Some patients in the focus groups shared that even though their partner had viewed the incision, they still found it difficult to participate in sexual intimacy unclothed. The nudity problem can be solved by purchasing and wearing a lacy camisole. Mastectomy patients should purchase one that has pockets to hold a lightweight prosthesis. A lacy camisole preserves feelings of femininity during the sexual relationship.

During the period surrounding your diagnosis and surgery, it is normal for stress and fatigue to affect your sexual functioning. Remember that during periods of stress, the need for emotional closeness usually increases. Most women expressed that they needed and wanted more touching, hugging and emotional closeness after surgery, but they often did not know how to express this need. I encourage you to speak up and share your needs. Do not allow walls of silence to separate you from the emotional closeness you need. Often, a partner does not physically reach out because they are not sure of how to treat you. Let your partner know that you still desire to be close and to cuddle, but that you may not feel up to sexual intercourse. Your honesty will be appreciated. Remember, your partner is also having to sort through this new experience.

Radiation Therapy Impact on Sexuality

If you require external radiation therapy, the side effect that impacts sexuality is fatigue. You may notice around week three of treatment that you begin experiencing increased fatigue, resulting in diminished sexual interest. External radiation does not cause you to be radioactive during treatments, and sexual contact can continue with no danger to your partner. When radiation treatments are completed, you will find there is no lasting impact on the sexual relationship if you have not, or will not, be taking chemotherapy or hormonal therapy.

Hormonal Therapy Impact on Sexuality

Hormonal medications are prescribed after breast cancer surgery at the completion of radiation or chemotherapy to reduce recurrence for women who are estrogen positive. The majority of ER/PR positive women will receive hormonal therapy for 5 – 10 years after other treatments are completed. Although hormonal therapies do not cause the acute side effects of chemotherapy, they do have sexual side effects that impact sexual functioning to a lesser degree. Approximately 30 – 40 percent of patients taking tamoxifen and 50 percent of patients taking an aromatase inhibitor report sexual problems.

Chemotherapy Impact on Sexuality

Side effects from surgery and radiation are short-term. However, sexuality changes caused by chemotherapy are the most problematic and become a long-term challenge, due to the lasting impact of the drugs on female hormones. Most patients undergoing chemotherapy are prepared for the well-known side effects of fatigue, nausea, vomiting and hair loss. However, very few patients are forewarned about the impact on their sexual functioning, other than the potential for premenopausal women to become infertile.

Chemotherapy usually causes instant menopause in premenopausal women and increases symptoms for menopausal women. This directly impacts sexual functioning. There is a vast difference in natural menopause and chemically induced menopause. Menopause caused by chemotherapy is different because it occurs suddenly, unlike normal menopause which occurs over a period of years. The symptoms of chemically induced menopause are more intense because the drugs diminish the hormones made in both the ovaries and the adrenal glands. Natural menopause impacts the hormones produced in the ovaries, while the adrenal glands continue to supply some hormones, causing natural menopausal symptoms to be less severe.

An important fact to understand about chemically induced menopause is the production of testosterone. Testosterone is predominantly a male hormone, but women also make it in much lower amounts in the ovaries and also convert hormones made by the adrenal glands into testosterone. Testosterone is the hormone that produces sexual desire and the ability to experience an orgasm; it also governs the intensity of the orgasm. When a woman takes chemotherapy, she has an instant reduction of all of her hormones, including testosterone, from both the ovaries and adrenal glands. Low testosterone causes a decrease in sex drive, increases the time needed for sexual arousal and decreases the ability to experience an orgasm. Because these sexuality side effects are experienced by only the patient and her partner, they are very rarely addressed. Yet, the impact on the sexual relationship can be great. In this chapter, we will discuss interventions to help deal with changes you may experience.

Menopausal Side Effects That Impact Sexuality

Women who receive chemotherapy for breast cancer experience menopausal side effects during and after treatment because the drugs lower hormonal levels. Menopausal side effects are not dangerous to your health, but they impact your quality of life. The most common symptoms are mood swings, vaginal dryness, fatigue, hot flashes, low sex drive and decreased ability to have an orgasm. After treatment is over, many premenopausal women remain in a menopausal state, causing symptoms to continue. Some women may have their periods return but usually experience an earlier onset of menopause.

Mood Swings

When women experience a significant drop in their estrogen, whether through natural or chemical menopause, one of the first things they notice is a change in their emotions. Before menopause, these mood swings are experienced for several days before the menstrual period begins and is referred to as premenstrual syndrome (PMS). You are probably well aware that this time is emotionally different.

Mood Swings
Mood swings increased:
■ 56% during treatment
■ 44% six months after treatment ended
■ 22% one year after completion of treatment

PMS occurs when estrogen and progesterone levels fall to allow menstruation. During these few days, increased moodiness, tearfulness, nervousness and outbursts of anger are common symptoms in many women. The same symptoms occur during the reduction of female hormones from chemotherapy. The low hormonal state causes a patient to experience the same emotional limbo as in PMS, but the emotional limbo continues day after day because the hormones continue to remain low. It is almost a certainty that your mood will fluctuate during treatments. You may find that you swing from normal to sad, then to angry, then to depressed, all with no apparent cause. It is important to understand that this emotional roller coaster is caused by the chemotherapy drugs and not by your inability to deal with cancer.

Mood Swing Treatments

What can you do about mood swings? If you find that mood swings are negatively impacting your life and relationships, talk to your physician and ask about a medication called an SSRI (Selected Serotonin Reuptake Inhibitor), which increases the levels of serotonin and elevates your mood. The trade names are Celexa®, Paxil®, Seroxat®, Prozac®, Luvox®, Zoloft® and Lustral®.

Vaginal Dryness and Painful Intercourse

Estrogen is the hormone that causes the vaginal walls to be soft and pliable. It is also responsible for the lubrication of the vaginal canal during foreplay, which makes intercourse more pleasurable. With the reduction of estrogen, the vagina becomes very dry and will not lubricate adequately during sexual arousal. Lack of lubrication combined with vaginal dryness can result in painful intercourse. If vaginal dryness is severe, intercourse can potentially cause a small amount of bleeding afterward, which can frighten both partners.

Vaginal Dryness Treatments

The initial treatments for vaginal dryness are vaginal moisturizers and vaginal lubricants. Both products can be purchased over-the-counter in the personal care section. Unlike most side effects of chemotherapy, vaginal dryness continues long past chemotherapy administration. Most focus group patients experienced escalating vaginal dryness after chemotherapy treatment ended. The good news is that most women can successfully manage their symptoms with over-the-counter products.

Vaginal Dryness
Vaginal dryness increased:
■ 123% during treatment
■ 134% six months after treatment ended
■ 160% one year after completion of treatments*
Vaginal dryness continued to increase.

■ **Vaginal Moisturizers** are designed to treat vaginal dryness by replenishing moisture, similar to a facial moisturizer. Brand names include Replens®, Fresh Start®, K-Y Silk-E®, Moist Again® and K-Y

Liquibeads®. Vaginal moisturizers are applied inside the vagina on a regular basis, several times a week, to restore and hold moisture. They are not designed to be used as a lubricant before intercourse. Most women find a vaginal moisturizer helpful in reducing dryness.

■ **Vaginal Lubricants** are designed to be applied just before intercourse. Products available include Astroglide®, FemGlide®, Just Like Me®, K-Y Jelly®, Slippery Stuff®, Summers Eve®, ID Millennium®, Pink®, Pjur® and Pure Pleasure®. A vaginal lubricant should be generously applied inside the vagina and on the external genitals just prior to penetrative intercourse. Applying it to your partner also increases effectiveness. Some couples find that lubricant application can be a part of sexual foreplay with partners applying the lubricant to each other. It is important that the lubricant be reapplied as frequently as needed during intercourse.

Approximately 20 percent of women have a chemical sensitivity to lubricants that have glycerin or paraben in the formula, which causes burning and irritation. If you experience irritation, look for a lubricant that is labeled glycerin-free and paraben-free. Liquid Silk® is a brand highly recommended by healthcare professionals. It is glycerin-free and also formulated to be bio-static, which means that if it is exposed to any bacteria, yeast or fungal spores, it will stop them from spreading. Liquid Silk® can be ordered online.

Avoid oil-based lubricants, such as petroleum jelly (Vaseline®) or baby oil, because they may promote vaginal infections and are not recommended for use with latex condoms.

Partner Understanding of Vaginal Lubrication

It is very important for your sexual partner to know that a lack of vaginal lubrication is not from your lack of desire, but is a side effect of chemotherapy. Often, a partner may mistake the reduction of vaginal lubrication during foreplay as a lack of desire for them as a sexual partner, and feel rejected. A partner may also feel that the use of lubricant is a sign that they are not sexually stimulating to their partner. Neither is true. Lack of vaginal lubrication is caused by chemical menopause. This is something that you, the patient, cannot control.

Participating in penetrative intercourse without adequate lubrication can cause pain. Experiencing pain will negatively impact your desire for future sexual encounters. It is suggested that you purchase and start using a moisturizer and vaginal lubricant early in your chemotherapy treatment to prevent any possibility of experiencing painful intercourse.

> **Painful Intercourse From Vaginal Dryness**
>
> **Painful intercourse increased:**
> ■ 137% during chemotherapy treatment
> ■ 147% six months after chemotherapy treatment
> ■ 163% one year after treatment completion
>
> These figures reveal that vaginal dryness with the potential to cause painful intercourse increases after treatment is completed. Therefore, couples should be prepared to deal with the lingering side effects.

Urinary Problems

Low estrogen levels may also cause urinary symptoms. Estrogen receptors are found in the lining of the bladder and urinary tubes. When estrogen levels are low, the lining becomes thinner and the muscles that support the bladder weaken. Patients often experience burning during urination, urinary urgency or urinary stress incontinence (loss of urine when walking fast, running or sneezing). Women find the sudden urge to urinate and the inability to hold their urine a source of embarrassment, which may limit their participation in some activities. The treatment for problematic urinary problems requires a physician's intervention. The first treatment option is a prescription for local estrogen (explained on the next page) or for medications designed to treat urinary urgency. For urgency or leaking that is not resolved with local estrogen therapy, a referral to a urologist or a gynecologist is needed to determine the exact cause of your problem.

Prescription Medications for Vaginal Dryness and Urinary Symptoms

Some patients, despite their liberal use of moisturizers and lubricants for vaginal dryness, find they still struggle with discomfort. During natural menopause, women are often prescribed estrogen replacement to relieve their symptoms. However, estrogen replacement is usually not an option during breast cancer treatment. After treatment is completed, if your vaginal dryness continues, discuss other options for local (not systemic) vaginal estrogen with your healthcare provider.

Localized estrogen medications relieve vaginal dryness and decrease urinary symptoms while keeping systemic estrogen levels in safe menopausal range. After several months of usage, the vagina increases in moisture and elasticity, making intercourse far more comfortable. Local estrogen therapy also replenishes the lining of the bladder and urinary tubes, causing urinary symptoms to decrease. Talk to your healthcare provider to determine if local estrogen therapy is an option for you. Vaginal estrogen therapies require a prescription and include:

- **Estrace®, Premarin®:** An estrogen cream that is applied to the external genital tissues and inside the vagina using an applicator. Requires daily application for several weeks and then is reduced to several times a week.
- **Estring®:** A ring of estrogen that is inserted and remains in the vagina for three months.
- **Vagifem®:** A tablet made from soy that is inserted into the vagina using an applicator. Requires daily application for two weeks and then is reduced to twice per week.

Vaginal Laser Rejuvenation for Vaginal Dryness and Urinary Stress Incontinence

A new treatment for vaginal dryness and urinary stress incontinence is vaginal laser rejuvenation. A CO_2 laser (similar to those used in facial rejuvenation) is inserted into the vagina and the laser treats the tissues for five minutes. The treatment is virtually painless and a patient is able to return to normal activities the same day. A series of three treatments, spaced six weeks apart, is recommended. The treatment increases the production of fibroblasts, which stimulates the production of collagen. Collagen production increases the elasticity of the vaginal wall and increases vaginal lubrication, which decreases vaginal dryness, laxity and urinary stress incontinence. The treatment is most often available from a gynecologist.

Vaginal Infections

Vaginal dryness can also cause vaginal itching and increase the potential for a vaginal infection (vaginitis) to occur. The two most common infections are:

- **Bacterial Vaginosis:** Caused by an overgrowth of bacteria which causes a discharge that has a thin, grayish discharge and a fishy odor.
- **Candida:** Caused by an overgrowth of a fungus which causes a thick, white discharge that forms cottage cheese-like clumps. The discharge causes itching, internal and external swelling. It is commonly called a yeast infection.

If you experience a vaginal discharge that is irritating or has a foul odor, promptly report it to your healthcare provider for treatment recommendations. Both of these vaginal infections can be effectively treated with medications. Neither will get better without treatment.

Sexuality After Treatment

After chemotherapy, most women experience a reduced sex drive, a reduced ability to become sexually aroused and may have problems reaching an orgasm. This often comes as a complete surprise. Understanding that a reduced sexual response is an **expected** side effect will help you to prepare for the changes and keep you from feeling that they are from a personal response to cancer treatment.

To address the problem of reduced sexual response, it is necessary to understand the basic differences in female and male sexual arousal before and after chemotherapy. Arousal time for a male is rapid, as illustrated in the chart. From the first sexually stimulating touch, a male can progress to orgasm with ejaculation in approximately three minutes. The female arousal time is much slower. A female requires about five minutes of sexually stimulating touch for vaginal lubrication and congestion to occur, creating sexual readiness. After female sexual stimulation occurs, it then requires an average of ten more minutes of uninterrupted sexual activity for the average female to reach orgasm. Not understanding the arousal time gap is a frequent cause of female complaints about painful sex. This is because penetration is attempted before full sexual arousal is achieved. Mutual awareness of the time required for sexual arousal is necessary.

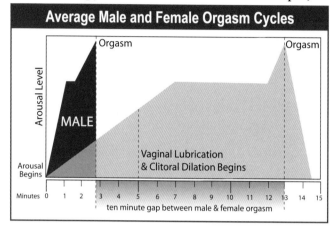

The sexual arousal time chart is presented as a norm; the time required may vary among individuals. However, the chart clearly points out the big difference in time required for arousal and orgasm of males compared to females. It is necessary to understand this difference for mutually satisfying sex to occur. Just as there is a vast difference between the cooking times required for a crockpot versus a microwave, the same principle applies to males and females in sexual arousal and orgasm. There is a large gap in time.

Cancer treatment causes sexual changes that require even more time for arousal and orgasm. This requires that both partners understand the changes and learn ways to compensate for them. Same-sex partners also need to discuss the impact of treatment on increasing arousal time. Full arousal makes sexual contact more comfortable and exciting. Plan to have this discussion with your partner.

Even with adequate arousal, you may find that you do not achieve an orgasm, or if you do, the intensity is reduced. Remember, if you are having difficulty, it is not a reflection on you but is a common side effect of treatment.

Orgasm Ability Before and After Chemotherapy					
Orgasm Frequency	**Never**	**Rarely**	**Occasionally**	**Most of the Time**	**All of the Time**
Before Treatment	1%	8%	19%	55%	17%
During Treatment	24%	27%	28%	16%	5%
One Year After Treatment	10%	23%	29%	30%	9%
Before treatment, 72% of women would experience orgasms, varying from most of the time to all of the time. During treatment, this fell to 21%. Following completion of treatment, this number rose only slightly to 39%, translating into a 46% reduction in ability to experience orgasms most or all of the time, one year after treatment.					

Addressing Arousal Problems

It is important to understand that the loss of testosterone—the hormone that causes interest, arousal and orgasm—is the basic problem. What can be done about these side effects? The testosterone level can be brought back into normal range by a trained, experienced healthcare provider who understands the complexity of hormonal balance. Women who have had their levels brought back into therapeutic range with testosterone cream report that this helped to restore the quality of their sexual life.

Ask your healthcare team if they check hormonal levels and if they prescribe supplemental testosterone cream. If they do not, contact the International Academy of Compounding Pharmacists (1-800-927-4227) and ask for the nearest compounding pharmacy. Your local compounding pharmacy can refer you to the providers in your area who are skilled at testing levels of existing testosterone and prescribing testosterone cream.

Another option that has proven helpful in increasing libido and orgasmic ability is Wellbutrin®, an anti-depressant that requires a prescription. If you have a history of anxiety or other disorders, this medication may not be appropriate. Ask your healthcare provider if you are a candidate for this medication.

A Sexuality Expert's Recommendation For Low Desire

Dr. Rosemary Basson, a specialist in sexuality, studied the issue of low desire and low sexual arousal in women. Her recommendation for a woman with low desire is to agree to submit to a partner's sexual stimulation (foreplay) **before** experiencing any sexual desire. After adequate sexual stimulation, desire can be created.

> ### Sexual Interest and Arousal
>
> **Sexual thoughts prior to diagnosis:**
> - 88% of women reported having sexual thoughts and fantasies before chemotherapy
> - 32% had sexual thoughts and fantasies during treatments
> - 41% reported sexual thoughts and fantasies one year after treatment completion
>
> **When questioned about the need for extra time to achieve sexual arousal after chemotherapy:**
> - 86% replied that the time required for sexual arousal had increased
> - 49% reported decreased nipple sensitivity from sexual arousal
> - 80% reported lack of vaginal lubrication during foreplay

Dr. Basson recommends that you agree to participate in sexual foreplay with your partner, even if you have no sexual desire. Most often, after adequate stimulation, desire for sexual activity is created. Participating in sexual stimulation to create sexual desire has worked well for chemo-treated women and for women who find their desire is all but absent.

Participating in sexual stimulation also helps maintain and preserve the health of the nerves and muscles of the genitals by increasing blood flow. Lack of blood flow to the genitals decreases the sensitivity of the nerves, which decreases sexual arousal. For this reason, routine sexual arousal helps maintain healthy functioning of the genital tissues.

The return of your sex drive and the ability to have an orgasm are quality of life issues. Since they have nothing to do with life and death, they may be ignored. For some women, the return of sexual satisfaction is important to their quality of life. For others, this is not an issue of importance. Only you can decide what is best for your relationship. There are no right or wrong answers, only what best meets your needs. If you find that this is an important issue, keep seeking a healthcare provider who addresses your problems, offers interventions and works to improve your quality of life.

Summary of Cancer Treatment Side Effects on Sexuality

Sexuality side effects after cancer treatment vary according to the type of treatment you receive. The following chart lists the most common side effects caused by different breast cancer treatments.

Cancer Treatment Side Effects on Sexuality								
	Fatigue	Mood Swings	Hot Flashes and Night Sweats	Urinary Changes	Vaginal Dryness	Nausea	Decreased Libido	Decreased Orgasm
Surgery	✓♦							
Radiation Therapy	✓♦							
Chemotherapy	✓	✓	✓	✓	✓	✓	✓	✓
Tamoxifen	✓	✓	✓		✓	✓	✓	
Aromatase Inhibitors	✓	✓	✓	✓	✓	✓	✓	✓
Menopause	✓	✓	✓	✓	✓		✓	✓
Key: ✓ Occurs	♦ Limited Time Surrounding the Time of Treatment							

Birth Control After Breast Cancer

Getting pregnant immediately after a breast cancer diagnosis or during chemotherapy is not recommended. Chemotherapy drugs may cause birth defects. If you are premenopausal, discuss birth control options with your physician.

The anti-estrogen drug tamoxifen (Nolvadex®) is often prescribed after treatment is over. Tamoxifen may increase ovulation (release of the egg from the ovary) when therapy is started, making a woman more fertile. Since pregnancy is not recommended during tamoxifen therapy, you need to discuss birth control options with your physician.

Chemotherapy usually stops your menstrual periods. They may or may not return after treatments are completed. If you are near menopause, they may never come back; if you are young, they may return. For some women, several years may go by before normal menstruation begins again. It is important to remember that you may be able to get pregnant before evidence of a menstrual period. Because of this, you may want to discuss birth control options with your physician after treatment is completed.

Partner's Understanding

Sex will change during cancer treatment. The majority of focus group patients, 89 percent, said they would have liked for their healthcare provider to have explained to their partner the changes caused by treatment. It is essential that your sexual partner understand the changes that chemotherapy may bring to your sexual relationship. Your partner's understanding will greatly enhance your return to sexual functioning. If you feel a discussion that includes your partner would be helpful, ask your healthcare provider for an appointment to discuss sexuality issues. You can also ask your partner to read this chapter.

Restoring Sexual Function

There are many things you can do to ensure that you are taking steps to reclaim your sex life. Read through the list below to identify areas that may need to be addressed.

Chapter 16

Body Image:

- Have I allowed my partner to see my scar?
- Am I still hiding in the closet to change clothes?
- Have I restored my body image with a well-fitted prosthesis or reconstruction? If not, am I considering either option?
  - Reconstructive surgery: Have I talked to a physician and received the information needed to make a decision?
  - Prosthesis: Have I made an appointment with a professional prosthesis fitter?
- If I am having problems adjusting to my body image or sexuality, have I asked to speak to a counselor?

Communication With Partner:

- Have I talked openly about my fear that our relationship will change because of cancer treatment?
- Have I expressed my desire for our sexual functioning not to be affected?
- Does my partner understand the potential side effects from chemotherapy on sexual arousal?
- Have I shared openly about what is physically comfortable or uncomfortable during intimacy?
- Have I discussed my need for increased time for foreplay?
- Have I explained that my lack of lubrication during foreplay does not reflect on my attraction for them as a partner, but is a side effect of treatment?
- Have I discussed my willingness to participate in sexual foreplay to create my desire?
- Am I honest when I am physically fatigued and would like to be held and cuddled without intercourse?
- Have I explained to my partner that when I do not feel up to the sexual act it is because I either need time to adjust or feel fatigued from treatment and not because I am rejecting them?

Personal Self-Care:

- Have I treated myself to something special to enhance my feeling of femininity after surgery, such as a lacy camisole, perfume, an item of clothing or a new haircut?
- Have I planned a special time and saved energy for the sexual relationship to be resumed?
- Have I been honest and asked for family assistance with household duties during treatments to allow myself more time and energy for pleasurable events?

Communication With the Healthcare Team:

- When I have a problem, such as hot flashes, vaginal dryness, painful intercourse or lack of sexual desire, do I ask my healthcare team how to manage the problem?

Reclaiming your sexuality requires that you take action to have your needs met. If you have identified any area that you have not addressed, plan to do so. Some patients think that their physicians are only interested in medical issues and not in issues such as sexuality. This is **not** true. Physicians are well aware that quality-of-life is one of the main components of a successful recovery. They may not ask about sexuality problems, but this does not mean that they will not discuss them with you. Don't hesitate to ask questions and report any side effects. If necessary, ask for a referral to a gynecologist.

The Emotional Struggle of Sexuality Changes

Women often emotionally struggle with sexuality changes after breast cancer. They often question their sexual attractiveness to their partner and fear that the changes will negatively affect their relationship. It is important to remember that breast cancer has not changed you. You are still the same loving person your partner selected. Even though you and your partner may experience sexuality changes after your surgery and treatment for cancer, they are challenges that many couples have overcome. Many couples share that the experience of breast cancer brought them closer together, and the meaning of the sexual relationship was enhanced because of the realization of how valuable they were to each other. Don't let your emotional fears interfere with reaching out to reclaim your sexuality.

The Single Woman and Future Intimacy

If you are single, a cancer diagnosis can add additional stress by impacting your view of future emotional, physical and sexual intimacy. Like many patients, you may find it difficult to imagine how you will handle a future intimate relationship. Some women in our sexuality focus groups reported that after their diagnosis and treatment, they felt as if they were damaged goods and they would not be sexually attractive as a partner. This is not true! Many women have successfully developed intimate relationships after a breast cancer diagnosis.

Single women often need help understanding the impact of diagnosis on developing future relationships. The first thing necessary is for you to rethink the subject. Cancer does not define who you are. You are still the same you. Most often a cancer diagnosis causes a person to become a stronger and more sensitive person. This life experience makes you a more attractive person. Unlike some diseases, breast cancer is treatable, and after treatment most women return to a normal state of physical and emotional health.

The first step is to make peace with yourself and take the steps needed to rebuild your self-image, whether by reconstruction, getting into shape physically or developing new skills. This is an opportunity for you to decide how you would like to change or improve.

Future Dating Reminders:

- Dating was not always successful before your diagnosis. Dating after cancer will be the same; sometimes the relationship is not the right one, but it has nothing to do with your cancer diagnosis.
- Most people have things they would like to change about themselves (overweight, balding, etc.).
- One third of Americans will have a cancer diagnosis. Ask yourself, *"If this person had a history of cancer, would I reject them?"*

One of the best ways to prepare for a future relationship is to talk to other breast cancer patients about their experiences in developing intimacy after their diagnosis. Support groups are a great place to talk to other women. The Young Survival Coalition, listed in the reference section of this book, is a nationally recognized resource. Professional counselors are also an excellent resource to have your fears and concerns addressed and to make plans for how to deal with them in the future. You need to prepare how you will share your diagnosis when you do find a new partner. Understanding how other women have handled the issue will give you a sense of preparedness and allow you to develop your own plan.

Sharing Your Diagnosis

Sharing your diagnosis with a new partner should not occur on the first date. The best time is when the relationship has passed the mutual friendship stage and is progressing. However, it is important to share before the relationship becomes serious or intimacy may occur. Only you know when this is happening. When you feel the time is right, select a time and place where you feel comfortable discussing your diagnosis. If you should become upset, you need to be in a place where you would not feel embarrassed.

Tips for Sharing the Details:

- State that you desire respect and honesty in your relationship, and that you have something to share.
- Share the facts about your diagnosis honestly and openly: *"In (year) I was diagnosed with breast*

cancer. This required that I have a (mastectomy/lumpectomy) that was followed by (type of treatments). I have been cancer-free for (time) or at the present I am dealing with (problems). I feel that what I went through has allowed me to become a stronger person by having to deal with a lot of hard issues. I wanted to be very honest with you before this relationship progressed. I will be happy to answer any questions you have about my diagnosis, treatment or present health."

- Do not appear as a victim; you do not want pity!
- Ask for feedback about what you just shared. Allow them to talk freely.
- If the person is hesitant to discuss your revelation, simply suggest that you know the information may have come as a shock: *"Why don't you call me in the next couple of days after you have had a chance to think about this, and we will discuss your feelings?"*

Remember, if this person ends the relationship after this conversation, this is a person who would have deserted you in the future if things did not go well. You did yourself a favor and prevented future heartaches. The nature of relationships is that some work and some don't. Your goal is to protect yourself emotionally by sharing early enough to find out if this will impact the relationship before you fall in love.

As a single woman at diagnosis, Lisa DelGuidice shared, *"Yes, I will admit I was self-conscious about how my chest looked after bilateral reconstruction. A guy friend of mine was so supportive and encouraging when he said, 'They are just boobs. They don't make you who you are. Anyone who looks at you differently because of a cancer diagnosis and subsequent scars is not worthy of you.' Will I feel uncomfortable when nude and keep my lingerie on during intimate moments? Probably. But, I know that won't last forever. My passion comes from within and my affectionate side comes from within. Surgery did not change that."*

Single Woman's Goals

As a single woman, you need to be prepared to discuss your diagnosis confidently with future partners. Surround yourself with understanding peers as you work through the process of preparing what you will say in the future. Cancer has not damaged you; it has been a tool for expanding your ability to love and appreciate life.

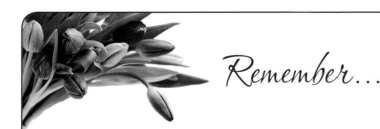

Remember...

- *Surgery and radiation therapy cause short-term interruptions in sexual functioning due to stress and fatigue. Chemotherapy can decrease sexual desire, sexual arousal and orgasmic ability, and also cause vaginal dryness. Hormonal therapy can decrease sexual desire and increase vaginal dryness.*

- *It is essential that your sexual partner understand that these sexual side effects are caused by treatment and not a lack of desire for them as a partner. Open, honest communication with your partner helps in making adjustments to any sexuality changes.*

- *Consider asking your partner to read portions of this chapter if you have difficulty expressing yourself in the area of sexuality.*

CHAPTER 17

Future Fertility

One of the issues least thought about during a cancer diagnosis is the impact of cancer treatments from chemotherapy and hormonal therapy on future fertility. Most thoughts naturally focus on selecting the most appropriate treatment for control of your cancer. However, one of the most important issues for younger couples who have not started or completed having their family is taking the time to discuss the potential impact on their future fertility. It is essential for couples to ask questions to protect their fertility or plan for future alternative fertility methods **before** treatment begins.

For women, infertility is the inability to start or maintain a pregnancy. Infertility can occur because of the inability of the ovaries to produce mature eggs (oocytes) for ovulation. It can also occur from the inability of the body to successfully allow implantation of a fertilized egg into the uterine wall or to maintain growth after implantation.

Fertility Threatened by Chemotherapy

Surgery has no effect on fertility, other than creating stress that causes a change in the hormonal balance, which may temporarily alter ovulation and possibly menstruation. This usually resolves itself in several months. Radiation therapy to the breast alone has only temporary effects, similar to surgery, because of stress and fatigue temporarily altering hormonal functioning. The major cause of infertility comes from chemotherapy.

Chemotherapy drugs work to treat cancer by killing rapidly dividing cells throughout the body. Chemotherapy drugs are cytotoxic (cyto=cell, toxic=poison). These drugs kill cancer cells, but they also kill healthy, rapidly dividing cells. Shortly after chemotherapy administration, the drugs drastically reduce the level of female hormones to a menopausal range. This hormonal reduction causes a large majority of premenopausal women to experience irregular or complete stoppage of the menstrual period during treatment.

It is very difficult for an oncologist to predict who will suffer the side effect of infertility. Some women have their fertility return after chemotherapy drugs are discontinued, but for others, infertility may be permanent.

"We were newlyweds when I was diagnosed. This raised a lot of questions about our future for becoming parents. Would chemotherapy rob us of the anticipated joy of one day having our own children?"
—*Anna Cluxton*

Factors That Help Predict Future Fertility:
- **Patient's Age:** The nearer a patient is to menopause, the less likely she is to have hormonal function (menstruation and ovulation) return.
  - Women under 40 are more likely to have hormonal functioning return than women over 40.
  - Women over 40 whose hormonal functioning returns may experience an earlier menopause, which decreases their window of fertility.
  - Return of the menstrual period is a sign of potential fertility, but it is not proof of fertility.
- **Drugs:** The chemotherapy drugs and length of administration have a great impact on fertility. A class of drugs, called alkylating agents, has an especially destructive effect on hormonal functioning. The most common drug used in breast cancer treatment is cyclophosphamide (Cytoxan®). Another drug that increases the potential for infertility is doxorubicin (Adriamycin®).

Addressing Fertility Issues

Since physicians cannot predict with absolute certainty whose fertility will be permanently affected, there are steps you may want to take to preserve your future ability to have children.
- The most essential step is letting your healthcare team know **before** treatments begin that having children in the future is a top priority.
- Ask about your treatment recommendations and the potential for causing infertility.
- Ask for a referral to a fertility specialist soon after your diagnosis if you have questions or concerns.
- Ask if there are treatment protocols that reduce the potential for infertility.
- Explore alternative fertility preservation options.

Fertility Preservation Options

Embryo Freezing

Hormones (like tamoxifen, proven safe to use in breast cancer patients) are used to stimulate egg production. Mature eggs are removed by a physician in a minor surgical procedure, fertilized in vitro (in a glass test tube) with sperm, frozen for future use and then stored. This procedure is called in-vitro fertilization (IVF). Pregnancy rates average 10 to 25 percent with each frozen embryo.

Egg (Oocyte) Freezing

Hormones (like tamoxifen) are used to stimulate egg production. Mature eggs are retrieved by the physician, frozen for future use and then stored (not fertilized). This method is new and currently has an estimated three percent pregnancy success rate.

Fertility Preservation Research in Progress

Ovarian Retrieval and Transplantation

Ovaries are surgically removed by a laparoscope (instrument that allows surgery to be performed through a small incision in the abdomen), divided into small strips, frozen and later transplanted back into the body when fertility is desired. Drugs are then given to stimulate ovulation. Some researchers call the process ovarian grafting. This method is experimental, but appears to have a potential for success in women who need to have chemotherapy that will damage their ovaries. A successful birth after chemotherapy with ovarian retrieval and transplantation has occurred. Check with your healthcare team about the progress of this research.

Ovarian Suppression

Hormones that suppress ovarian function and protect eggs from treatment toxicity are administered before and during chemotherapy treatments. This procedure to preserve fertility is currently in clinical trials. Recent reports offer promise for this new method, especially in women who need to proceed with chemotherapy and do not have time to undergo ovarian stimulation for egg retrieval. Ask your healthcare team for the latest information.

Expense and Time Requirements

The procedures for fertility preservation are expensive and usually require several months for egg retrieval, which may delay cancer treatments. At this time, most of the cost is not covered by insurance. While making treatment decisions, this adds another difficult choice for some couples who still desire to have a family of their own, but this is an important consideration if future fertility is desired.

It is important to understand that some cancers require immediate attention and do not allow time for fertility preservation procedures. One of these is inflammatory carcinoma, a cancer that is already systemic because of the involvement of the lymphatic system and requires that treatment start within days of diagnosis. If fertility is a concern, ask your physician if any type of treatment delay would reduce your chances for survival.

Alternative Parenthood Choices

Some couples find that their priority during the diagnostic period is optimal cancer treatment and that preserving fertility is not the most important issue for them. In this case, you may want to consider donor eggs, a surrogate or adoption in the future.

Questions To Ask Before Chemotherapy:

- What is the predicted impact of the drugs on fertility?
- What percentage of women who take these drugs experience permanent infertility?
- Are there drugs with less potential for infertility that can be used?
- What options do I have to preserve my fertility?
- Do you make referrals to physicians specializing in fertility preservation, if I am interested?
- If I decide to pursue embryo freezing as an option, will the time required to collect the eggs impact my survival outcomes by delaying treatment for several months?
- If my fertility returns, how long do you suggest I wait before becoming pregnant?

Pregnancy After Breast Cancer Facts:

- Pregnancy does not reduce patient survival or trigger recurrence.
- Women who have had systemic chemotherapy have been able to conceive and deliver healthy, normal children with the chance of birth defects near that of the normal, untreated population.
- Developing eggs exposed to chemotherapy may suffer genetic damage. Some physicians suggest waiting six months after regular menstrual periods return before pregnancy is attempted. However, the time recommendation varies according to many other variables. Ask your healthcare team for their recommendations.
- Some lubricants can reduce sperm motility. The lubricant Pre-Seed® has a pH which causes minimal decrease in sperm motility and is recommended for women trying to conceive.

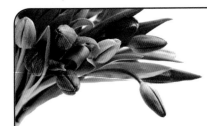

Remember...

- *Issues of future fertility are often not thought of during a cancer diagnosis when the emphasis is on effectively treating your breast cancer.*

- *If you have not yet completed your family, it is essential to bring up your desire for having children in the future when talking to your physicians.*

- *Discussion of future fertility should be made **before** any treatment decisions are made. Ask your oncologist about the effect of recommended chemotherapy drugs on your fertility.*

- *If future fertility is important to you, ask for a referral to a fertility specialist to discuss options for you and your partner.*

Additional Information

Young Survival Coalition
www.youngsurvival.org
1.877.972.1011

CHAPTER 18

Care of the Surgical Arm

"I give a great deal of credit to my Reach to Recovery visitor for my physical recovery. She provided me with a wealth of information. For the first time, I had something I could read and re-read. I was discovering fast the necessity of education in this new and strange world."

—*Harriett Barrineau*

"Doing my exercises gave me an immediate sense of control. I could feel my body getting stronger each day."

—*Anna Cluxton*

After surgery for breast cancer, it is important to begin your journey to physical recovery by restoring the normal function of your surgical arm. This can be accomplished through an arm exercise program and learning to protect and care for your arm in the future. In this chapter, we will refer to the surgical arm as the arm on the side of your surgery, and the non-surgical arm as the opposite arm.

Surgical Arm Changes

After your surgery, sensation in the area of your incision will be diminished, and your arm may feel numb or tingly. The area under the arm (if the lymph nodes are removed) contains nerves that, if injured or cut, can cause different types of sensations. The area under your arm and the back of your arm is where the numbness usually occurs. If the nerve is stretched or injured during surgery, these sensations may improve in a few months. If the nerve is cut, the numbness will be permanent; however, this will not affect the use of your arm.

After surgery, the surgical arm will feel very tight when you attempt to stretch it up over your head. Removing your lymph nodes also requires the removal of an area of fat around the lymph nodes. This causes the area to feel pulled and tight after surgery. The feeling is temporary and will improve as you begin your arm exercise program and gradually stretch this area.

After surgery, your surgical arm needs to be exercised to restore your normal range of motion. However, do not begin any exercises until your surgeon gives you permission. Most physicians prefer that all drains and sutures or staples be removed before you attempt an arm exercise program.

"Dealing with the restrictions to my arm movement was tough. Progress was slow, but steady. Staying active and doing my arm exercises made a tremendous difference in how quickly I regained my full range of motion."
—*Anna Cluxton*

"Working in medical records, I had problems with this side of my body (surgical arm), lifting up charts. It was so painful just to reach up, but I had to do it."
—*Earnestine Brown*

Ask your physician when to begin range of motion exercises. Additional instructions as to types of arm exercises may be provided by your physician.

Arm Exercise Program

Graphically illustrated arm exercise worksheets begin on page 279. Tear the sheets out and use them as your arm exercise guide.

When you begin your arm exercise program, you may find that you tire easily and have some discomfort as you attempt to perform the movements. You should continue to perform the exercises to the point of slight discomfort but not until it becomes painful. It may take several weeks before you are able to complete some of the exercises. Work at your own pace. Your progress will be gradual. Some women find the routine is more comfortable if they take their pain medication, aspirin, Advil® or Tylenol® an hour before starting, or if they take a warm shower just prior to beginning the exercises.

Exercises should be performed on a regular basis—preferably two or more 10 to 15 minute sessions a day. Persistence is the key to regaining complete range of motion. Do the arm exercises slowly, and hold the position when you get to the end of the range. This helps to stretch and strengthen the muscles.

If you are having difficulty performing the exercises or feel you are not making progress, tell your surgeon or oncologist. Some women need the assistance of a physical therapist to regain complete range of motion, or they may need the motivation of an exercise group led by a professional.

After breast surgery, it is not uncommon for some women to favor the use of their non-surgical arm and become one-armed as they resume their daily activities. Weakness in the surgical arm, which most women experience to some degree, will cause this to happen. However, it is helpful if you remember that normal use of the surgical arm will gradually increase arm strength.

Assessing Range of Motion

After having performed your arm exercises for several months following your surgery, ask these questions to determine whether you have regained adequate range of motion in your arm.

If You Could Perform the Following Prior to Surgery, Can You Now Easily:

- Brush and comb your hair?
- Pull a t-shirt or sweater over your head?
- Close a back-fastening bra?
- Completely zip up a dress that has a long back zipper?
- Use your surgical arm to wash the shoulder blade area on the opposite side?
- Reach over your head into a cabinet to remove an object?
- Make a double bed?

When you master the full range of motion exercises, congratulate yourself on the hard work required to stick with your routine arm exercise program to accomplish this task. Ask your surgeon or oncologist to refer you to a physical therapist for help if you cannot perform your full range of motion approximately eight weeks after surgery. It is advantageous that you regain your range of motion early in your recovery.

Surgical Scar Massage

During the first four weeks after surgery, your surgical incision will heal and will eventually turn into a scar. Scars form fibrous (thickened) tissues that are firm and do not stretch or move easily. The goal of surgical scar massage is to soften and restore pliability (movement) to the scar area. This is especially important if you are planning delayed reconstructive surgery.

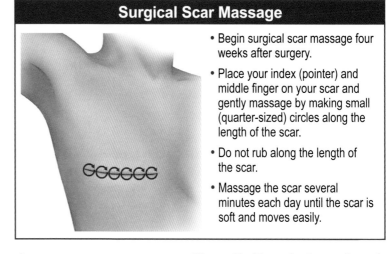

Surgical Scar Massage

- Begin surgical scar massage four weeks after surgery.
- Place your index (pointer) and middle finger on your scar and gently massage by making small (quarter-sized) circles along the length of the scar.
- Do not rub along the length of the scar.
- Massage the scar several minutes each day until the scar is soft and moves easily.

Lymphedema

Removal of the lymph nodes under your surgical arm or radiation therapy to the underarm area may cause a swelling called lymphedema (lymph, from lymphatic fluid; edema, swelling from fluid accumulation). Having only sentinel nodes removed will greatly reduce this potential. However, radiation therapy may cause fibrosis (excessive development of scar-like connective tissue) in some women, which increases the potential for lymphedema.

Lymphatic fluid is high in proteins. When the lymph fluid in the vessels is blocked from leaving the arm, because of node removal or radiation fibrosis, the lymph vessels leak proteins into surrounding tissues. The leaked protein then draws water into the tissues. This accumulation of protein and water causes swelling. Only a small percentage of women experience lymphedema after surgery, but all women need to know of the potential risks and available treatments if it should occur. Lymphedema can occur anytime from shortly after surgery to years later. To monitor your arm, it is suggested that you have someone measure your arm three inches above and three inches below the elbow prior to surgery. This will help to more accurately monitor any possible swelling.

Arm lymphedema can cause pain; restrict movement of the shoulder and arm; and increase susceptibility to an infection, called cellulitis. Lymphedema treatments are often limited in their effectiveness; therefore, the best strategy is to prevent the problem before it occurs.

Lymphedema Management Begins By:

- Understanding the causes
- Knowing how to prevent it
- Recognizing symptoms early if they occur
- Understanding the need for early reporting of swelling
- Being familiar with the signs of cellulitis (inflammation/infection)

Causes of Lymphedema:

- Surgical removal of lymph nodes (axillary dissection)
- Poor range of motion in your surgical arm
- Infection
- Obesity
- Radiation therapy to the breast and underarm area causing fibrosis
- Constriction caused by clothing or jewelry

- Long periods of positioning the arm below the level of the heart
- Repetitious tasks using the surgical arm

Lymphedema Prevention:

- The first line of defense against the development of lymphedema is regaining your full range of motion by using the arm exercises suggested in this book or by your physician. These exercises may seem dull and unnecessary, but they serve to increase the flow of lymphatic fluid from the arm area.
- For several weeks after surgery, prop your arm up on a pillow, above the level of your heart, when lying down. Elevating the arm helps reduce swelling and prevents additional accumulation of fluid.
- Avoid using your arm and hand in a dependent position (below the level of the heart) for long periods of time. If you need to perform a task of this sort, periodically hold your arms above your head to promote drainage.
- Squeeze a small rubber ball in your hand or make a fist repetitively for two to three minutes several times a day to assist the accumulated fluid in returning to general circulation.

Injury and Infection Prevention:

- Do not allow the surgical arm to be used for blood pressure checks, blood samples or injections. Remind your healthcare provider to use your non-surgical arm if possible.
- Do not wear anything tight on the surgical arm or hand, such as rings, watches, bracelets or tight elastic in sleeves.
- Do not cut your cuticles; avoid nail salons that use rotary files which could injure your cuticles. Keep hands soft by using hand lotion regularly.
- Do not carry heavy packages or purses on the side of your surgery.
- Wear protective gloves when working in the garden, washing dishes or using irritating chemicals (hair dye, cleaning products, etc.).
- Avoid burns and cuts when cooking.
- Avoid sunburn. Wear long sleeves or sunscreen when in direct sunlight for a period of time.
- Use a thimble when sewing.
- Avoid insect bites by wearing insect repellent.
- Be careful with animals. Avoid scratches.
- Use an electric razor to shave under your arm.
- Wash all cuts or injuries with antibacterial soap, apply an antibiotic medication and cover the area with sterile gauze or a Band-Aid® until the wound heals.

Notify Your Physician If You Have:

- Persistent swelling several weeks after your surgery
- Localized pain, redness, swelling and tenderness in the surgical arm or breast
- Skin that resembles an orange peel (peau d'orange)
- Red streaks that appear on the arm
- Fever, chills or fatigue

Early intervention is essential to prevent the spread of infection to other parts of your body. If you have any symptoms of cellulitis, your healthcare provider needs to be notified as soon as possible. Cellulitis is a problem that needs immediate attention. Antibiotics are necessary to treat the infection.

Lymphedema Treatments

Elastic Sleeve for Lymphedema

A special elastic sleeve, designed to reduce swelling, may be ordered by your physician. The sleeve looks like support hose and can be worn under long-sleeved clothing. A professional fitter will measure your arm and order a customized sleeve to fit you.

Elastic Sleeve Tips:

- Ask your physician to write a prescription for insurance reimbursement.
- Purchase two sleeves so that you can wash one while wearing the other one.
- Wash the sleeve in lukewarm water and allow the sleeve to air dry thoroughly. Do not wring out while wet. Do not put the sleeve in the dryer.
- Do not wear a sleeve that does not fit well. Improper fitting causes skin irritation and can increase your swelling after wearing it.
- Ask for a water-soluble adhesive lotion to apply under the top of the sleeve if you have a problem with the top of the sleeve rolling down on the arm. This adhesive washes off easily with soap and water when the sleeve is removed.
- Ask the fitter to measure your arm periodically to see if the sleeve is still the appropriate size. To be effective in reducing swelling, sleeves must fit properly.
- Replace your sleeve about every six months because it will stretch and lose elasticity from repeated use. Contact your insurance provider and ask how often they will pay for a sleeve replacement.
- Plan to wear an elastic sleeve on long airline flights. Pressure changes can cause an increase in lymphedema.

Lymphedema Massage

To treat lymphedema, a gentle, specialized massage technique, Manual Lymphatic Drainage (MLD), also known as complex decongestive physiotherapy, is performed by a trained physical therapist or massage therapist to remove swelling from the arm. This method stimulates the skin and underlying lymphatic vessels by a special technique that is different from traditional massage therapy. Because it is so vigorous, traditional massage may increase, rather than decrease, swelling.

MLD therapists are trained to delicately move their hands over the surface of the skin slowly, in circular or pumping motions, to move fluid toward the shoulder. These sessions last approximately one hour. At the conclusion of the massage, the arm is wrapped in a special bandage to prevent reaccumulation of fluid in the arm. Instructions are given on how to massage the arm with the bandage in place. This method of massage and bandaging is performed several times a week for several weeks, or until the swelling has been reduced to a manageable level. Patients and family members are often instructed in the massage and bandaging techniques so that treatment may be continued at home.

When seeking treatment for lymphedema, always ask if the therapist is trained in or has certification in manual lymph drainage for breast cancer. If your physician does not have a recommended therapist, you can find a list of specialists online at the National Lymphedema Network (www.lymphnet.org).

Compression Pumps for Lymphedema

Your physician may order a special sleeve that is connected to an air pump that compresses your arm. A compression pump needs to be used several hours a day to manually remove the accumulated fluid. Pumps are expensive, and their progress is often not monitored by a trained therapist, but rather by a salesperson for the company. It is recommended that you use a pump **only** with a physician's order and that a trained professional monitor your progress throughout use of the pump. Overuse or too much pressure may increase swelling.

Diuretics: Not Generally Recommended for Lymphedema

Diuretics (medications that remove excess water from your entire body) are **not** generally recommended for treating lymphedema. Swelling is caused by leakage of protein from the vessels in the arm. Diuretics cannot remove the protein that has seeped out into the arm. They may remove some of the water temporarily, but once you stop taking the diuretics, swelling returns because the excess protein in the arm pulls the fluid back.

Lymphedema and Weight Lifting

Previously, it had been recommended that women with lymphedema avoid weight lifting. However, a study from the University of Pennsylvania School of Medicine was conducted with breast cancer patients who had pre-existing lymphedema. The study concluded that patients who participated in progressive weight-lifting exercises for 13 weeks had a reduction in symptoms, compared to women who did not lift weights during that time. This study showed that participating in a safe, structured, weight-lifting routine, which is supervised by a certified fitness professional, can help women with lymphedema reduce symptoms. Weight-lifting increases bone density and helps control weight.

It is recommended that a well-fitting, elastic compression sleeve be worn during workouts and that a trained professional supervise correct techniques for weight-lifting. Consult your healthcare team for their advice regarding weight-lifting.

Additional Information

Tear-out Worksheet

Surgical Arm Exercises - page 279

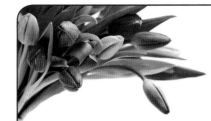

Remember…

- *Taking care of your surgical arm begins with restoring your pre-surgical range of motion by performing arm exercises.*

- *Regular arm exercises should be started as soon as your surgeon gives you permission.*

- *Perform the arm exercises to the point of discomfort, but not pain. Taking Tylenol®, Motrin® or Aleve® one hour before exercising may reduce discomfort.*

- *Lymphedema is caused when lymph vessels are blocked from surgical removal or by radiation fibrosis in the underarm area. Protein in the blocked lymph vessels seeps into the surrounding tissues, and the protein attracts water, which causes swelling.*

- *Patients who had sentinel lymph node biopsy, without breast radiation, are at a low risk for lymphedema. Axillary dissection or breast radiation to the underarm area increases the potential for lymphedema to occur.*

- *A break in the skin can allow bacteria to enter and cause an infection in the trapped fluid, called cellulitis. If a break in the skin occurs, wash the area, apply an antiseptic and cover the area until it is healed.*

- *Any signs of cellulitis, such as redness, pain or a streak going up the arm, should be reported to your physician immediately. Cellulitis requires treatment with an antibiotic.*

- *Protect your surgical arm from injury to decrease your potential for swelling and infection.*

- *Lymphedema can also occur in the lumpectomy breast, which causes swelling and the potential for cellulitis if the skin is broken.*

- *Lymphedema is not related to your cancer, but is a side effect of surgery or radiation therapy.*

- *Prevention of swelling is the best treatment for lymphedema.*

161

Thoughts To Ponder...

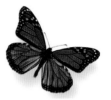

We cannot prevent an unexpected illness, stop accidents or avoid the loss of some relationships in life. Loss is a component of being human. It is a universal experience experienced by all. After we face a painful experience, it is natural to be severely disappointed. It also is not unusual to want to emotionally give up because the loss is hard to face. However, no matter what loss comes into our lives, we still have the personal power over how we confront the painful times. Personal power comes not from quitting, but from having the courage to go on with life. This is not just positive thinking, but proactively seeking what we can do now that loss is our reality.

—Judy Kneece

Use everything that comes into your life for your upliftment, learning and growth. Everything! No matter what you do, no matter how stupid, dumb or damaging you judge it to be, there is a lesson to be learned from it. No matter what happens to you, no matter how unfair, inequitable or wrong, there is always something you can take from the situation and use for your upliftment, learning or growth.

Remember the Writer's Creed: When the world gives you lemons, write the Lemon Cookbook.

—Peter McWilliams

It is a fact that there is no way to rewrite our past. What has happened has happened. Acceptance is the only way to make peace with our past and move on after a cancer diagnosis.

Our goal should be to become designers of our future life. We need to add to our life things or events that make us smile, inspire us to keep going and let us experience a deep, inner sense of peace. What do you plan to add to your life in the future?

A major sign of emotional recovery is when we reach out to help others in need. It is in serving others that we rediscover our worth as a human being and recapture the best we can be.

Helping other people is a powerful secret for healing ourselves.

—Judy Kneece

Health Insurance and Employment Issues

"Nothing prepared me for the magnitude of the responsibility I would have in seeing to it that I received the insurance benefits to which I was entitled. I was overwhelmed by the number of bills I received following surgery. Good recordkeeping was essential."

—*Harriett Barrineau*

When you are diagnosed with breast cancer, inform your insurance provider and ask for guidelines for filing and payment of claims. The following questions may need to be answered. Some of the answers may be found in your insurance policy manuals.

- What is my co-pay or out-of-pocket deductible?
- Do I need a second opinion for any procedures?
- Do I need pre-approval for diagnostic tests or hospital admissions?
- How do I file claims?
- What is the name of a representative at the company who can answer questions about my case?
- Are there any limits on the amount that will be paid for surgery, radiation therapy, chemotherapy, reconstruction or treatments offered in a clinical trial?

Insurance After Diagnosis

After diagnosis of a major illness, insurance concerns can add additional stress. Recent healthcare laws are designed to protect individuals concerning insurance coverage. You can find information about the Affordable Care Act on the U.S. Department of Health & Human Services website at www.hhs.gov/healthcare/rights/law/.

Financial Assistance

If your illness is going to be a financial burden to you, ask to speak to the social worker in the cancer treatment center. Social workers are trained to

"So much to do—so little time. I made the effort to write down the name, time and date every time I spoke with someone regarding my benefits. Don't take 'no' for an answer. Keep everything!"
—*Anna Cluxton*

"My co-pay was fifty dollars for every specialist visit, and sometimes I'd see three or four specialists a week. I hit my insurance maximums and ended up owing $14,000 out of pocket. I pay what I can."
—*Earnestine Brown*

help you with the social issues of your illness, including helping you to secure financial help for needed medical services. There are a variety of services available, but you will need to apply for them. The earlier you can make your need known, the more effective the social work team can be in helping you file the forms. People often feel embarrassed to ask for help, but it is important to ask for it early. Many people find that an unexpected illness drains their financial reserves. You are not alone. A listing of health insurance and financial assistance is available at www.cancer.org by searching "Health Insurance and Financial Assistance for the Cancer Patient."

Financial Tips:

- If your insurance requires a co-payment for each office visit, pay it at the time of each visit, if possible. These charges accumulate quickly and can seem overwhelming if they are not kept current.

- If you have an annual insurance deductible and cannot afford to pay out-of-pocket, speak with the business office at the cancer treatment center about a monthly payment plan. Make sure the payment is reasonable and is an amount that you can afford to pay each month. Begin making these payments before you receive your first bill. The treatment center will reimburse you if you overpay.

- If you are on a payment plan with the hospital or cancer treatment center and you cannot make your payment one month due to an unexpected change in your monthly budget, contact the business office to discuss the problem.

- Some pharmaceutical companies offer programs to aide in the cost of medications. Grant programs may also be available. Check with your healthcare provider to see what options you may have.

- Check with your hospital about patient assistance for your surgery or other treatments. Most hospitals are obligated, by law, to provide some patient assistance in their budget. Their funds tend to run low by the end of the year, so check as soon as you think you need help.

Reimbursement Recordkeeping

During breast cancer treatment, it is very important that you keep records to receive payment for services covered under your insurance. Many patients find this task overwhelming. If you need help, ask a partner or a friend for their assistance in this area. Keeping accurate records will make the task much easier.

Recordkeeping Tips:

- Keep a calendar record of all appointments (a pocket calendar is helpful).
- Write on the calendar the physician you visited, procedures performed and medications purchased.
- Provide physicians with appropriate information for filing claims.
- Ask for copies of all charges at the time of service, or ask to have copies mailed to you.
- Keep copies of all medical bills in one place (a box, a notebook or file folder).
- Check frequently to see if appropriate payment is made to medical providers.
- Ask your healthcare facility or provider to help you understand or assist you in providing information for adequate repayment, if problems arise.
- Ask your Human Resources Department for assistance in filing claims if your insurance is through your employer.
- Call your insurance provider and talk with a representative about unpaid claims. Offer additional records or assistance for getting information from your medical providers. Always write down the date of contact and the person's name with whom you spoke.
- Keep all premiums current; do not allow your insurance to lapse.

Employment Issues During Treatment

Breast cancer surgery and treatment will require some time away from your job. You will need to give notice of your absence and expected time away from your job. Most employers are very understanding and offer their support during this time.

Occasionally, however, a breast cancer patient will be discriminated against because of illness. If you have reasons to believe that your employer has treated you unfairly because of your illness, there are laws to protect you. There are federal laws and varying state laws that offer protection against discrimination or unfair practices. Listed in the *Resource* section of this book are names and telephone numbers you can call for information on how to best manage your situation.

Family and Medical Leave Act

In 1993, the Family and Medical Leave Act (FMLA) granted certain employees up to 12 weeks of unpaid, job-protected medical leave per year. It also requires that the employee's group health benefits be maintained during the leave. As a cancer patient, your illness meets the requirements if you are employed by a public agency, a public or private elementary/secondary school or a company with 50 or more employees. You may be eligible for medical leave if you have:

- Worked for your employer at least 12 months.
- Worked at least 1,250 hours over the past 12 months.

Documentation Needed for Medical Leave

To receive medical leave, you will be required to provide a form signed and dated by a doctor, stating:

- You have a cancer diagnosis
- When the illness started
- Whether absences are expected to be continuous or in short blocks of time
- When you may be expected to return to work
- Whether further treatment will be required after the absence

To learn more about FMLA provisions and rules, read the FMLA Fact Sheet posted on the United States Government's Department of Labor website at: www.dol.gov (enter "FMLA" in the search box), or call the Wage and Hour Division's referral and information line at the Department of Labor at 1-866-487-9243. They can give you other helpful information and tell you how to reach the Department of Labor division office nearest you.

What To Tell Your Co-Workers

It is necessary for you to decide how much to tell your employer, fellow employees and friends about the details of your illness. Some women are very open about their illness and treatments. Others feel that this is a private matter and would rather not share the details with everyone. Decide what you wish for others to know. If you inform your support partner or family members of your wishes, it will be helpful when people call or drop by.

You do not have to constantly share your illness story with others if this makes you uncomfortable. The simple reply, *"I appreciate your concern, but right now I am not up to talking about it. Thank you for understanding,"* allows you the right not to share. You need to communicate, but you do not need to feel that you have to talk with everyone who asks about your illness. It may be helpful to allow family members to answer the phone and screen your calls if you would rather not talk. Plan to do what best suits your particular personality.

When Co-Workers Don't Call or Visit

Often, women find that their co-workers or friends don't call or come to see them after their diagnosis. This can be emotionally painful because these are people that you saw and worked with every day. Why does this happen?

- They don't know what to say.
- They don't know what to do.
- It distresses them to see you in emotional or physical pain when they can't do anything about it.
- Your diagnosis serves as a reminder that they, too, could be diagnosed with cancer. It becomes easier for them to avoid you than to face their own vulnerabilities.

Breaking the Silence:

- Be sure that you have not sent out unspoken messages that you want your illness to be a private affair.
- Call your friends and co-workers. Let them know that you are handling your diagnosis as well as you can and that you miss them.
- When they ask if they can help, be specific: pick up the children, take me to lunch, pick up a prescription, drive me to the doctor, etc. They want to know that they will not add to your burdens but can truly help you during this time.
- Invite them over for a cup of coffee or tea.
- Ask them to join you for a walk.

"Before breast cancer I was a very healthy person, so I didn't know the ins and outs of insurance coverage and reimbursement. I purchased a journal that I called 'All Things Breast Cancer' for my recordkeeping. After each phone call to my insurance company, my Human Resources department or my disability provider, I would write down all pertinent facts and things I needed to do. It was helpful to have everything documented in one place. It helped me stay organized."

—Lisa DelGuidice

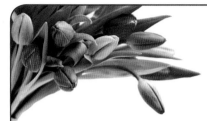

Remember ...

- *Ask a partner or friend to help you keep records for insurance reimbursement.*

- *Review your insurance policy for coverage, shortly after diagnosis.*

- *Determine the name and contact number of the insurance representative who will be handling your claims.*

- *Ask any questions you have about your coverage.*

- *Contact the social workers at your cancer center, as early as possible, if you determine that you will have financial needs during treatment.*

- *Recordkeeping will help take the hassle out of filing for insurance claims. A dedicated calendar to record all appointments or treatments is helpful. Ask for a copy of all charges, and keep records in one place.*

- *Discuss with your physicians the expected time you may need away from your job for treatment. Share your expected absence with your employer.*

- *Understand that co-workers or friends often do not know what to say or how to respond to someone with a cancer diagnosis. If you miss their friendship, reach out to them.*

Thoughts To Ponder...

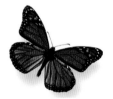

During cancer treatment, some of my friends bailed. Some went, "Um, no, you're just not fun anymore. You're sick and talk about cancer. I don't want to hear any talk about cancer. I want to talk about me." It was heartbreaking. But, at the same time, that's when I would think, "God, cancer is a godsend in a lot of ways because, boy, did it clean house in my life."

—Shannen Doherty

When I was going through chemotherapy, instead of feeling mad at my body for failing me, I tried to give myself permission to take it easy. Easier said than done—I'm still struggling with being kind to myself. I couldn't help but feel frustrated with my body when I was overly tired or when my mind was fuzzy from chemo brain. Sometimes I would beat myself up over sleeping late. It was a daily struggle not to view these as personal weaknesses. Isn't it interesting, during the time we should be the easiest on ourselves, I found that we can often be the most judgmental and harsh?

—Suleika Jaouad

After a cancer diagnosis, living with uncertainty during treatment is common. You may feel as if you have lost complete control of your schedule. Making plans is difficult because you never know when you will be scheduled for treatment or if you would even feel up to doing anything. One approach that works well for many patients is to decide to live spontaneously. Forget the scheduling, take the opportunity to seize the moments when your energy is up. This period of uncertainty is time-limited; it will soon come to an end.

—Anonymous

We never think that painful or upsetting experiences are worth it, and yet those are often the main events through which we grow and expand. Pain grows us. If we saw pain as a natural teacher, maybe then pain wouldn't be our enemy. We can learn courage, strength, persistence, grace, compassion, and tools to face something seemingly impossible from our life experiences.

—Judy Tatelbaum, LCSW

Most of our lives have been spent learning to postpone our happiness until "I can do or achieve." We deny gratification, waiting for the future. We have to retrain ourselves to grasp the happiness each day brings and not feel guilty. This is the power of living in the present. Cancer has taught you a valuable lesson— don't waste a happiness opportunity.

—Anonymous

CHAPTER 20

Diet and Exercise

A breast cancer diagnosis can provide the perfect opportunity to slow down and reevaluate every area of your life. Part of this evaluation should include how you fuel your body to achieve maximum health and immunity and how you move your body to stay strong physically.

As you recover, it is helpful to keep in mind that chemotherapy and radiation treatments kill cancerous cells and, in the process, destroy normal, healthy cells that have to be replaced. New cells are rebuilt from what you eat and drink. Therefore, it is important you have the nutrients necessary to rebuild healthy cells for recovery to occur. What you eat and drink are extremely important.

Maintaining as much energy as possible is also vital. New research shows that physical movement during treatment and recovery can contribute to a sense of well-being and can increase energy.

This chapter is not about restrictive diets and gym workouts, but is about suggestions that are flexible and easily incorporated into your normal lifestyle. I encourage you to consider your diet and exercise as a vital part of your recovery. You alone can make these decisions. This is a gift only you can give yourself.

Healthy Eating

Your goal during cancer treatment should be to eat a nutritious, balanced diet, which maintains your body weight, while not making you feel hungry or deprived. This is not the time for fad diets, which often cut out certain food groups. You should not attempt any diet that causes extreme hunger or is highly restrictive. Restrictive diets do not promote recovery; they only increase stress, which is definitely not good for you. The focus in this chapter is to provide tips that will help you to make better nutritional choices without the stress of a restrictive diet. Remember that every time you make a food selection, you have the opportunity to give your body the fuel needed to rebuild healthy cells.

"As soon as possible, I got out of the house to get into the fresh air and sunshine. I asked how soon I could start doing arm exercises, and then I did them every day. I was training to get back into life."
—Anna Cluxton

"Before my breast cancer diagnosis, my busy work schedule didn't leave much time for exercise. I realized I needed to focus on me, my health and my well-being. The change started the day after surgery. I began walking the hospital corridor and progressed to a 5K walk. Now I walk five days a week, teach a fitness class and attend strength and cardio classes. It feels great!"
—Lisa DelGuidice

Weight Gain During Treatment

Some women undergoing chemotherapy for breast cancer experience weight gain, and some do not. Like other side effects, weight gain is usually time-limited. Weight gain may be caused by:

- Hormonal changes caused by chemotherapy or hormonal medications
- Fluid retention from chemotherapy medications
- Keeping food in the stomach to relieve nausea
- Increased eating caused by stress
- Decreased activity during treatments

If you find that you gain weight during treatment, do not panic and go on a restrictive diet, which could impact your recovery. Don't allow the numbers on a scale to determine how you feel. Avoid daily weighing during this time because medications can cause wide fluctuations in weight. Think of this time as temporary—your body will undergo changes you don't like, but they are time-limited.

Dietary Tips During Breast Cancer

While going through treatment, it is helpful to evaluate your dietary habits to ensure that you are eating nutritious foods from all food groups and not adding empty calories that could add to weight gain. The goal is to incorporate as many of the following dietary tips as possible to maintain your energy and prevent unwanted weight gain.

Controlling Hunger

It takes fewer calories to prevent hunger than it does to deal with it once it occurs. Tips to control hunger:

- Plan to eat smaller food portions five to six times a day. Reduce portions at meal times to spread your calories throughout the day. Plan to include nutritious snacks between meals.
- Eat frequently to prevent low blood sugar (hypoglycemia), which causes fatigue, increases your potential for nausea and slows down your metabolism. When blood sugar is low, it causes an increase in appetite and is often the cause of uncontrolled (binge) eating.

Staying Hydrated

Drink lots of water. Water (fluid intake) is crucial to your health. Water makes up about 60 percent of your body weight, and every system in your body depends on water to function properly. Lack of water can lead to dehydration, a condition that occurs when you don't have enough water in your body for your cells to carry on normal functions. Even mild dehydration can drain your energy and make you tired. That is why it is important to report to your physician any nausea, vomiting or diarrhea that you cannot control within 12 – 24 hours. It is essential that you are able to drink and retain adequate amounts of fluid to maintain your energy.

Early Signs and Symptoms of Dehydration:

▪ Thirst	▪ Dry mouth	▪ Dizziness
▪ Fatigue	▪ Muscle weakness	▪ Lightheadedness
▪ Headache	▪ Little or no urination	

How Much Water Do You Need?

There are different recommendations for water intake. The National Institute of Health recommends that women drink about 9 cups (72 ounces) a day to maintain water balance. This recommended amount increases when activities cause excessive sweating.

Making Water More Tasteful

Some people dislike drinking plain water. The goal is to drink fluids that are not calorie dense and loaded with sugar. Sugary drinks do not rebuild cells but can add weight. Tips to make water more tasteful include:

- Squeeze lemon into water.
- Add whole strawberries or slices of cucumber, orange or lime to a pitcher of water and allow flavor to permeate.
- Add products like Emergen-C® (found in discount or health food stores). These flavored products come in individual packages and can easily be added to a bottle or glass of water to provide a healthy, energizing drink containing extra vitamin C, B vitamins and electrolytes.

Eliminating Empty Liquid Calories:

- Avoid all sugary drinks when possible—soft drinks, sweetened tea, sweetened coffee or sports drinks. These drinks are full of calories and cause a quick rise in blood sugar. You may get a rush of energy, but the down side is that your blood sugar drops quickly afterwards, leaving you feeling fatigued. A good alternative is Propel, a flavored water without carbonation or artificial sweeteners.
- Avoid diet drinks; they have been associated with weight gain in some people and add no nutritional value to your diet.
- Monitor the amount of fruit juice you drink because it is also high in calories. Choosing to eat the whole fruit with fiber is a better choice when possible.
- Select 100 percent vegetable or tomato juice, one percent or skim milk, soy milk, unsweetened tea or coffee for lower-calorie beverage choices.

Understanding Carbohydrates in Your Diet

Carbohydrates (carbs) are foods that when eaten and digested break down into glucose (sugar), which gives you energy. In the past few years, some of the fads in dieting have promoted low-carb diets for weight control. The goal during cancer treatment is to avoid fad diets and eat foods from all food groups, including carbohydrates. However, some carbohydrates are healthier choices than others for maintaining energy and weight control. Healthy carb choices are identified through the glycemic index.

The glycemic index ranks carbohydrate foods by how much and how quickly they raise glucose levels, which is called the glycemic response. Foods that raise glucose levels quickly have a higher glycemic index rating than foods that cause a slower rise. The lower the rating, the better the carbohydrate is to help control your appetite and lower your risk of diabetes. Lower-rated carbs are healthier choices, because they are usually lower in calories and higher in fiber, nutrients and antioxidants. Choosing low glycemic index foods may help you control your appetite because they tend to keep you feeling full longer. Other health benefits of low glycemic index foods include:

- Controls your blood glucose levels by maintaining a more constant level of energy
- Controls your appetite by maintaining your blood sugar level
- Lowers your risk of getting heart disease by helping control your cholesterol levels
- Lowers your risk of getting type 2 (adult-onset) diabetes by keeping blood sugar levels lower

Glycemic Index Rating

Carbohydrates on the glycemic index are rated as low (55 or less), medium (56 – 69) or high (70 and up). Your goal is to select lower glycemic foods.

Low Glycemic Foods (55 or less):
- Skim milk
- Plain yogurt
- Apples/plums/oranges
- Sweet potato
- Oatmeal (slow-cook oats)
- Oat bran bread
- Bran cereal
- Converted or parboiled rice
- Pumpernickel bread
- Pasta
- Lentils (beans)
- Honey

Medium Glycemic Foods (56 – 69):
- Bananas, pineapples, raisins
- Popcorn
- Brown rice
- Shredded wheat cereal
- Whole wheat bread
- Rye bread

High Glycemic Foods (over 70):
- Dried dates, watermelon
- Instant mashed potatoes
- Baked white potato
- Instant rice
- Bagel, white
- Soda crackers
- Jelly beans; candies
- French fries
- Corn Flakes®, Rice Krispies®
- Ice cream
- Cookies
- Table sugar

Maximize Good Carbohydrates

Good carbs are lower on the glycemic index and include beans and grains. The fiber content will fill you up while promoting healthy blood sugar levels.

Beans

- Beans are filled with nutrients and phytochemicals (plant chemicals) that have been shown to be active in prevention of diseases.
- Beans are inexpensive, easy to prepare and last for several days when refrigerated. They can be eaten alone, over brown rice or added to soups, salads or stews. Aim for one half cup serving or more of beans each day.
- Best choices for beans include: soybeans, lentils, kidney beans, chickpeas (garbanzo), butter beans, navy beans, black beans, white beans or split peas.

Grains

- Do not deprive yourself of breads and cereals; just make sure that you choose 100 percent whole grains—whole wheat, whole oats, brown rice, rye, barley, etc.
- When buying grain products look for the word whole in front of grain.

Vegetables and Fruits

- Vegetables are low in calories and high in fiber. Vegetables are natural appetite suppressants because they are very filling and are packed with vitamins, minerals and phytochemicals.
- Best choices for vegetables include: cabbage, kale, broccoli, cauliflower, Brussels sprouts, collards, carrots, leeks, tomatoes, asparagus, spinach, dark varieties of lettuce and red or orange bell peppers.
- Limit or avoid the high glycemic index or starchy vegetables, such as corn, white potatoes, parsnips and rutabagas, which raise your blood sugar quickly.
- Fruits are highly nutritious. Strive to include two servings a day.
- Best choices for fruit include: berries (any variety), cherries, plums, any whole citrus, cantaloupe, grapes, peaches, apples, pears and dried or fresh apricots.
- Limit higher glycemic fruits, including: bananas, mangoes, papaya, pineapple, raisins and dates.

Healthy Proteins

- Proteins provide a steady, prolonged blood glucose level with minimal insulin response and will keep you feeling satisfied longer between meals.
- Best choices for healthy proteins include: fish (oily varieties such as salmon, tuna, mackerel, sardines, herring and trout), shellfish, skinless poultry, nuts, seeds, soy, wild game, lean dairy products (cottage cheese and yogurt), beans/legumes and eggs.
- Limit other protein sources such as red meat or pork to several servings a week.
- Eating protein at breakfast is especially important for energy and weight control.

Fats

The most recent dietary studies have shown the importance of dietary fat. The body requires fat to repair cells during and after chemotherapy. It is important to eat good sources of dietary fat.

- Dietary fat makes food taste better, satisfies your appetite and reduces hunger.
- Many of the good fats are found in the sources of protein listed above. Additional sources of good fats include extra virgin olive oil, canola oil, nuts, seeds and avocados.
- Green salads with olive oil dressing are an excellent way to get a healthy serving of fat.
- Avoid trans fats (vegetable oils that have been processed, such as margarines and shortenings).
- Minimize saturated fats found in fatty cuts of beef, pork and lamb.

Nuts

- Unsalted, unprocessed nuts are a great source of protein. They make an easy, healthy snack and can aid in weight loss.
- Best choices for nuts include: walnuts, almonds, cashews, pistachios, hazelnuts, Brazil nuts and pecans.
- Include 1 – 1.5 ounces of nuts in your daily diet. Buy raw nuts in bulk and divide into smaller packages to carry as a handy snack.

Portion Control

When eating a meal, limit portion sizes to no more than the equivalent of your hands cupped together. The exception to this rule is non-starchy vegetables, which can be consumed in unlimited amounts.

Healthy Eating Preparation

Eating right requires being prepared. When you are hungry, or when your energy is low from treatments, it is easy to eat the most convenient food, rather than the healthiest food. Tips for healthy eating include:

- Purchase and have healthy foods, snacks and drinks available.
- Stock your pantry and freezer with an assortment of healthy foods before you begin chemotherapy. Use the week before your next treatment to replenish your supplies.
- Cook several meals and freeze them for the days when you don't feel up to cooking.
- Buy large packages of nuts and whole grain crackers and divide them into small plastic bags.
- Keep small amounts of food in your stomach to help prevent nausea and to prevent fatigue, which is caused by low blood sugar.
- Carry water and a healthy snack of nuts, fruit or whole wheat crackers with you to avoid getting hungry when away from home. Don't get caught without something nutritious to eat.

Nutrition During Chemotherapy

If you take chemotherapy drugs, you may experience side effects that alter your dietary intake. Taste changes, nausea, vomiting, diarrhea or constipation may all change how, when and what you eat. Some people find that they need to adjust their diets to maintain their calorie intake during chemotherapy.

Tips for Eating During Chemotherapy:

- Make every spoonful and every drink you take count nutritionally. Your body is building healthy, new cells to replace those damaged by chemotherapy.

- Eat five to six small meals a day rather than three large ones. Small meals are better tolerated.

- Because your body is building new cells, it is essential to get adequate protein. You need more protein when you may least feel like eating. Good protein choices during this time include: whole wheat bread or crackers combined with peanut butter or almond butter (tastes like peanut butter and is highly nutritious), hard-boiled eggs, yogurt, liquid yogurt or cottage cheese.

- Limit the amount of fluid you drink with meals to avoid getting full too quickly. Drink between meals instead. Adequate fluid intake and hydration are essential. Monitor your intake to be sure you are getting enough fluids. Filling a bottle with your daily intake at the beginning of the day will help you monitor how much you are drinking.

- Make your own high-protein smoothies in a blender with yogurt, fresh fruit or peanut or almond butter. This is a smart way to get calories and protein while avoiding the hassle of food preparation.

Remember, chemotherapy is time-limited, and problems affecting your eating and nutrition will come to an end. Additional dietary information is available from the American Cancer Society.

Staying Physically Fit

Recovery from breast cancer is a time to consider an exercise program as part of your personal fitness plan. Your hospital or clinic may offer or recommend exercise classes with a focus on regaining the range of motion of the surgical arm. These programs are very beneficial. I encourage you to join if there is one available. If not, refer to *Chapter 18: Care of the Surgical Arm* and perform the *Surgical Arm Exercises* beginning on page 279 until the full range of motion is restored to your surgical arm. In addition, take a serious look at how physical exercise can increase your physical stamina, reduce treatment side effects and shorten your recovery time.

Why Should I Exercise When I'm Already So Tired?

Most people who have not participated in regular exercise think of exercise as an additional activity that will decrease their available energy. The opposite is true. Physical exercise has been proven to restore energy and reduce many side effects during cancer treatment and recovery.

Normal fatigue is expected after surgery, radiation therapy and chemotherapy. The traditional recommendation in years past was you need to rest, and many patients reverted to bed rest to manage their fatigue. It was believed that the more you rested, the more quickly you would recover. However, newer studies have shown that bed rest can actually promote physiological changes that **increase**, rather than decrease, fatigue.

Fatigue
When patients were asked how chemotherapy impacted energy levels:
■ 62% reported a decrease in energy **during** treatment
■ 40% reported a decrease in energy **six months** after completion of treatment
■ 22% reported a decrease in energy **one year** after completion of treatment

Studies by Greenleaf and Kozlowski revealed, *"Maintenance of optimal health in a person requires a proper balance between exercise, rest, and sleep, as well as time in an upright position."*

Bed Rest Versus Activity Study Revealed:

- Too much rest promotes fatigue (imbalance).
- Too little activity promotes fatigue (imbalance).
- A dynamic balance between rest and activity decreases fatigue.

The study conclusion was that patients need to remain as active as possible during periods of physical recovery. There needs to be a balance of activity and rest in order for maximum energy to be maintained.

Clinical Study of Cancer Patients Revealed Benefits of Exercise:

- Exercise functioned as a stress relief mechanism in coping
- Patients maintained a feeling of control over their lives
- Increase in internal control (ability to make decisions)
- Increase in mood elevation
- Decrease in tension and anxiety
- No harmful or debilitating effects reported
- 40 percent gain in functional capacity at end of 10 weeks
- Decrease in complaints of nausea and vomiting

Another interesting study outcome involved those who did not participate in regular exercise. Unlike those who exercised, those who did not exercise reported a worsening of mood as treatment progressed.

It is important that you understand the newer concepts of energy building, especially after a cancer diagnosis. The older recommendations for bed rest need to be replaced with the new facts:

- Too much rest can decrease available energy.
- Exercise can build energy.
- Decreased movement may make a person feel worse.
- Excessive bed rest and inactivity are enemies of recovery.
- Too much rest can cause increased fatigue, constipation, pneumonia and deep vein thrombosis (DVT).
- Activity and rest must be balanced to maintain or build energy.
- Maintaining or starting a moderate exercise program based on your present ability can speed recovery and reduce symptoms of treatment; it will not harm you.
- Exercise can reduce the need for pain and nausea medications that have fatigue as a side effect.

This is your opportunity to make recovery a time of balance between appropriate rest and appropriate exercise. If you did not participate in an exercise program prior to your cancer diagnosis, now is the time to build energy by adopting moderate physical movement as a part of your complete recovery plan.

Whatever exercise you select and consistently do will raise your energy levels and speed your psychological recovery by decreasing depression. In addition, exercise reduces pain by promoting the release of natural painkillers referred to as endorphins, or natural morphine, into the body.

Exercise Programs During Cancer Treatments

Before beginning any exercise program, ask your physician if you have limitations. While it is important to maintain physical activity, it is also necessary that you understand that your tolerated level of activity may change during treatment. Strive to maintain your activity at a level that allows you to exercise regularly without exhaustion. Enjoy the activity and look at this as a special time set aside to take care of your own needs. The rewards will be increased physical stamina and psychological well-being.

What Type of Exercise Program Is Best?

Some women prefer group/peer exercise, and others prefer to exercise alone, or with a family member or friend. The goal is for you to decide what type of physical activity is suitable for you and take steps to start. The right exercise for you is something you can physically do, you have the time to do, is convenient for you and you enjoy. You do not need to join a gym or health club. Walking programs, Pilates, yoga, biking, swimming or gardening are all good choices.

Walking Program

Starting a regular walking program is a good choice because you can walk anytime you choose, it does not cost anything and it can be adapted to your present physical condition. A walking program can be easily modified to meet your changing needs during treatment; it can be started, suspended, decreased or accelerated according to your physical energy.

Recommendations for a Walking Program:

- **Frequency:** Four times a week minimum, six times a week maximum; try not to skip more than one day in a row if your health allows.
- **Goal:** Gradually increase and maintain your heart rate at 100 to 120 beats per minute.
- **Duration:** Brisk walking at your own pace; start at 10 minutes per session and increase gradually to 30 minutes per session, as tolerated.
- **Place:** Preferably outdoors, when weather permits; indoor mall or treadmill.
- **Attire:** Comfortable shoes designed for walking and layered, loose, cotton clothing to absorb perspiration. Consider purchasing a pedometer or Fitbit® that measures the distance you walk and monitors your heart rate.
- **Evaluation:** Use the talk test to determine if the activity is too strenuous. During your exercise, you should be able to talk in sentences without feeling out of breath. If you cannot say a sentence without losing your breath, reduce your exercise level. Stop any exercise if it causes or increases pain.

Walking Routine:

- Five minutes of slow walking to warm up.
- Increase walking to a brisk pace to increase heart rate to 100 to 120 beats per minute (take your pulse for 6 seconds and multiply by 10 to check your heart rate).
- Gradually increase the time your pulse remains at your target heart rate by extending your walk as tolerated. Do not exercise to a point of causing fatigue; this is not healthy or recommended.
- For the last five minutes, reduce your pace to allow your heart rate to return to normal gradually.

Walking Tips:

- Walk with a partner, if possible.
- Listen to inspirational CDs or your favorite music if you walk alone.
- Keep an exercise log or diary to monitor your progress.
- Exercise at the same time each day, if possible, to make walking routine.
- Drink a full glass of water before and after you walk.

- Carry personal identification with you.
- Carry a cell phone to call for assistance if you run into a problem.
- Walk in a safe area, away from traffic.

Exercise Evaluation

The ultimate test to evaluate whether you are overdoing your exercise is to wait one hour after completion and then ask yourself, *"Do I have more energy and feel more relaxed?"* If the answer is yes, you are exercising in a range that is building energy. If the answer is no, you are over-taxing your body's physical reserves, and you need to reduce the intensity or duration of your exercise.

Do Not Exercise if You Have:

- Fever
- Nausea or vomiting
- Muscle or joint pain with swelling
- Bleeding from any source
- Irregular heart beat
- Dizziness or fainting
- Chest, arm or jaw pain
- Intravenous chemotherapy administration on the same day
- Blood drawing on the same day (may exercise afterwards, but prior exercise may alter counts)
- Any restrictions placed on exercise activities by a physician

Exercise Precautions During Treatment

If you are receiving chemotherapy, your nurse or physician will alert you if your counts are in a range where exercise is not advised. When you have your blood drawn, ask if your counts are still in a safe range.

Diet and Exercise Summary

What you eat and how you move your body are predictors of how you will feel during treatment and recovery. Eating nutritious food and getting regular exercise are keys to increasing your energy and improving your mood. When your body has nutrients from food available and the ability to transport oxygen to all its cells, it increases its capacity to heal, increases available energy, elevates mood, decreases pain, lowers anxiety, decreases depression and boosts immunity.

Plan to incorporate changes that will enhance your recovery and that can easily fit into your lifestyle. These are changes that no one can make for you. Food and exercise are habits. The good news is that bad habits can be broken, and new habits can be implemented. If you recognize that there are changes that may benefit you, now is the time to plan what you need to change and when you want to get started. If you find change hard to stick with, enlist a friend or support partner to join you or to be your cheerleader. Friends can help motivate you to keep your commitment. You will never regret making these positive changes. This is a gift that you can give yourself.

Exercise and Diet Plan

- My support person for change:

  _____

- Change(s) I plan to make in my diet:

  _____
  _____
  _____
  _____

- Exercise(s) I plan to start:

  _____
  _____
  _____

- Date I plan to start:

  _____

- Equipment or supplies I may need:

  _____
  _____

- My goal(s):

  _____
  _____
  _____
  _____

Additional Information

Tear-out Worksheet

Surgical Arm Exercises - page 279

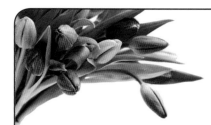

Remember...

- *Chemotherapy kills cancer cells, but also kills normal, healthy cells that have to be replaced. Rebuilding cells requires that adequate nutrients be available for the process. Making healthy choices of food and drink can supply these needed nutrients. What you eat and drink during recovery are important.*

- *Weight gain during breast cancer treatment may occur due to medications and decreased activity. If you gain weight, do not allow this to cause you to go on a restrictive diet. Restricting certain food groups could cause inadequate nutrients that are needed to repair your cells.*

- *Eating a small amount of food five to six times a day helps to control hunger. Controlling hunger helps to control binge eating.*

- *Staying hydrated with water is essential. Dehydration causes headache and fatigue. Adequate hydration assists with the elimination of chemotherapy medications from your body. The body requires about 9 cups of water a day to stay hydrated.*

- *Eliminate sugary drinks like soft drinks; they add calories and provide no nutritional benefit.*

- *Maintain adequate levels of dietary protein, which is required for rebuilding cells.*

- *Include healthy fats in your diet. Fats are needed for rebuilding cells. Fats also increase your energy.*

- *Plan to carry healthy snacks when you are away from home. Raw nuts or whole fruits are good choices.*

- *Stock your pantry with nutritious foods. Cook and freeze several meals the week before your treatment to use on days when you don't feel like cooking.*

- *Staying physically active during treatment rather than staying on bed rest has proven to elevate the mood, increase energy and decrease anxiety. Daily walking is a good choice.*

- *Recruit a partner for your planned exercise. The shared commitment increases your motivation to continue the exercise.*

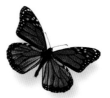

Thoughts To Ponder...

It is a fact that there is no way to rewrite our past. What happened has happened. Acceptance is the only way to make peace with our past and move on after a cancer diagnosis.

Our goal after a cancer diagnosis should be to become designers of our future life. We need to add to our life things or events that make us smile, inspire us to keep going and let us experience a deep, inner sense of peace.

What do you plan to add to your life in the future?

—**Judy Kneece**

From the earliest days of my diagnosis, one of the casualties of cancer was the feeling that I had to shelve my dreams and goals. These paused plans— interrupted dreams —weighed on me every day. I was constantly thinking of everything I could be doing. Then, I decided that I didn't want to let cancer put my life entirely on hold. It had always been my goal to become a writer of some kind. So now I'm going after that goal.

—**Suleika Jaouad**

A major sign of emotional recovery is when we can start reaching out to help others in need. Our pain and loss allows us to recognize others' pain and uniquely prepares us to reach out to help.

It is in serving others that we rediscover our worth as a human being and recapture the best we can be. Helping other people is a powerful secret for healing ourselves.

—**Judy Kneece**

Since my diagnosis, I've begun to send letters and care packages to other cancer patients and friends of mine going through a difficult time. By reaching out, I'm paying it forward for all the help and care I have received. I have found that small acts of gratitude or connectedness to other people who are suffering rescues me from my own self-pity and makes me feel like I'm capable of helping, and not just being helped.

—**Suleika Jaouad**

Monitoring Your Future Health for Recurrence

"They found more calcifications (thankfully, benign) in my breast during follow-up, so I had to have another biopsy. Before cancer I would have rushed back to work. Now I'm learning to take care of myself. People take time off to go to the beach, time off to do whatever. This is my health. I can take time off to take care of me."

—Earnestine Brown

At the conclusion of your cancer treatment, your oncologist will discuss a plan to monitor your future health for a potential cancer recurrence. The follow-up care recommended by your oncologist is usually from the American Society of Clinical Oncology (ASCO) and is the most effective method known to monitor your future health.

When cancer treatments end, it is a happy time for you as a patient. This is the time you have been waiting for. Your cancer treatment is concluding, and there is no evidence of cancer. Yet, in the back of every patient's mind lingers the fear that her cancer could come back one day. Survivors report that their number one fear after breast cancer treatment is the possibility of recurrence. One patient summed up her fears as:

> *Fear of recurrence is like a black cloud in my blue sky. Some days it is right over my head, causing everything to appear dark and gloomy. Some days it is far away, and my day is sunny. But I'm always aware it is there.*

Not talking about recurrence is like seeing a pink elephant standing in the middle of the room and having everyone ignore it—everyone sees it, but they're afraid to mention it. Failing to mention it only creates more anxiety for everyone involved. A better solution is to talk about the potential for breast cancer recurrence and to learn how you can take appropriate steps to monitor your own health. Having worked with breast cancer patients for over twenty-nine years, I can tell you that most patients overestimate their potential for recurrence. Talk to your doctor and find out about your

"Being so involved in the cancer community, I am acutely aware of the potential for recurrence. To protect my future, I keep up with my appointments and keep a list of questions to discuss with my doctors."
—Anna Cluxton

"I think it's very normal to think about recurrence; however, I can't let it consume me. No one knows what the future holds. I must live in the here and now."
—Lisa DelGuidice

particular risk. Then, remember that you are an individual, not a statistic. In this chapter, we will discuss breast cancer recurrence and provide you with the information you need to guard your health.

Breast Cancer Recurrence

The majority of breast cancer recurrences occur within the first five years after treatment, with approximately 60 to 80 percent occurring in the first three years. Therefore, it is very important that you keep your appointments with your physician for close monitoring of your health. Breast cancer recurrence is highly unpredictable—no one can say if, or when, it will happen.

Types of Recurrence:

- **Local Recurrence:** When cancer returns to the local area of removal. This type of recurrence occurs because surgery or radiation left behind microscopic cells. A local recurrence does not change the stage of your cancer.
- **Regional Recurrence:** When cancer spreads outside the breast. This spread may be to the underarm lymph nodes, chest muscles, internal mammary nodes located underneath the breastbone or in the nodes above the collarbone.
- **Distant Recurrence:** When the cancer is found in a distant site such as the bones, lungs, liver, brain or other sites in the body.

Regional or distant cancer recurrence may require your cancer to be restaged.

Potential Local Recurrence Signs and Symptoms:

- Change in size, shape or contour of the lumpectomy breast
- Nipple discharge that is clear or bloody
- New onset of breast pain
- A new lump that may feel like a small pea
- Thickening in breast tissues or on mastectomy chest wall
- Changes in the skin: nipple inversion, dimpling (pulling in of skin), scaly appearance, rash, redness or any discoloration on breast or mastectomy chest wall
- A lump or thickening in the underarm area

Potential Regional or Distant Recurrence Signs and Symptoms:

- New lump or thickening in the area above the collarbone
- Chronic bone pain
- Tenderness in any area of the body
- Chest pain with shortness of breath
- Chronic cough with or without sputum production
- Headaches, dizziness or fainting
- Persistent abdominal pain or swelling
- Vision changes
- Increasing fatigue unrelated to treatments
- Yellowing of the skin or eyes
- Inability to control urine or bowels
- Persistent nausea or loss of appetite
- Changes in weight, especially weight loss

If you have any of the above symptoms, do not hesitate to report them to your healthcare team between office visits. If you have a new symptom that lasts longer than two weeks, or an old symptom that is progressively getting worse, contact your oncologist. Do not ignore any change as being unimportant. Instead, let your physician or nurse make the decision. What may seem unimportant to you may be important to your healthcare team.

Surveillance Guidelines

A plan for future surveillance will be recommended by your oncologist. Oncologists usually follow the Surveillance Guideline recommendations of the American Society of Clinical Oncology (ASCO), which is composed of oncologists who treat breast cancer. These guidelines are carefully researched and are updated regularly. It is very important that you keep these visits with your doctor.

Other physicians involved in your care may also require return visits in their area of specialty. Some patients may be referred back to their primary care provider for cancer surveillance. Understanding your recommended surveillance guidelines, along with the signs and symptoms that should be reported to your physician(s) between visits, is vital.

ASCO Recommendations for Surveillance:

- Patient history should be updated at each physician visit
- Physical and breast clinical examination should be performed at each physician visit
- Patient should receive instructions on signs and symptoms of recurrence
- Breast self-exam should be recommended for all breast cancer patients
- Breast imaging should continue on a regular, individualized schedule
- Pelvic exam is recommended for all patients; frequency should be based on individual history of tamoxifen therapy, hysterectomy or oophorectomy (removal of ovaries)
- Diagnostic/surveillance tests (bone, CT, MRI, PET, liver scans, etc.) should be recommended **only** when symptoms indicate a need for additional study

Physician Exams

Returning to your physician for a physical exam and update of your history is the most important thing you can do to monitor for recurrence. It has been proven that a physician's exam and review of your recent physical changes is the number one way that most recurrences are detected.

Recommended Physician Exam Schedule:

- 1 – 3 years past treatment, every 3 – 6 months
- 4 – 5 years past treatment, every 6 – 12 months
- 6 years or more past treatment, every 12 months

Make the most of your appointment by preparing to report any changes you have experienced since your last visit. Write down any changes before you go to the exam so that you don't forget to let your doctor know. To help you prepare to report your symptoms, use the *Health Symptoms Record* on page 291. Report any changes early in the visit so that the physician will have time to evaluate the changes.

What To Expect During Follow-up Visits

At each follow-up visit, your doctor will ask about any changes in your health and perform a physical and breast exam. During the exam, your lymph nodes will be checked for enlargement, your heart and lungs will be listened to and your abdomen, liver, spleen, neck and other areas will be checked for swelling or tenderness. Your doctor will also check for any changes in your neurological (nerve) functioning.

Potential Diagnostic Tests

If your reported symptoms or your physical exam warrant the need for more diagnostic information, your physician will order needed tests. Diagnostic tests may include: blood chemistries, MRI, breast MRI, PET scan, computed tomography (CAT scan), chest X-rays, bone scans, liver ultrasound, tests for breast cancer tumor markers such as CA 15-3, CA27.29 or CEA, or other tests as determined by your physician.

Understanding ASCO Surveillance Recommendations

Breast Self-Exam

ASCO recommends breast self-exams (BSE) as part of routine follow-up care after any type of breast surgery (mastectomy, with or without reconstruction; or lumpectomy). It is suggested that you perform a breast self-exam each month. This includes a careful check of your breast(s) or surgical site for any new lumps, redness or swelling. Breast self-exam provides interval monitoring that may detect changes that need to be reported before your next scheduled mammogram or physician's exam. Refer to *Appendix D: Understanding Breast Self-Exam*, page 215, for breast self-exam information and instructions.

Breast Self-Exam Schedule:

- **Premenopausal Women:** One week after monthly period begins
- **Postmenopausal Women:** The first day of every month or a day easily remembered

Breast Imaging

Your oncologist will recommend the frequency and type of breast imaging to monitor your breast(s). Mammography is the most common. Breast MRI may be recommended for high-risk women.

Breast Imaging Schedule:

- **Lumpectomy:** You should have your first post-treatment mammogram six months after completion of radiation therapy, and then annually or as indicated by your doctor. Some physicians prefer to follow a six-month schedule for lumpectomy patients for several years.
- **Mastectomy:** You should have a yearly mammogram of the non-surgical breast.
- **Silicone Implants:** The FDA recommends that patients have a breast MRI three years after implant placement and then every 2 years to detect any non-symptomatic ruptures. Mammography is performed during alternate years.

Pelvic Exam

Every woman should have a pelvic exam at regular intervals. For most women, this will be yearly. If you have had a total abdominal hysterectomy and oophorectomy, the exam may be done less often. Your periodic pelvic exam should include a Pap test as well as a rectal exam. If you take, or have taken tamoxifen, your physician will ask you specifically about vaginal discharge or bleeding.

Bone Density Scan

Treatment with chemotherapy accelerates the loss of bone density during treatment and during the first year after treatment. Decreased bone density puts survivors at higher risk for osteoporosis, a bone-thinning disease that can increase the risk of bone fractures. The most common sites for fractures are the hips, spine and wrists. However, osteoporosis causes progressive bone loss throughout the skeleton, causing fractures in any site. Osteoporosis can be difficult to fight because it is a silent disease. It is often undetected until a person suffers a fracture.

ASCO Recommends Bone Density Scanning Every Two Years For:

- All breast cancer patients who received chemotherapy
- All patients who experienced premature menopause
- Premenopausal women taking tamoxifen
- Postmenopausal women of any age taking an aromatase inhibitor

The recommended diagnostic test to evaluate bone density is the dual energy X-ray absorptiometry (DEXA) measurement of the spine and hip. Osteoporosis has no cure, but women diagnosed with the condition can usually prevent further loss by following their healthcare provider's treatment plan.

Recommendation for Prevention or Treatment of Bone Loss:

- Diet or dietary supplement: 1,200 mg of calcium along with 400-800 IU of Vitamin D daily
- Medications to prevent or slow additional bone loss include: Fosamax®, Miacalcin®, Evista®, Actonel®, Boniva®, Reclast® and Prolia®
- Weight-bearing exercise on a regular schedule
- Estrogen replacement therapy may be an option if your tumor was estrogen negative

Colorectal Screening

The American Cancer Society recommends colorectal cancer screening after the age of 50 for all breast cancer patients.

Your Future Health

It is very important to remember that you will still experience the same illnesses, aches and pains after breast cancer that all people experience. Not every physical symptom is a sign of recurrence. Don't be over-vigilant, automatically fearing that every ache and pain is a sign of cancer. A good guideline is that if a symptom lasts longer than two weeks, you should give your healthcare team a call and report the change. Their experience can provide guidance about whether you need to have additional evaluation of the symptom. Monitoring for recurrence is a partnership with your healthcare team.

Dr. David Spiegel addresses the subject of patient anxiety about aches and pains experienced after cancer. These aches cause patients much concern about potential recurrence, but people wrestle with whether they should call the doctor or ignore it. In *Living Beyond Limits*, he writes:

> *My rule of thumb is, if it is on your mind, do something about it. You treat anxiety by doing something. Even if you are just humoring yourself, you are still reducing your anxiety, and that in and of itself is worthwhile. If your doctor thinks you are worrying about nothing, he or she can tell you so. Doctors count on their patients to be good reporters of what they feel in their bodies.*

You report; let your healthcare provider decide.

Questions About Your Follow-up Care:

- How often will I need to return for a check-up?
- Do I call to make follow-up appointments, or will your office call me?
- What should I expect as normal, long-lasting side effects of my treatment?
- What changes should I report to you between office visits?
- Are there any things that I should do, or that I should avoid (activities, medications, food, etc.)?

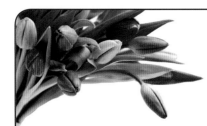

Remember…

- *The fear of recurrence is the number one fear of breast cancer survivors.*

- *Local recurrence does not change the stage of your cancer. If you have a regional or distant recurrence the stage of your cancer may change.*

- *A plan for your surveillance will be provided by your physician at the end of treatment. The plan is usually based on breast cancer recommendations from the American Society of Clinical Oncology (ASCO).*

- *Surveillance guidelines recommend that your physician provide you with information about recurrence symptoms, along with updating your history and performing a physical and breast exam at each office visit. The physician should also recommend an individualized schedule for breast imaging procedures, pelvic exams, bone density scanning and colorectal screening.*

- *Breast self-exam is recommended. Detailed instructions are located on page 215.*

- *Diagnostic tests such as bone, CT, MRI, PET and liver scans are **only** recommended when your symptoms indicate a need for additional study.*

- *Follow-up physician visits are recommended every 3 – 6 months for three years. The frequency of the visits decreases the fourth and fifth year to every 6 – 12 months, and then to once a year thereafter.*

- *The major way physicians detect recurrence is by a patient reporting a recent change in their health. The reported symptom is evaluated by the physician and, if needed, diagnostic tests are ordered.*

- *Reporting changes in your health to your physician, without judgment as to their importance, ensures that you have your best chance of detecting a recurrence early. You report changes; your physician determines their importance.*

- *Monitoring your health is a partnership of open communication between you and your physician.*

Additional Information

Tear-out Worksheets
Health Symptoms Record - page 291
Survivorship Surveillance Guidelines - page 295

Appendix
Appendix D: Understanding Breast Self-Exam - page 215

Facing the Future After Breast Cancer

What about my future after breast cancer treatment is over? What do I need to do to get back on track with my life? How do I plan? What can I do? These are all legitimate questions about your future. How do you take what has happened and rebuild your life?

Eileen Crusan said in *Coping* magazine:

> "To me, cancer was like a tornado. There is no warning before a tornado strikes. There is very little time to prepare for the destruction it leaves in its path. It's hard to find a safe place to hide. It sucks you into its terrible motion and tosses you about like a toy. When the storm has run its course, some things are left standing and others are totally flattened. The landscape is significantly changed."

No woman would ever choose to have breast cancer. Breast cancer changes your life, and there are some things that will never be the same after your diagnosis. Many women have shared, though, that their breast cancer experience added a new dimension to their lives—one that allowed them to enjoy life even more than before. If you are reading this chapter shortly after your cancer diagnosis, you may find this unbelievable. However, as time passes and side effects subside, many women find that their diagnosis presents an opportunity to reevaluate their lives and make positive changes that they had postponed because they were waiting for the right time.

"There comes a time after you grieve your losses that you have to choose if you want to live your life as a memorial service around the event or learn from the horrible things sent your way and build a new and even better life."
—Brenda Harmon,
Breast Cancer Patient

If you are like most women, your life has centered on doing for others. Take it from other patients who have survived cancer—change is needed. It is time to look at your life closely and incorporate things you always wanted to do, but didn't, because you were too busy putting others first. Not to plan means that you leave decisions up to others or to chance. To plan means that you chart your own course and take steps to build the life that you would like. This is not being selfish; it is becoming the best version of yourself.

Journaling as a Recovery Tool

One of the most effective tools to promote your recovery is journal writing. Writing in a journal is an effective way to handle the emotions that living with cancer has triggered. Journal writing empowers you to express your difficult feelings in a safe and private way. It allows you to come to terms with cancer at your own pace and in your own way. Your journal is always there to receive your thoughts and feelings. It helps you make sense of life events, find meaning in them and learn the lessons they have to teach. Because journal writing forces you to look inward, it helps to clarify your fears and thoughts. By writing, you will realize that your illness is only a part of you, not the whole person. It helps you put your illness into perspective.

Prepare by getting a journal or by creating a document on your computer. Select a quiet time for daily journaling. Devote a page to each of the following topics. Add to your lists gradually, and you will be amazed at how journaling keeps you focused and centered on your healing path. Suggested topics include:

- Ways that cancer has changed your life.
- Ways that you have learned to cope.
- Ways to nurture yourself.
- Things in your life that you are grateful for.
- Your "bucket list" of things that you have always wanted to do in life.

Encouragement Box

Collect inspirational sayings, poems and stories that inspire you, as well as pictures of your friends and family. Place these items in an encouragement box. When you begin to feel sad or anxious, go to your encouragement box and read the items you have collected and look at the pictures of those you love. Learning to encourage yourself is a valuable tool for emotional healing. Replacing negative thoughts and fears with grateful thoughts causes a swift change in your body chemistry, which promotes healing.

Survivorship Attitudes

I began my work over twenty-nine years ago as a Breast Health Navigator in a hospital working with women throughout the entire breast cancer experience. I learned that women facing a challenge are strong and resilient if they are given information about what they need to know and what they can do to make a difference in their own lives. From those women, I observed the coping skills and survivorship attitudes that can help build an even richer life after a breast cancer diagnosis. These skills and attitudes are not new. There are no secrets revealed here. Sometimes, though, in the midst of a crisis it can be helpful if someone reminds you of what has worked for others who have encountered a similar experience.

Survivorship attitudes and coping skills lead to happiness in spite of the event that paid an unexpected visit to your life. Survivorship attitudes do not deny the loss and pain you've endured, but rather encompass the loss as a learning and motivating experience. Breast cancer survivors have used these lessons to make changes in their lives, including taking care of themselves emotionally and physically. Survivorship is mostly attitude—the attitude that I CAN take charge of my decisions and become the best survivor ever!

As you read through the remainder of this chapter, think of how these attitudes may help to add a sense of control and bring joy back to your life. This is what this final chapter is all about, learning how to maneuver the ups and downs of treatments and recovery to emerge a stronger, happier person.

Cancer Recovery Tips

Recovery Timetable

Recovery from breast cancer is a gradual process for the mind, just as it is for the body. Physical healing usually comes long before psychological healing. Your treatment team will focus on your physical healing; you must manage your psychological recovery on your own timetable. Some women are eager to put the experience behind them, while others need time to absorb the impact of the changes that cancer brings. Only you can decide what is best for you. Just as your treatment team has plans for you to recover physically, you need to chart a mental recovery plan.

Dealing With Emotions and Fears:

- Some people get emotionally stuck trying to figure out "why." In the field of breast cancer, we don't know why most women have breast cancer. Instead of focusing on why, concentrate on what you can do now. Do not concentrate on the what ifs. Thinking about what you could or could not have done differently will not change anything. The past is the past, and yesterday cannot be changed.

- Do not suppress your emotions. Strong emotions are expected after a cancer diagnosis. Cry when you need to, and talk about your experience. Grieve over your loss. Grief is not a sign of emotional weakness; it is a normal response to a loss. Talk to someone you can trust about your feelings and fears. You may have to find this person outside of the family unit—a professional counselor or peer.

- Identify your fears. Write them down and take action to disarm them. Fear is a paralyzing factor. Our fears rob us of peace in the moment and torment us about future decisions. Fear can only be mastered by naming the fear and facing it with action. Fear causes anxiety, and long-term anxiety weakens the body's immune system, which allows all types of illnesses to occur. Seek help for anything that causes you to feel anxious. Dealing with your fear is essential for your good health to return.

- Acknowledge that there are going to be days when things don't go well and you won't feel well physically or psychologically. Remember to reach out, ask for help if you need it, and know that this, too, will pass. Don't try to be a superwoman. Prepare yourself for emotionally trying days (treatment, medical tests, anniversary dates, etc.) with a stress-free schedule as often as possible. Recruit a friend to share this time, or plan a special treat to soften the experience. Be proactive in planning for your own mental health.

- If your emotions turn into continuous anxiety or overwhelming depression, ask your physician about counseling or medication. Do not suffer emotionally without seeking help; delaying only slows down your physical recovery. If you had diabetes, you would seek help. Depression and chronic anxiety can be helped as well. Remember, you have to reach out to your treatment team to get emotional help. It is available, but you have to ask.

Stress Management Tips

Planning is the first step to eliminating unnecessary stress in life. The second step is to be realistic and expect certain things to be stressful. Determine to accept the things you can't change, and work to change the things you can.

- Plan a schedule for daily living. The body performs better when it sleeps the same hours each day. Schedules help you avoid a lot of unknowns.

- Plan, in order of importance, what you want to accomplish daily. Do one thing at a time. You don't have to do everything for everyone. There are no rewards for over-commitment!

- Spend some time meditating or having a devotional period before you begin each day. Prepare your mind for the day by reviewing your reasons to be grateful, even in your present circumstances. Get mentally dressed before tackling your day.

- Reduce the noise in your environment. Use voice mail to control a constantly ringing phone. This lets you talk when you feel you are physically or emotionally up to it.

- Take mini breaks. Take a series of deep breaths when you feel yourself getting stressed. It sends oxygen to the brain, reduces tension in your body and elevates your mood. Plan time for a walk. Exercise is good medicine for the mind and body.

- Avoid people who are stress carriers or those who are negaholics. Say "no" to the things you don't want to do or that cause you stress. Saying "no" to others is saying "yes" to yourself. One patient said, *"I finally realized that I can say 'no' and feel guilty for thirty minutes, or I can say 'yes' and feel resentful for thirty days."* Plan something good for yourself every day. Remember, no one else can do this for you.

- Monitor your self-talk, the internal conversation you have with yourself daily. Is it positive or negative? Remember, you can't prevent negative thoughts coming your way, but you can stop them from camping out. Refuse to entertain them. Replace them with positive affirmations, scriptures or meditations.

- When you feel like your last nerve has been used, put a big smile on your face and hold it. (You may need to leave the room to try this.) A smile can reduce stress. Try being angry with a smile on your face—it won't work!

- Avoid being a TVaholic. The majority of television shows are depressing. Spend some of your time reading, writing in a journal, taking up a new hobby, volunteering at your local nursing home or healthcare facility or doing things that bring you pleasure and satisfaction.

- Learn to express your needs and to communicate your feelings. Use *"I feel..."* or *"I need..."* statements. Don't make others guess what you need. Ask. Unmet needs create stress.

- Shy away from criticizing, condemning, blaming, pouting and getting even. These are all energy drainers and accomplish little except to increase your stress. Practice letting it go. Choose to be happy and at peace rather than fighting to be right.

- When something happens that causes you stress, examine the event and determine what you can do to reduce or stop it. Practice saying, *"I refuse to let something like this bother me." "This is not worth my getting upset." "What difference will it make in a month anyway?" "I don't have to win to be happy." "Some people are just naturally unhappy and negative, but I refuse to participate in their pity party."*

- Laugh every chance you get. Rent old movies. Watch comedy shows. Laughter is as good as medicine for elevating the spirit.

- Look for beauty in the small things that come your way daily—the people, the smells, the colors and the sounds. Savor the moment.

- Set up your own personal reward system. After getting chemotherapy or completing radiation therapy, go out to eat, see a movie, do some shopping or visit with a friend. Plan to celebrate the milestones in life. It helps when you have something to look forward to.

- Share your own oil of kindness with others who cross your path. Speak, smile and say, *"I appreciate you." "I love you." "You are such a wonderful help." "You do such a good job." "I always enjoy seeing you." "You certainly did a good job." "I hope you have a blessed day."* Recognize their value as a person. When we give the oil of kindness away, it automatically spills onto us in the process. We feel better.

- Plan special times for yourself and those special to you. Enjoy life together whenever possible.

- End each day remembering the reasons you have to be grateful. Our happiness in life is more dependent on what we think about our life than on our circumstances. Keep the reasons for your gratefulness in the forefront of your mind. Record them in your journal.

Places To Find Encouragement

- Participate in a support group. Find a group that provides education as well as support. Women who attend support groups tend to adjust better than those who do not.

- Use your spiritual faith as a source of strength, a place to find answers and a way to give meaning to the hard questions of life.

- Allow your family and friends to participate in your recovery by helping you. Tell them what is helpful. It is therapeutic for them to feel needed. Stop long enough to say, *"Thank you,"* or *"I appreciate you,"* to your caregivers, whether they are the healthcare staff, family or friends. Like you, they need to know that they are appreciated and valued. Being a caregiver is not always easy, and most people forget to share what they feel.

Diet and Exercise

- Eat nutritious foods, exercise regularly, rest when needed and get adequate sleep. These are the foundations for physical and emotional health.

- Don't resort to covering your anxiety with alcohol or recreational drugs. This postpones your psychological recovery and can lead to depression.

Monitoring Your Health

- Follow your physician's guide for medical monitoring after cancer. Keep your appointments, perform monthly breast self-exams and get your mammograms, Pap smears and bone density scans—but don't make a career out of monitoring for cancer. Don't let it dominate your thoughts and actions. If a lingering symptom is bothersome, call your nurse and ask if it should be evaluated.

- It is vital to remember that you are not a breast cancer statistic. You are an individual. Do not look at your future purely through statistics. If only one person has ever beaten the odds, you have the right to become the second.

Charting Your Future

- Look at the breast cancer experience as a caution light in your life that allows you to slow down and examine your real needs and wishes for the future.

- Take time to do the things that make you feel good, whatever they may be. Plan your own fun times. Don't wait for happiness to come. Go and find it!

- Decide that you are going to make this a time of intensive personal growth. Start a journal and list the things you have always wanted to do and never gotten around to. Writing your goals down is essential. This list will serve as your road map for personal recovery. Chart new courses for yourself—take a class or go back to school, change careers, read a long book, take a trip, plant a flower garden, get physically fit or do whatever you have always wanted to do "when I have time." Beginning a new project will give you new energy and facilitate recovery.

- Surround yourself with things that you love and cause your spirit to soar … music, books, pets, hobbies, whatever makes you smile. You deserve it.

- Cancer can be the reason you decide that your goals and dreams are important. Remember that you, and you alone, can start making your heart's desires a reality. Today is the day!

Reflections on My Journey . . .

"I consider myself a survivor, not a victim. I think about recurrence, but it no longer consumes me. I do not fear death, nor do I fear life after having had breast cancer. My life will never be the same as before, but any negatives breast cancer has brought have been matched by positives."

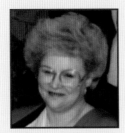

Harriet Barrineau

"The most important thing about cancer is learning you can say 'no' to others. I couldn't before. I couldn't say 'no' to my kids, I couldn't say 'no' to my mother, but I can say 'no' now. It's a very important thing to be able to do."

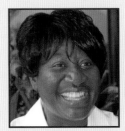

Earnestine Brown

"When we had been married for 12 days, we were shocked when I was told, 'You have breast cancer.' Our hopes and dreams for our future had been hijacked. We were facing a new, unplanned future of surgery, reconstruction, chemotherapy and years of hormonal medication. Later, when we realized having children of our own was not possible, Brian said, 'It's okay. We can adopt dogs and travel. I'd rather have that!'

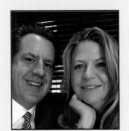

Anna Cluxton

Cancer changed our lives. Out of my passion, I co-founded the Central Ohio Young Survival Coalition (YSC). I was appointed to the national YSC Board, became vice-president and then national president.

Now, fifteen years later, we have travelled the world together talking about breast cancer in young women, the importance and uniqueness of their issues and the amazing way that YSC helps young women. Our hopes, hijacked by breast cancer, have been replaced with an extraordinary life."

"My cancer diagnosis came as a negative surprise that changed me. Cancer changed the way I live my life and how I think about my future. I realized my work/life balance

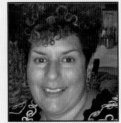

Lisa DelGuidice

was NOT in balance and I needed to make changes. I reduced my work week from 60–70 hours per work to 40–50. I made more time for me, not in a selfish way, but in an empowering way; I needed to rebuild my health and my life. I now use that reclaimed time for self-care and nurturing. Fitness has become a big part of my healing journey.

My advice to other survivors is to try to find the silver lining while being grateful that we live in a time when we have many medical choices to treat our cancer. Remember, 'Knowledge is power'. . . Be your own advocate. You will not know how strong you are until strong is the only choice you have.

Today, I am a cancer survivor and I couldn't be happier. Cancer helped me find my balance in life."

Dear Survivor,

*Breast cancer is an unwelcome visitor in any woman's life. You have found yourself forced to embrace an enemy. Yet, even in the midst of this frightening and often lonely experience, you **do** have the capacity to find new strength as you work through this challenge.*

Recovery is not a one-size-fits-all journey. It is an individual journey. Only you can decide what you need to master the challenge of living well with breast cancer. It takes time. Be patient. Becoming a triumphant survivor is achieved by taking life one day at a time and learning to live with the uncertainty cancer brings—it is a gradual process, not an event.

As I said on the first page of the book, "There may be scars on your chest, but there need not be scars on your heart." It takes longer to heal the heart; but, like thousands of other women, you, too, can turn this unexpected crisis into a time of personal growth and emerge stronger, emotionally and physically.

It has been my privilege to share this part of your journey with you. I hope you have found needed information to make decisions. But, most importantly, I hope you have found the encouragement you needed to make your journey with breast cancer a little easier.

My love and best wishes for a happy and healthy future,

Judy

Additional Information

Tear-out Worksheet
Personal Plan for Recovery - page 289

Reading
Breast Cancer Survivorship Handbook
Author: Judy C. Kneece, RN, OCN
Available at www.EduCareInc.com

APPENDIX A

Understanding Diagnostic Tests

BLOOD COUNTS

Your doctor will monitor your blood counts by drawing blood from your finger, arm or implanted vascular port on a regular basis. This blood test evaluates how you respond to the effects of chemotherapy, monitors for infections and detects changes in your blood chemistry.

Main Counts Monitored Will Be:

■ Red blood cells (RBCs): Carry oxygen to all parts of your body

■ White blood cells (WBCs): Combat infection and provide immunity

■ Platelets: Determine how your blood will clot

■ Electrolytes (potassium, magnesium, calcium, sodium, chloride, glucose and carbon dioxide)

■ Hemoglobin (iron): The portion of the red blood cells (RBCs) that attaches to oxygen

Remind the technician drawing the sample not to use your surgical arm. If you had bilateral mastectomies, the technician will need to use special procedures to reduce the potential for infection.

BONE SCAN

A bone scan is a nuclear medicine test that uses special cameras and a radioactive contrast agent to determine if cancer from another area of the body has spread to the bones. After injection of a radioactive contrast agent, the agent accumulates in the organ or area of your body being examined, where it gives off a small amount of energy in the form of gamma rays. Special gamma cameras detect these rays and, with the help of a computer, create pictures offering details of the structure. The gamma camera does not emit any radiation.

Inform Your Physician Prior to Exam:

■ If you have difficulty lying still or if you are highly anxious or claustrophobic.

■ If you have an iodine or seafood allergy.

■ If you have had a test using barium contrast material within the past four days or if you have taken a bismuth-containing medicine like Pepto-Bismol. Barium and bismuth can interfere with bone scan results.

Prior to the Exam:

■ You will sign an informed consent form.

■ Medication for anxiety, if ordered, will be administered.

■ An I.V. will be placed in your arm, and the radioactive substance will be administered.

■ After the injection, you will drink lots of fluids to help distribute the substance throughout your body.

■ After the injection, there will be a wait-time of 2 – 4 hours before the scan begins.

What To Expect During the Scan:

- You will lie on an examination table.

- The table will slide in between parallel gamma camera heads suspended over the examination table and beneath the examination table.

- The camera may rotate around you or stay in one position. You will be asked to change positions between images. You will be required to remain still for brief periods of time.

- In some cases, the camera may move very close to your body.

After the Scan:

- You may resume your normal activities, unless otherwise directed by your physician.

- Drink lots of water to flush the radioactive agent out of your body. It will naturally leave through your urine or stool.

BREAST CANCER GENETIC TESTING

Breast cancer genetic testing determines if a person carries a mutated breast cancer gene, either BRCA1 or BRCA2 (BR=breast; CA=cancer) that puts them at the highest risk known for breast or ovarian cancer. These two genes prevent cells from becoming breast cancer by helping to repair damages to a cell. When these cells are damaged and suffer mutation, the probability of malignant transformation and cancer is very high.

These mutated genes are passed on at conception from either the mother or the father. If one parent has a mutation, each child has a 50 percent chance of inheriting the mutation from that parent.

A man or a woman may inherit and carry a BRCA mutation without ever developing cancer. This may cause the disease to look as though it has skipped a generation. In smaller families or families with more men, it may be harder to see the hereditary cancer risk because there are fewer women to develop cancer. It was once thought that the number of relatives with cancer was the highest predictor of a hereditary syndrome. We

now know that other important factors, such as young age at diagnosis, triple negative breast cancer, a history of more than one cancer in the same person or male breast cancer in the family are also strong clues that may indicate the presence of a mutation existing in a family. Certain ethnic groups have a greater likelihood of carrying a BRCA mutation. For instance, 1 in 40 Jewish persons of Northern and Central European descent (Ashkenazi) may be carriers of a mutation.

What Are the Cancer Risks?

Women who inherit a BRCA mutation have a 56 to 87 percent risk of developing breast cancer by age 70. They also have a 27 to 44 percent risk of developing ovarian cancer. Women also face increased risk of developing a second breast cancer if they carry a mutation. Increased risks for other cancers exist but are much lower than the risk of developing breast or ovarian cancer.

Hereditary Breast Cancer Genetic Testing

After a breast cancer diagnosis, a close evaluation of family cancer history and personal cancer characteristics will determine if a patient meets the criteria for genetic testing. (Refer to *Chapter 6: What Is Breast Cancer?* for Hereditary Breast Cancer testing criteria). Genetic testing requires that a small sample of blood or saliva be sent to a lab for testing.

Potential Outcomes of Genetic Testing:

- **Negative** test result shows that you do not have a detectable mutation and allows you to move forward with treatments as recommended by your physician, including breast conservation, if recommended. A negative test is not always definitive. Discuss test results with your physician.

- **Positive** test result for either a BRCA1 or BRCA2 gene may limit your surgical options. Breast conservation followed by radiation therapy may not be a recommended option. Other recommended options include: bilateral mastectomy; high risk ovarian surveillance (transvaginal ultrasound exam and CA-125 testing) or oophorectomy (ovary removal).

- **Uncertain** test result reports that a "variant of uncertain significance" was found. This means that an unusual change or variant is present in your breast genes, but at this time it has not been clearly associated with an increased cancer risk. Even though you do not get a clear negative answer, you do not have any limitations on treatment options. It is suggested that you keep in touch with your genetic counselor to find out if additional information becomes available about the particular change that was found in your genes.

Positive Gene Impact on Your Family

If a person is diagnosed with a positive mutation in either BRCA gene, it can be passed equally to either sons or daughters. It also means that your brothers and sisters are at risk (50 percent chance) for having inherited the gene and may now be carriers of the mutation. A positive diagnosis places your children and siblings at increased risk of developing breast, ovarian and, to a much lesser extent, prostate, colon and pancreatic cancer. Knowing you are a carrier allows you to tell your children and siblings so that they can pursue genetic testing (after age 18) to see if they have inherited the gene. If they are identified as positive carriers, they can take steps of high-risk surveillance.

High-Risk Surveillance Recommendations:

- Perform monthly breast self-exams and have an annual clinical exam beginning at age 25
- Begin screening mammograms or breast MRIs between ages 25 – 35
- Begin transvaginal ultrasound exams and CA-125 testing between ages 25 – 35

Chemoprevention Recommendations:

- Drugs such as tamoxifen or Evista® may be prescribed
- Oral contraceptives may be prescribed for ovarian protection

Prophylactic Surgery Considerations:

- Prophylactic bilateral mastectomy (after breast-feeding desired children) to prevent occurrence
- Prophylactic bilateral ovary removal (after age 35 or after number of children desired) to prevent occurrence

BREAST MRI / BREAST MRI BIOPSY

Breast MRI (magnetic resonance imaging) uses a powerful magnetic field, radio frequency pulses and a computer to produce detailed pictures of the breasts. In comparison, mammography uses X-rays to create images. MRI does not use radiation. MRI is performed on a special table that has openings that allow the breasts to fall through for the exam. The openings contain special MRI coils (antennas) that circle the breasts and receive the imaging data during the exam to create the images.

Breast MRI may be used to more closely evaluate breast abnormalities first seen on a mammogram or to study the extent of the breast cancer after a diagnosis. It allows physicians to easily visualize the muscle and chest wall in the vicinity of the breast, along with the breast tissue. It may also be used to examine implants for leaking. Recently, researchers have studied MRI as a screening tool for women who are at high risk for breast cancer, are young or have dense breasts.

Benefits of Breast MRI:

- Highly sensitive to identifying and characterizing hard-to-assess abnormalities found on mammography
- Helpful in evaluating the extent of breast cancer before lumpectomy
- Determines if breast cancer has spread to the chest wall
- Visualizes dense breasts for abnormalities
- Evaluates inverted nipples for evidence of cancer

- Visualizes breast implants for ruptures
- Evaluates abnormalities found in the breast after lumpectomy
- Evaluates breast after neoadjuvant chemotherapy
- Screens high-risk women for breast cancer

Inform Your Physician Prior to Exam:

- If you have difficulty lying still on your abdomen.
- If you are claustrophobic (fear of enclosed spaces), medication for anxiety can be ordered before the exam.

What To Expect During an MRI Breast Exam:

- Medication for anxiety, if ordered, is administered prior to exam.
- Patient is positioned on table face-down with breasts falling through openings in the table.
- Compression of breasts is not required; there is no pain during the exam.
- The MRI machine makes loud humming and thumping sounds; ear plugs may be provided.
- A series of images is taken, which causes tapping sounds.
- Exam typically takes 30 – 60 minutes.
- If you receive medication to relax, you will need someone to drive you home; otherwise, you can drive yourself.

MRI Breast Biopsy

Your physician may recommend an MRI biopsy of an abnormality found in your breast. MRI locates the abnormality by creating images using a large, powerful magnet instead of an X-ray. The biopsy is performed on a special table that has openings which allow the breasts to fall through for the biopsy. The openings contain special MRI coils (antennas) that encircle the breast and receive the imaging data during the exam to create the images that are used by the physician to locate the abnormality for biopsy.

Inform Your Physician Prior to Your Exam:

- If you have difficulty lying on your stomach.
- If you have an iodine or seafood allergy and are scheduled to receive a contrast agent.
- If you are taking any prescription or over-the-counter medications, to evaluate the potential for increased bleeding.

Prior to the Exam:

- You will sign an informed consent form.
- You will have an I.V. inserted into your arm.
- Medication for anxiety, if ordered, will be administered.

What To Expect During the Biopsy:

- You will lie face-down on a table. The breasts are allowed to fall through a cushioned opening where they are visualized by a special coil that encircles the breast.
- The breast being biopsied will be placed in a compression device which has small grid-like openings.
- You will enter a cylinder-shaped machine where you will hear tapping sounds as the images are taken.
- You will receive a contrast material (gadolinium DTPA) through your I.V. to improve the quality of contrast between the tissues, which highlights the abnormality for the physician.
- Your images will be reviewed to determine the entrance site and lesion depth for placement of the biopsy needle.
- The skin is cleansed with an antiseptic and numbed at the site for the needle entrance.
- The biopsy needle guide is inserted through the grid on the compression device into the area of the breast abnormality. After the correct positioning is confirmed, the biopsy needle is inserted, and samples of the lesion are removed. The samples are sent to a pathology lab for evaluation. A small biopsy marker is placed in the area for identification during future imaging.

- When the biopsy is completed, compression of the area (example: Ace bandage) will be used, along with an ice pack to reduce the potential for bleeding.

- No pain is involved other than the needle stick for the I.V. and the injection of the anesthesia to numb the breast. You will feel a slight pressure on the breast from the compression device used to stabilize the breast, and some pressure as the biopsy needle enters.

- When the anesthesia wears off, you may have local discomfort, and there may be discoloration of the breast from the procedure.

- The biopsy procedure usually takes less than one hour.

After the Biopsy, Report the Following:

- Any pain that is sudden or severe.

- Bleeding that soaks through your bandage.

- Appearance of a hard lump at the biopsy area (sign of internal bleeding).

- Signs of infection at biopsy site, such as fever over 100.5° F, redness of biopsy area or a colored drainage (infection is rare).

COMPUTED TOMOGRAPHY SCAN (CT OR CAT SCAN)

Computed tomography (CT or CAT scan) is a diagnostic imaging test that produces multiple images of the inside of the body (organs, bones, soft tissue and blood vessels) using X-rays. These images can be viewed on a computer monitor, printed on film or saved onto a CD.

The CT scanner looks like a large, box-like machine with a short tunnel in the center. The patient lies on a narrow exam table that slides into and out of the tunnel. When the table is inside the scanner, the machine's X-ray beam rotates around the patient, creating images.

Inform Your Physician Prior to Exam:

- If you have an iodine or seafood allergy and are to receive a contrast agent before the exam.

- If you are claustrophobic (fear of enclosed spaces), medication for anxiety can be ordered before the exam.

Prior to Exam:

- Your physician will tell you if you will receive a contrast agent and whether you can eat, drink or take medications on the day of your scan.

- Remove any metal objects, including jewelry, eyeglasses, bra with hooks or underwires, hearing aids and dental appliances.

- Take anxiety medication, if prescribed.

- Use the restroom just prior to the exam.

- If contrast material is used, it will be swallowed, injected through an I.V. or, rarely, administered by enema. If administered through a vein, you may feel a warm, flushing sensation during administration, especially in the perineal area (between vaginal opening and anus), which is followed by a metallic taste in the mouth.

What To Expect During a CT Scan:

- A CT scan is painless.

- You are positioned on the exam table and asked to lie still while the table is in the scanner. Movement will blur images. Your technologist may ask to hold your breath for short periods of time.

- A built-in communication system enables you to communicate with the technologist at all times while in the scanner.

- If you receive medication to relax, you will need someone to drive you home; otherwise, you can drive yourself.

After the Scan:

- If you are given a contrast agent, it will naturally leave your body within 24 hours. Drink lots of water to flush the contrast agent out of your body.

- Contrast agent may cause diarrhea.

- CT scans give off no more radiation than a series of regular X-rays. You will not be radioactive.

LIVER SCAN

A liver scan is a nuclear medicine exam that uses a contrast agent to highlight the liver. It is used to check for liver diseases such as liver cancer, abscesses or cysts of the liver.

Inform Your Physician Prior to Exam:

- If you have an iodine or seafood allergy.
- If you have difficulty lying still because of pain or anxiety.

Prior to the Exam:

- There is no preparation prior to the scan. You can eat, drink or take any medications the day of the exam, unless otherwise instructed by your physician.
- Remove any metal objects, including jewelry, eyeglasses, bra with hooks or underwires, hearing aids and dental appliances.
- You will be asked to sign an informed consent form.
- Use the restroom just prior to the exam.
- Medication for pain or anxiety will be administered, if ordered.
- Injection of the contrast agent will be given by I.V. prior to your exam, usually into a vein in the hand or arm.

What To Expect During a Liver Scan:

- A technologist will instruct you to change positions during the exam while the machine moves above your body taking images.
- There is no discomfort from the exam, unless you have difficulty lying still or turning as requested.
- The level of radiation during a liver scan is minimal and is not considered significant enough to cause harm.

After the Scan:

- Drink lots of water to flush the contrast agent out of your body.

MAGNETIC RESONANCE IMAGING (MRI)

MRI is a non-invasive exam that uses powerful magnets and radio waves to take pictures of your body. No radiation is used in an MRI. The MRI scanner contains a powerful magnet that causes the hydrogen atoms in the body to line up in a certain way, similar to the way the needle on a compass works. When the radio waves are sent to these lined-up atoms, they bounce back, and a computer records the signals made, creating the images. Different types of body tissue send back different signals. Each signal sent back is called a slice. The images can be stored on a computer, printed onto film or saved onto a DVD for your physician to interpret.

Inform Your Physician Prior to Exam:

- If you have body implants, including: inner ear (cochlear) implants, brain aneurysm clips, artificial limbs or joints, artificial heart valves or implanted infusion ports.
- If you have ever had metal fragments lodged in your body.
- If you have a pacemaker (not a candidate for an MRI).
- If you have difficulty lying still because of pain.
- If you are claustrophobic (fear of enclosed spaces), medication for anxiety can be ordered before the exam.
- If you have an iodine or seafood allergy and are to receive a contrast agent before the exam.

Prior to the Exam:

- You will be asked to remove any metal items such as jewelry, hearing aids, eyeglasses, dentures or a bra with hooks or underwires.
- You will sign an informed consent form.
- Medication for pain or anxiety will be administered, if ordered.
- The contrast agent is administered through an I.V into a vein, if ordered.

What To Expect During an MRI:

- You will be placed on a narrow table that slides into the MRI machine.
- There is no pain from the exam. It is important that you remain completely still because movement blurs the images.
- The MRI machine makes loud humming and thumping sounds; ear plugs may be provided.
- The technologist will watch from outside of the room. A two-way audio system allows you to communicate during your exam.
- Time in the MRI scanner varies according to the area being scanned.

After the Exam:

- You are free to return to normal activities. If you have received a sedative, you will need someone to drive you home.
- The contrast material, if used, is naturally excreted with your urine.
- Results of the exam will be given to the physician ordering the exam.

PET SCAN
(POSITRON EMISSION TOMOGRAPHY)

A PET scan is a nuclear medicine diagnostic imaging test based on the detection of positrons, which are tiny particles of a radioactive sugar substance injected into the patient prior to the exam. During the scan, the machine creates images based on how the positrons collect in the body. PET scans are used to detect cancer, determine the stage of cancer and evaluate the effectiveness of cancer treatment, such as chemotherapy or radiation therapy.

The PET machine looks like a large doughnut because it has a hole in the middle of the machine. Inside the machine are multiple rings of detectors that detect the positrons and show the images on a computer outside the room.

Inform Your Physician Prior to Exam:

- If you are highly anxious or find it difficult to lie still.

Preparation for a PET Scan:

- Do not eat for four hours before the scan.
- Drink lots of water prior to the exam.
- Your physician will instruct you on taking any regular medication before the procedure (ask specifically about insulin, pain medication, blood pressure or heart medications).

Prior to the Exam:

- You will sign an informed consent form for the exam.
- Medication for anxiety or pain, if ordered, will be administered.
- An I.V. will be placed in your arm, and a radioactive substance, mixed with a natural substance like glucose (sugar), is administered.
- You will be asked to rest during this time; avoid significant movement and talking. After approximately 30 – 60 minutes, when the substance has traveled throughout your body and been absorbed, the exam will begin.

What To Expect During the Exam:

- The PET scan will begin and requires approximately 30 – 45 minutes of lying on a table in the open area of the machine for image acquisition.
- The images of a PET scan reflect the accumulation of the substance in different colors. For example, a glucose substance may be attracted to organs that use a lot of glucose. Because cancer requires a lot of glucose to divide and grow, these areas will show up with brighter colors. The images will be shown on a computer outside of the room.
- The testing physician may compare previous CT or MRI scans with the PET scan images.

After the Exam:

- Drink plenty of fluid to flush the radioactive substance from your body.

- There are no restrictions on daily routines after an exam is completed.
- The testing physician will send a report to your physician.

ULTRASOUND / ULTRASOUND BIOPSY

Ultrasound may be ordered after mammography to further evaluate a lump or abnormality. Ultrasound is not recommended by the American College of Radiology as the best method of screening for breast cancer, but rather as an additional procedure. Ultrasound is especially helpful in determining whether a lump is solid or fluid-filled. Ultrasound is safe for a pregnant woman. Ultrasound is also used to provide a physician with real-time guidance when performing a fine needle aspiration (FNA), a hand-held core biopsy or a vacuum-assisted biopsy. Using ultrasound allows the physician to see the movement of the biopsy instrument and the fluid movement in the breast on the screen and to capture still pictures, when needed, to document the procedure.

What To Expect During an Ultrasound:

- There is no advance preparation for the exam.
- The ultrasound exam is painless.
- You will lie on a table. The examiner will apply a gel that allows the transducer to move smoothly over your breast while evaluating the area of concern.
- There is no discomfort, unless lying on your back is difficult.
- Your referring physician will inform you of the ultrasound finding.

What To Expect During an Ultrasound Breast Biopsy:

- You will lie flat on your back with your arm raised.
- The physician will apply the gel and move the transducer across the suspicious area.
- When the area is located, a local medication is given to numb the area.
- A small surgical nick is made in the skin where the biopsy needle is to be inserted.
- Using ultrasound guidance, the needle is inserted and advanced to the location of the abnormality as the physician watches on the screen.
- Tissue samples are removed using one of two methods:
  - **Core biopsy** inserts a large, hollow needle to remove three to six core samples of the tumor.
  - **Vacuum-assisted biopsy** inserts a hollow needle attached to a vacuum-powered instrument to collect eight to ten core samples without removing the needle.
- A small marker may be placed at the site before the biopsy device is removed from the breast so that the biopsy site can be easily identified on mammography in the future.
- The needle is removed, and pressure is applied with a cold compress to stop any bleeding. The biopsy site is covered with a dressing. No sutures are needed.
- The procedure takes approximately one hour.
- If you receive medication to relax, you will need to have someone drive you home; otherwise, you can drive yourself.
- Avoid strenuous activities for 24 hours. You can then return to normal activities.

After the Breast Biopsy:

- Bruising and some swelling are normal and expected after the biopsy.
- For discomfort in the biopsy area, apply a cold pack for 20 – 30 minutes at a time and take an over-the-counter pain reliever.
- Report to the physician any bright red bleeding from the site that does not stop after pressure and a cold compress are applied for 15 minutes.
- Your referring physician will receive the biopsy pathology report and give you the results.

APPENDIX B

Understanding Chemotherapy Drugs

There are many drugs used to treat breast cancer. The drugs listed below are the most common. Your physician and nursing staff will provide you with the names and side effects of the drugs you will receive.

Chemotherapy drugs are often given in combination. Often your treatment team will refer to the combination of drugs by the initials of each drug.

Most Common Drug Combinations:

- **CMF** (Cytoxan®, Methotrexate®, 5-FU®)
- **CAF** (Cytoxan®, Adriamycin®, 5-FU®)
- **FAC** (5-FU®, Adriamycin®, Cytoxan®)
- **AC** (Adriamycin®, Cytoxan®)
- **ACT** (Adriamycin®, Cytoxan®, Taxol® or Taxotere®)
- **FEC** or **CEF** (5-FU®, Epirubicin®, Cytoxan®)
- **EC** (Epirubicin®, Cytoxan®)
- **AT** (Adriamycin®, Taxol® or Taxotere®)
- **GT** (Gemzar®, Taxol®)
- **TCH** (Taxotere®, Carboplatin®, Herceptin®)
- **TCH+P** (Taxotere®, Carboplatin®, Herceptin®, Perjeta®)

Initials Used for Drug Administration:

- **P.O.** (Per Orally); given by mouth
- **I.M.** (Intramuscular); given by injection into a muscle
- **I.V.** (Intravenous); given by a needle into a vein
- **S.Q.** or **S.C.** (Subcutaneous); given by injection into the fatty tissues of the body

Dose-Dense Chemotherapy

Dose-dense chemotherapy is a term used for giving the same amount (dose) of chemotherapy drugs over a shorter period of time. Traditionally, administration time has required a three-week schedule because blood counts needed to return to their near-normal level before the next dose. Dose-dense therapy combines special drugs to promote blood cell recovery when needed, so that the administration schedule can be shortened to every two weeks.

CHEMOTHERAPY DRUGS

ABRAXANE (ALBUMIN-BOUND PACLITAXEL)

Brand Name: Abraxane®

Method Administered: I.V.

Side Effects: Decreased white (WBC) and red (RBC) blood cell counts; fatigue; nausea and vomiting; diarrhea; tingling in hands and feet; muscle aches starting 2 – 3 days after administration

Notify Physician of These Side Effects: Fever over 100.5° F; chills with or without fever; shortness of breath; tingling or numbness in hands or feet; nausea and vomiting not controlled with medication

Precautions: Tell your doctor of any over-the-counter medications you are taking.

CAPECITABINE

Brand Name: Xeloda®

Method Administered: P.O.

Report to Physician: If pregnant; taking a blood thinner such as warfarin (Coumadin®); taking Dilantin®; taking the vitamin folic acid; if you have a history of kidney or liver problems

Side Effects: Diarrhea; nausea; vomiting; constipation; weakness; fatigue; dizziness; headache; sleeplessness; dry or itching skin; dehydration; mouth sores; tenderness and redness of hands and feet

Notify Physician of These Side Effects: Severe diarrhea; loss of appetite; severe vomiting; tingling; numbness; pain; redness or swelling of the hands or feet; sores or pain in the mouth or throat; fever over 100.5° F or infection; chills; sore throat; chest pain; rash

Precautions: Take within 30 minutes of a meal. Use barrier-type (condom) method of birth control. Do not breastfeed while taking.

CARBOPLATIN

Brand Name: Paraplatin®

Method Administered: I.V.

Side Effects: Decreased blood cell counts (WBCs, platelets, hemoglobin); nausea; vomiting; numbness of hands and feet; hearing changes; allergic reaction (esp. after 6 – 7 doses)

Notify Physician of These Side Effects: Fever over 100.5° F; chills; signs of infection; unusual bleeding or bruising; nausea not controlled with medication within 24 hours; tingling or loss of feeling in hands or feet; changes in hearing

CISPLATIN

Brand Name: Platinol-AQ®

Method Administered: I.V.

Side Effects: Decreased blood cell counts (WBCs, platelets, RBCs); nausea; vomiting; potential kidney damage; potential hearing loss; diarrhea

Notify Physician of These Side Effects: Fever over 100.5° F; chills; signs of infection; unusual bleeding or bruising; dizziness or fainting; diarrhea not controlled with medication; blood in urine or stools; decreased urine output; changes in hearing

CYCLOPHOSPHAMIDE

Brand Names: Cytoxan® and Neosar®

Methods Administered: P.O., I.V.

Side Effects: Decreased blood cell counts (WBCs, platelets, RBCs); nausea; vomiting; loss of appetite; hair loss; stopping of menstrual periods; darkening of skin

Notify Physician of These Side Effects: Blood in urine; fever over 100.5° F; chills; painful urination; unusual bleeding or bruising

Precautions: Drink lots of fluids while taking this medication. One to two quarts a day is recommended during the 24-hour period following administration. If the drug is given by mouth, take in the morning and follow with adequate fluids during the day.

DOCETAXEL

Brand Name: Taxotere®

Method Administered: I.V.

Side Effects: Temporary hair thinning or loss; rare reports of permanent hair loss; decreased white blood cell count with increased risk of infection; decreased platelet count with increased risk of bleeding; diarrhea; loss of appetite; nausea; vomiting; rash; numbness and tingling in hands or feet; edema

Notify Physician of These Side Effects:
Redness; swelling and pain in hands or feet; swelling in the ankles; shortness of breath; weight gain; clothes feel too tight at the waist

Precautions: Some drugs increase toxicity. Consult your physician or pharmacist. Take dexamethasone (Decadron®) medication, as ordered by your physician, prior to chemotherapy.

DOXORUBICIN

Brand Names: Adriamycin PFS®, Adriamycin RDF®, ADR®

Method Administered: I.V.

Side Effects: Hair loss; sore mouth; nausea; vomiting; decreased blood cell counts (WBCs, platelets); changes in heart rhythm; darkening of nail beds; red urine; painful urination; flu-like symptoms; sensitivity to sun; inflammation of eyes

Notify Physician of These Side Effects: Fast or irregular heartbeat; fever over 100.5° F; chills; redness or pain at injection site; shortness of breath; swelling of feet and lower legs; diarrhea for over 24 hours; unusual bleeding or bruising; wheezing; joint pain; side or stomach pain; skin rash or itching; sores in mouth

Precautions: If burning or pain occurs at I.V. site or in nearby veins when the drug is being administered, notify your nurse immediately. If drug leaks into tissues, necrosis (cell damage) may occur in area of infiltration. Causes urine to turn reddish in color hours after administration and may last for one to two days after administration. May stain clothing.

EPIRUBICIN

Brand Names: Ellence®, Pharmorubicin PFS®

Method Administered: I.V.

Side Effects: Stopping of menstrual periods; nausea and vomiting; diarrhea; hot flashes; darkening of soles, palms or nails; loss of

appetite or weight loss; decreased white blood cell counts; hair loss; red urine; sore mouth

Notify Physician of These Side Effects: Severe vomiting; dehydration; fever over 100.5° F; evidence of infection; shortness of breath; injection site pain; fast or irregular heartbeat; chills; swelling of feet and lower legs; diarrhea for over 24 hours; unusual bleeding or bruising; wheezing; joint pain; side or stomach pain; skin rash or itching; sores in mouth

Precautions: If burning or pain occurs at I.V. site or in nearby veins when the drug is being administered, notify your nurse immediately. If drug leaks into tissues, necrosis (cell damage) may occur in area of infiltration. Causes urine to turn reddish in color hours after administration and may last for one to two days after administration. May stain clothing. Tell your physician if you are taking cimetidine (Tagamet®).

ERIBULIN MESYLATE

Brand Names: Halaven®

Method Administered: I.V.

Side Effects: Constipation; joint pain; fever; weight loss; appetite loss; headache; diarrhea; vomiting; anemia; decreased white blood cell count; fatigue; hair loss

Notify Physician of These Side Effects:
Numbness in hands or feet; fever over 100.5° F; chills; cough; painful or frequent urination

ETOPOSIDE (VP-16)

Brand Name: Vepesid®

Method Administered: P.O.

Side Effects: Decreased blood cell counts (WBCs, platelets); nausea; vomiting; hair loss; sore mouth and throat; low blood pressure

Notify Physician of These Side Effects: Fever over 100.5° F; chills; signs of infection; excessive bleeding or bruising; nausea not controlled in 24 hours with medications; difficulty eating or swallowing because of irritation; dizziness when standing

Precautions: Medication should be stored in refrigerator.

FLUOROURACIL

Brand Names: Adrucil® and 5-FU®

Method Administered: I.V.

Side Effects: Decreased blood cell counts (WBCs, platelets); sore mouth; nausea; vomiting; diarrhea; loss of appetite; some hair loss; sore throat; sensitivity to sunlight; darkening of skin; nail changes; dermatitis or rash; dark veins where drug was administered; tenderness, redness or peeling of hands and feet

Notify Physician of These Side Effects: Chest pain; cough; difficulty with balance; shortness of breath; black, tarry stools; diarrhea over 24 hours in duration; fever over 100.5° F; chills; sores in mouth; stomach cramps; unusual bleeding or bruising

Precautions: Avoid people with colds or infections. Avoid prolonged exposure to sunlight.

GEMCITABINE

Brand Name: Gemzar®

Method Administered: I.V.

Side Effects: Nausea; vomiting; fatigue; diarrhea; sores in mouth or on lips; flu-like symptoms with first treatment; skin rash; swelling in hands, ankles or face; thinning hair; itching

Precautions: Do not take aspirin or medications containing aspirin.

IXABEPILONE

Brand Name: Ixempra®

Method Administered: I.V.

Side Effects: Decreased white blood cell count; allergic reaction to medication; numbness in hands and feet; loss of appetite; taste alterations;

nausea; vomiting; sore mouth and throat; diarrhea; constipation; abdominal pain; hair loss; nail changes; skin rash; redness, pain and peeling of hands and feet

Notify Physician of These Side Effects: Fever over 100.5° F; chills; signs of infection; redness, tingling, pain or numbness in hands and feet; nausea or diarrhea not controlled with medication within 24 hours

LAPATINIB

Brand Name: Tykerb®

Method Administered: P.O.

Side Effects: Nausea; vomiting; diarrhea; redness, pain and peeling of hands and feet; skin rash; mouth sores; loss of appetite; indigestion

Notify Physician of These Side Effects: Vomiting or diarrhea not controlled in 24 hours with medication; red or painful hands or feet; mouth sores

Precautions: Take with food or within 30 minutes of eating. If you miss a dose, do not double the dose the next day.

METHOTREXATE

Brand Name: Folex PFS®

Methods Administered: P.O., I.M., I.V.

Side Effects: Sore mouth; nausea; vomiting; loss of appetite; diarrhea; hair loss; taste alterations; blurred vision; dizziness; fatigue; infertility; itching; sensitivity to sun

Notify Physician of These Side Effects: Black, tarry stools; bloody vomit; diarrhea over 24 hours in duration; fever over 100.5° F; chills; sore throat; sores in mouth; stomach pain or unusual bleeding or bruising

Precautions: Do not drink alcohol while receiving the drug. Avoid sun exposure, sun lamps and tanning beds. Do not take aspirin or ibuprofen without first checking with your physician.

PACLITAXEL

Brand Name: Taxol®

Method Administered: I.V.

Side Effects: Decreased blood cell counts (WBCs, platelets, RBCs); allergic reaction during administration; numbness in hands and feet; low blood pressure; body aches; nausea; vomiting; diarrhea; sore mouth and throat; hair loss

Notify Physician of These Side Effects: Fever over 100.5° F; chills; signs of infection; excessive bleeding or bruising; shortness of breath during drug infusion; tingling or numbness in feet or hands; body aches unrelieved by prescribed medication; nausea or vomiting not controlled in 24 hours with medication; inability to eat or swallow

PERTUZUMAB

Brand Name: Perjeta®

Method Administered: I.V.

Side Effects (During Infusion): Allergic reaction causing fast heartbeat, headache, fever over 100.5° F, chills, muscle pain or an unusual taste in the mouth

Side Effects (After Infusion): Heart problems; diarrhea; nausea; vomiting; fatigue; loss of appetite; dry skin; rash or itching; numbness or tingling in hands or feet; cold symptoms (stuffy nose, sneezing or sore throat); temporary hair loss may occur

Notify Physician of These Side Effects: Difficulty breathing; fever over 100.5° F or chills with upper respiratory tract infection

TRASTUZUMAB

Brand Name: Herceptin®

Method Administered: I.V.

Side Effects: Chills; pain at tumor site or in abdomen or back; shortness of breath; muscle weakness or stiffness; rash; headache

Notify Physician of These Side Effects: Difficulty breathing; nausea; vomiting; diarrhea; loss of appetite; sleeplessness; unusual bruising or bleeding; swelling of the feet or ankles; rapid heartbeat; upper respiratory tract infection; excessive coughing; fever over 100.5° F

VINCRISTINE

Brand Names: Oncovin® and Vincasar PFS®

Method Administered: I.V.

Side Effects: Hair loss; numbness in limbs; nausea; vomiting; decreased blood cell counts (WBCs, platelets); ovary suppression; constipation

Notify Physician of These Side Effects: Fever over 100.5° F; chills; unusual bleeding or bruising; blurred or double vision; confusion; constipation; difficulty walking; tingling in fingers and toes; sores in mouth; pain in stomach

Precautions: This medication can cause severe constipation. Eat lots of fiber, drink lots of water and ask your physician about using a stool softener or laxative.

VINORELBINE

Brand Name: Navelbine®

Method Administered: I.V.

Side Effects: Redness and tenderness at injection site; darkening of vein used; hair loss; nausea; vomiting

Notify Physician of These Side Effects: Difficulty walking; cramping in legs; redness and pain at site of I.V.; unusual bleeding or bruising; black, tarry stools; lower back or side pain; fever over 100.5° F; chills; painful or difficult urination

Precautions: Avoid people with infections.

HORMONAL DRUGS

ANASTRAZOLE

Brand Name: Arimidex®

Method Administered: P.O.

Side Effects: Weakness; fatigue; headache; nausea; mild diarrhea; increased or decreased appetite; sweating; hot flashes; vaginal dryness; decreased sexual libido; bone and joint aches

Notify Physician of These Side Effects: Pain in lower leg; redness or swelling of your arm or leg; shortness of breath; chest pain

EXEMESTANE

Brand Name: Aromasin®

Method Administered: P.O.

Side Effects: Fatigue; hot flashes; pain at tumor site; nausea; depression; difficulty sleeping; increased appetite; weight gain; increased sweating; decrease in sexual libido

Notify Physician of These Side Effects: Severe hot flashes; difficulty sleeping; depression

Precautions: Keep taking the drug even when you are feeling well. Take drug after eating.

FULVESTRANT

Brand Name: Faslodex®

Method Administered: I.M.

Side Effects: Nausea; feeling listless or tired; vomiting; constipation; diarrhea; abdominal pain; headache; back pain; hot flashes; sore throat; pain at injection site; flu-like symptoms; pain in chest or pelvis; decrease in libido

Notify Physician of These Side Effects: Bloating or swelling of face, hands, legs and feet; tingling in hands or feet; unusual weight gain or loss

Precautions: Notify physician if taking blood thinners such as Coumadin®.

GOSERELIN

Brand Name: Zoladex®

Method Administered: S.Q.

Side Effects: Light, irregular vaginal bleeding; stopping of menstrual periods; hot flashes; headaches; decrease in libido

Notify Physician of These Side Effects: Pelvic pain; burning, itching or dryness of vagina; anxiety; deepening of voice; increased hair growth; mental depression; mood changes; nervousness; fast or irregular heartbeat

Precautions: Your menstrual period may become irregular or cease, but you still need to use non-hormonal birth control methods (condoms or spermicides) if you are sexually active. Drinking alcohol while on goserelin increases risk of osteoporosis.

LETROZOLE

Brand Name: Femara®

Method Administered: P.O.

Side Effects: Back, bone, joint or muscle pain; hot flashes; loss of hair; weight loss; decreased appetite; sleepiness; anxiety; constipation; diarrhea; stomach pain; weakness

Notify Physician of These Side Effects: Shortness of breath; chest pain; increased sweating; severe nervousness; cough; light-headedness; sudden headache; slurred speech; sudden loss of coordination; swelling of hands; vaginal bleeding

LEUPROLIDE

Brand Names: Lupron®, Lupron Depot®, Viadur®, Leuprorelin®

Method Administered: I.M.

Side Effects: Light, irregular vaginal bleeding; stopping of menstrual periods; hot flashes; blurred vision; headache; nausea or vomiting; swelling of hands or feet; swelling and tenderness of breasts; trouble sleeping; weight gain; bleeding, bruising, burning or itching at injection site; decrease in libido

Notify Physician of These Side Effects: Fast or irregular heartbeat; trouble breathing; sudden, severe drop in blood pressure; swelling around the eyes; rash, hives or itching; numbness or tingling in hands or feet; anxiety; deepening of voice; increased hair growth; mental depression; mood changes; nervousness

Precautions: Your menstrual period may become irregular or cease, but you still need to use non-hormonal birth control methods (condoms or spermicides) if you are sexually active.

TAMOXIFEN

Brand Names: Nolvadex®, TAM®

Method Administered: P.O.

Side Effects: Hot flashes; nausea when first beginning drug; fluid retention; vaginal discharge; menstrual irregularities; vaginal dryness; bone pain during first few weeks of treatment; increased fertility; decreased libido

Notify Physician of These Side Effects: Excessive vaginal dryness; vaginal infection; changes in vision; continued bone pain

Precautions: Take medication with food. Ask your physician about the need for birth control. A yearly gynecological exam is recommended. Some SSRI antidepressants (Prozac®, Zoloft® and Paxil®) may interfere with Tamoxifen's function.

TOREMIFENE

Brand Name: Fareston®

Method Administered: P.O.

Side Effects: Nausea or vomiting; hot flashes; bone pain; dizziness; dry eyes

Notify Physician of These Side Effects: Blurred vision or changes in vision; change in vaginal discharge; confusion; increased urination; loss

of appetite; pelvic pressure or pain; unusual tiredness; vaginal bleeding

Precautions: Taking a thiazide diuretic will increase side effects of drug. Taking Coumadin® increases risk of bleeding.

MISCELLANEOUS DRUGS

BEVACIZUMAB

Brand Name: Avastin®

Method Administered: I.V.

Side Effects: Abdominal pain; diarrhea; gastrointestinal perforations; decreased wound healing; hemorrhage; blood clots; high blood pressure; congestive heart failure; kidney problems

Notify Physician of These Side Effects: Fever over 100.5° F; chills; signs of infection; abdominal pain; unusual bleeding or bruising; dizziness or fainting; shortness of breath; pain in chest or legs; diarrhea not controlled with medication; blood in stools; headaches

DARBEPOETIN ALFA

Brand Name: Aranesp®

Method Administered: S.Q.

Side Effects: Pain at injection site; elevated or lowered blood pressure; headache

Notify Physician of These Side Effects: Dizziness; fainting

DENOSUMAB

Brand Name: Xgeva®

Methods Administered: S.Q.

Side Effects: Reduced calcium levels; jaw pain; decrease in jaw density

Notify Physician of These Side Effects: Fever over 100.5° F; chills; cough; rapid breathing; painful or frequent urination

DEXAMETHASONE

Brand Names: Decadron®, Dexasone®, Dexone®, Hexadrol®

Methods Administered: P.O., I.M., I.V.

Side Effects: Euphoria; restlessness; insomnia; stomach irritation; increased appetite

Notify Physician of These Side Effects: Dizziness; fainting; shortness of breath; fever over 100.5° F; wounds that don't heal; swelling of feet or legs

Precautions: Take medication with food. Do not take more than prescribed. Do not stop taking medication without informing your physician.

DOLASETRON

Brand Name: Anzemet®

Methods Administered: I.V., P.O.

Side Effects: Diarrhea; abdominal or stomach pain; headache; dizziness; light-headedness; fever over 100.5° F; chills; fatigue

Notify Physician of These Side Effects: High or low blood pressure; blood in urine; painful urination; chest pain; rapid heartbeat; severe stomach pain; rash, hives or itching; swelling of face, feet or lower legs; trouble breathing

DRONABINOL

Brand Name: Marinol®

Method Administered: P.O.

Side Effects: Dizziness; drowsiness; nausea or vomiting; false sense of well-being; trouble thinking

Notify Physician of These Side Effects *(may be signs of an overdose)*: Amnesia; memory loss; confusion; hallucinations; delusions; anxiety; mental depression; fast heartbeat; severe drowsiness; decrease in motor coordination; slurred speech; constipation; problems urinating

Precautions: Avoid alcohol and central nervous system depressants (alcohol, pain medications, tranquilizers or sleeping medication).

EPOETIN

Brand Names: Epogen®, Procrit®, Eprex®

Method Administered: S.Q.

Side Effects: Fatigue and weakness; tingling, burning or prickling sensation; loss of strength or energy; muscle pain

Notify Physician of These Side Effects: Chest pain; shortness of breath; seizures; coughing; sneezing; sore throat; fever over 100.5° F; weight gain; swelling of legs, arms, feet or hands

Precautions: May cause seizures, especially during the first 90 days of treatment. Avoid driving, operating heavy machinery or any other activity that may pose danger if a seizure occurs.

EVEROLIMUS

Brand Names: Afinitor®

Method Administered: P.O.

Side Effects: Cough; skin rash; joint pain; loss of appetite; nausea; fatigue

Notify Physician of These Side Effects: Fever over 100.5° F; chills; cough; rapid breathing; wheezing; chest pain; painful or frequent urination; yellowing of skin; pain in upper right side of stomach

FILGRASTIM

Brand Names: Neupogen®, Leukine®

Method Administered: S.Q.

Side Effects: Rash or itching; headache; pain in arms, legs, joints, muscles, lower back or pelvis

Notify Physician of These Side Effects: Redness or pain at injection site; fever over 100.5° F; rapid or irregular heartbeat; sores on skin; wheezing

FOSAPREPITANT DIMEGLUMINE

Brand Names: Emend®

Method Administered: I.V.

Side Effects: Fatigue; diarrhea; neutropenia; anemia; numbness in hands and feet; urinary tract infection; allergic reaction during I.V. administration

Notify Physician of These Side Effects: Fever over 100.5° F; chills; cough; rapid breathing; painful or frequent urination

GRANISETRON

Brand Name: Kytril®

Methods Administered: I.V., P.O.

Side Effects: Abdominal pain; constipation; diarrhea; headache; agitation; dizziness; drowsiness; heartburn; indigestion; trouble sleeping

Notify Physician of These Side Effects: Fever over 100.5° F; severe nausea or vomiting; chest pain; fainting; irregular heartbeat; shortness of breath; rash, hives or itching

NETUPITANT AND PALONOSETRON

Brand Names: Akynzeo®

Method Administered: P.O.

Side Effects: Headache; fatigue; constipation; redness of the skin

Notify Physician of These Side Effects: Fever over 100.5° F; chills; cough; rapid breathing; painful or frequent urination; severe headache

ONDANSETRON

Brand Names: Zofran®, Zofran ODT®

Methods Administered: I.V., P.O.

Side Effects: Constipation; diarrhea; fever over 100.5° F; headache; abdominal pain; burning, prickling or tingling sensation; drowsiness; dry mouth; feeling cold; itching

Notify Physician of These Side Effects: Chest pain; burning, pain or redness at injection site; shortness of breath; rash, hives or itching; trouble breathing; wheezing

OPRELVEKIN

Brand Name: Neumega®

Method Administered: S.Q.

Side Effects: Red eyes; weakness; numbness or tingling of hands or feet; skin discoloration; rash at injection site

Notify Physician of These Side Effects: Fast or irregular heartbeat; sore mouth or tongue; white patches on mouth or tongue; shortness of breath; swelling of feet or lower legs; bloody eye; blurred vision; severe redness or peeling of skin

PALBOCICLIB

Brand Names: Ibrance®

Method Administered: P.O.

Side Effects: Decreased white blood cell count; blood clot in lungs; fatigue; nausea; anemia; headache; diarrhea; constipation; hair loss; vomiting; rash; decreased appetite

Notify Physician of These Side Effects: Fever over 100.5° F; chills; cough; rapid breathing; chest pain; painful or frequent urination

PALONOSETRON

Brand Name: Aloxi®

Methods Administered: I.V., P.O.

Side Effects: Headache; constipation; diarrhea

Notify Physician of These Side Effects: Headache not relieved with prescribed pain medication; diarrhea not controlled within 24 hours with medication; constipation not relieved with medication

PAMIDRONATE

Brand Name: Aredia®

Method Administered: I.V.

Side Effects: Abdominal pain; body aches or pain; bone pain; constipation; diarrhea; joint pain; kidney problems

Notify Physician of These Side Effects: Decrease in amount of urine; headache; muscle pain or cramps; jaw pain; nausea

PEGFILRASTIM

Brand Name: Neulasta®

Method Administered: S.Q.

Side Effects: Allergic reaction, which may include hives, difficulty breathing and swelling of face, lips, tongue or throat

Notify Physician of These Side Effects: Pain in upper stomach, spreading to shoulder; severe dizziness; skin rash; flushing of skin; rapid heart rate; rapid breathing; shortness of breath; signs of infection

PREDNISONE

Brand Names: Deltasone®, Liquid Pred®, Meticorten®, Orasone®, Panasol® and Prednicen-M®.

Method Administered: P.O.

Side Effects: Increase in appetite; indigestion; nervousness; restlessness; trouble sleeping; false sense of well-being; nausea; vomiting; fluid retention

Notify Physician of These Side Effects: Blurred vision; frequent urination; hallucinations; hives or skin rash; abdominal pain or burning; black, tarry stools; irregular heartbeat; unusual bruising; wounds that do not heal; nausea or vomiting over 24 hours in duration

Precautions: Take medication at same time of day, starting early in morning. Do not take at night or late in afternoon. Do not increase or decrease dose without physician's consent. Do not stop taking medication without notifying your physician.

ZOLEDRONIC ACID

Brand Name: Zometa®

Method Administered: I.V.

Side Effects: Fatigue; nausea; vomiting; bone pain; jaw pain; headache; decreased appetite

Notify Physician of These Side Effects: Nausea or vomiting not relieved within 24 hours with medication; headache or body pain not relieved with prescribed pain medication

Precautions: Take a daily multivitamin that contains 400 IU of Vitamin D and at least 500 mg. of calcium daily. Drink lots of fluids.

APPENDIX C

Understanding Clinical Trials

Clinical trials are new, investigational studies that research effective treatment and prevention strategies. Thousands of research studies are currently underway in the United States. Most clinical trials are conducted by the National Cancer Institute (NCI), major medical centers or pharmaceutical companies. If a new treatment is determined to be safe and effective at the completion of the trial, the U.S. Food and Drug Administration (FDA) grants approval for widespread commercial use by patients.

Four Phases of Clinical Trials:

- **Phase I:** New treatments tested to determine the acceptable dose and method of administration.
- **Phase II:** Studies the safety and effectiveness of the drug and how it affects the human body.
- **Phase III:** Requires that a large number of patients receive either the newer therapy or the standard therapy in order to compare beneficial survival results and quality of life during treatment. If the newer drug is found to be more effective than the standard one, the trial is stopped, and all participants are eligible for the more successful treatment. If there is any evidence that the newer drug is inferior or

has unusual toxic side effects, the experimental medication is discontinued.

- **Phase IV:** Studies are conducted to further evaluate long-term safety and effectiveness of the trial drug after approval for standard use.

Clinical Trial Informed Consent

Your doctor or nurse will explain in detail the type and purpose of the trial. You will be given an informed consent form to read and sign. This form must include the expected benefits, the negative aspects, other treatment options, assurance that your personal records will be kept confidential and a statement indicating that your participation is voluntary and that you may withdraw at any time.

Participating in the trial does not prevent you from getting any additional medical care you may need. If you decide to participate in the trial, you will need to contact your insurance provider to ask if it covers any charges. Be sure the researchers are aware if your plan does not cover the costs of clinical trials. Some trials are simply a comparison of two drugs or timing of administration to determine which is more effective. Your physician will explain the details of the trial.

Clinical Trial Questions:

- What phase is the clinical trial in now?

- Who is sponsoring the study? (It needs to be approved by a reputable national group like the NCI, a major teaching institution or the FDA.)

- What is the purpose of this study?

- What advantage does this trial have compared to standard recommended treatment?

- How long will the clinical trial last?

- Where will treatments be given and evaluated while on the trial?

- Is the drug or combination of drugs available outside of the clinical trial?

- How will the success of the treatment be evaluated (blood tests, scans, etc.)?

- How much additional time will participating in the trial require over standard treatment?

- Will there be any extra expenses, or will all costs of the trial be covered?

- Will my insurance cover the cost of the trial?

- What type of follow-up will continue after the trial is completed?

Understanding Clinical Trials

If you want to know more about clinical trials, the best place to start is with your oncologist.

Other Resources:

- **National Institutes of Health (NIH)**
  https://clinicaltrials.gov
  search "clinical trials".

- **American Cancer Society**
  Contact a clinical trials specialist at
  1-800-303-5691.

To Participate or Not to Participate

The decision whether or not to participate in a clinical trial is often not an easy one to make. This decision is very personal and one that can only be made after you discuss the advantages and disadvantages with your physician and clinical trial nurse. When the final decision is made, you need to feel that you have chosen what is best for you. Some women prefer the tried and true, while others feel that they are getting an even better chance by taking a newer drug or drug combination. Some feel that by their participation in clinical trials they will be helping other women in the future. Remember, no one has the right answer to the question of whether or not you should participate; there is not an absolute answer. That is why it is called a trial.

APPENDIX D

Understanding Breast Self-Exam

After breast cancer surgery, there is an increased risk that cancer may occur in the remaining breast tissue (lumpectomy) or in the other breast. Breast self-exams have long been a part of cancer education for detection. However, a recent debate among national organizations regarding the usefulness of breast exams has left many women confused. To clarify this issue for you, as a breast cancer patient, we refer to the organization of healthcare professionals who treat and monitor breast cancer patients for recurrence, the American Society of Clinical Oncology (ASCO). The ASCO breast cancer surveillance guidelines state, *"All women should be counseled to perform monthly breast self-examination."* This chapter provides instructions on how to perform a breast self-exam to follow their guidelines.

Normal Nodularity
The goal of breast self-exam is to carefully check your breast(s) for unique changes in your tissue, especially new lumps or areas of thickening. This check is **not** to find cancer, but rather to find and report any changes you may discover.

When To Perform a Breast Self-Exam
Check your breast(s) when they are least filled with fluid.
- **Menstruating women:** the last day, or several days past, the menstrual period

- **Menopausal or pregnant women:** the same date each month
- **Women receiving treatment, who are not having a regular menstrual period:** the same date each month

Breast Self-Exam After Surgery:
- **Mastectomy patients** should begin their exam of the surgical area after complete healing of the incision, usually two to three months after surgery.
- **Lumpectomy patients** should begin their exams of their surgical area after complete healing of the incision, usually two to three months after surgery, or at the completion of radiation therapy.
- **Reconstructive surgery patients** should begin their exams when their incision is completely healed, usually two to three months after surgery.

Normal Changes After Surgery
After surgery, you need to become familiar with how your incision area feels. It will feel different than the surrounding tissue; the scar will feel firm to your touch. Occasionally, an area in the incision will be slightly firmer. This is scar tissue formation. Areas where drains were placed may also feel firm. This firmness is normal. Breast cancer occurring in the scar area during the first few months after surgery is very rare. Knowing

215

what your normal scar feels like will help you to recognize suspicious changes, should they ever occur.

MammaCare® Method of Self-Exam

The exam described below has been taken from the MammaCare® method. This method was developed from research at the University of Florida and is considered the state-of-the-art breast self-exam technique.

Area To Be Examined (A)

The breast tissue extends beyond the breast mound. It covers a large portion of the chest wall. Examine the area from the middle notch of your collarbone, following under the collarbone until you reach mid-underarm, then straight down until you reach your bra line. Follow the bra line to the middle of the breastbone and then back up to the notch.

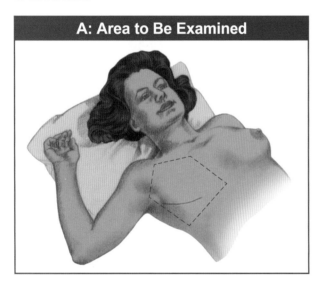

A: Area to Be Examined

Fifty percent of cancers occur in the upper, outer quadrant of the breast and eighteen percent under the nipple. Examine these areas carefully.

Finger Positions (B)

Use the flat pads of your three middle fingers, from the first joint down to the tips. Place flat pads of fingers in a bowing position on the breast tissue.

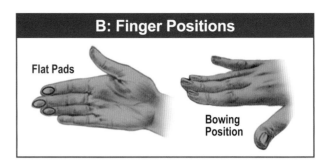

B: Finger Positions

Flat Pads

Bowing Position

Three Levels of Pressure (C)

Using three levels of pressure allows you to carefully examine the full thickness of the breast and not displace small lumps into fibrous tissues or into your rib area. Pressures do not injure your breast tissue.

- Position your fingers on the first spot to be examined.
- Use your fingers to make dime-sized circles using light pressure (barely moving the top layer of skin).
- Without lifting your fingers, repeat the circles using medium pressure (go halfway through the thickness of the breast).
- Again, without lifting your fingers, repeat the circles using deep pressure (go to the base of the breast next to the ribs).
- Lift your fingers. Move to the next position and repeat the process.

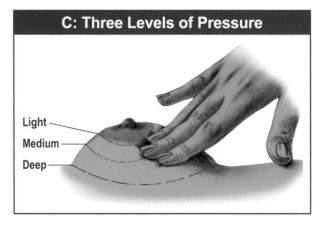

C: Three Levels of Pressure

Light

Medium

Deep

Remember: Do not lift your hand or release the pressure from your breast until you have completed the three sets of circles in each area.

Performing Your Exam

Step 1: Side-Lying Exam Positioning (D)

Use the following techniques to examine the lumpectomy breast or the mastectomy site:

- Lie down on the bed, roll onto your left side to examine your right breast.

- Pull your knees up slightly, rotate your right shoulder to be flat on the bed.

- Place your right hand, palm up, on your forehead. Your nipple should point directly toward the ceiling. Use your left hand to examine your right breast. You may place a small pillow under the arch of the back to increase comfort.

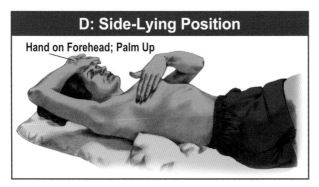

D: Side-Lying Position

Hand on Forehead; Palm Up

This position allows you to examine the outer half of the breast by spreading out the tissue. Fifty percent of all cancers occur in the area of the breast which extends from the nipple to underneath the arm. The side-lying position prevents breast tissue from falling into the underarm area.

Step 2: Side-Lying Exam (E)

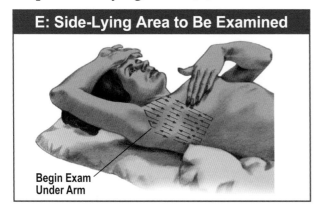

E: Side-Lying Area to Be Examined

Begin Exam Under Arm

- Using the flat pads of your three middle fingers in the bowing position (B), begin your exam under the arm. Make dime-sized circles using the three levels of pressure in each spot (C), following the up and down pattern of search. Do not release the pressure as you spiral downward. Ten to sixteen vertical strips will be needed. Continue the pattern of search until you reach your nipple area.

Step 3: Back-Lying Exam Positioning (F)

- When you reach your nipple area, roll onto your back; remove your right hand from your forehead and place this arm alongside your head on the bed.

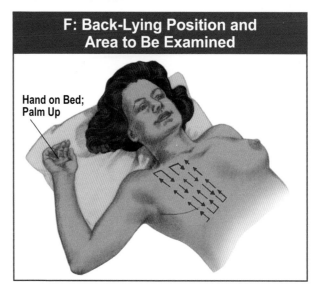

F: Back-Lying Position and Area to Be Examined

Hand on Bed; Palm Up

Step 4: Back-Lying Exam (F)

- Continue the exam of the nipple area using the same pressures (C). Do not squeeze the nipple.

- Report any discharge from your nipple that is not associated with the onset of a menstrual period, hormonal medications, sexual stimulation or excessive manipulation of the breasts. A bloody discharge or a discharge from only one breast needs to be reported promptly.

- Examine the remaining breast tissue with the same pressures and pattern of search until you reach the breastbone.

- Repeat steps 1 – 4, examining the opposite breast.

Step 5: Lymph Node Exam (G)

- Make a row of circles above and below your collarbone on each side.

- While standing, check the depressed area near your neck by rolling your shoulders upward and turning your face toward the side you are examining. With the opposite hand, place your fingers in the formed depression and check carefully.

- Feel under each arm for axillary lymph node enlargement.

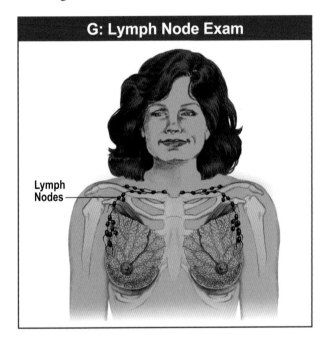

G: Lymph Node Exam

Lymph Nodes

Lymph nodes are soft to hard, pea-like areas in the lymphatic system. They may become enlarged from cancer or infection. Enlarged lymph nodes do not always indicate cancer, but you should report any lymph node enlargement to your healthcare provider for evaluation.

Step 6: Visual Exam (H)

A visual inspection of your breast(s) is important. Some cancers do **not** form a hard lump. The first indication of cancer may be one you can see, but not feel. Looking into a mirror, closely examine your breast(s) in the following four positions.

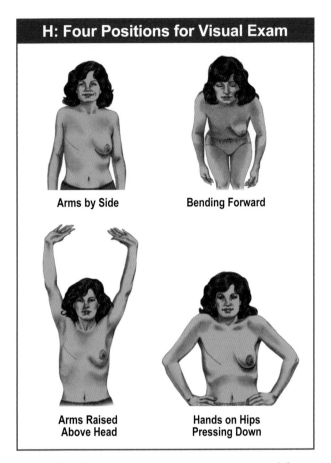

H: Four Positions for Visual Exam

Arms by Side

Bending Forward

Arms Raised Above Head

Hands on Hips Pressing Down

Carefully observe your incision. It is normal for it to be raised and red in the beginning. The color will gradually begin to fade to a light pink, and the scar area will flatten out. A lumpectomy scar area may have a depression or sinking in of the tissues.

Look for the Following Changes Surrounding Your Scar and the Non-Surgical Breast (I):

- Skin texture that resembles an orange peel
- Dimpling, bulging or pulling in of the skin
- Inverted nipple (not normally inverted)
- Difference in vein pattern over one breast
- Color changes in breast tissues
- Swelling or decreased size of the non-radiated breast
- Crusty material or irritation around the nipple
- Open sore or bump; red rash

I: Visual Signs to Report

1. Orange Peel Skin

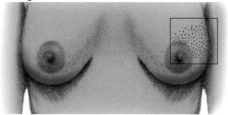

Texture of your skin may look like an orange peel

2. Dimpling

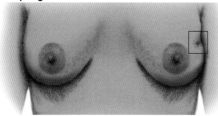

Dimpling or pulling in of the skin

3. Inverted Nipple

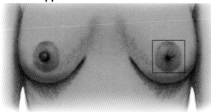

Inversion of previously normal nipple

4. Vein Pattern

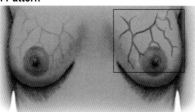

Difference in vein pattern on one breast; much larger veins or increased number of veins

What Cancer Feels Like

Ninety percent of cancers form a very hard lump, feel anchored in the surrounding tissues, are usually painless and do **not** change in degree of hardness during a menstrual cycle. Ten percent of cancers do **not** form a lump but may cause visual changes in the breast. Therefore, both a manual exam and a visual exam are needed each month to ensure the best surveillance of your breast health.

Breast Self-Exam After Surgery

When you complete your monthly exam, congratulate yourself for taking an active part in guarding your health. Then forget about it until the next month.

APPENDIX E

Recommended Reading

BREAST CANCER EDUCATION

**Breast Cancer
Support Partner Handbook**
Judy C. Kneece, RN, OCN
Publisher: EduCare Publishing Inc.; 2016
Available at www.educareinc.com

**Breast Cancer Survival Manual:
A Step-by-Step Guide for the Woman
With Newly Diagnosed Breast Cancer**
John Link, M.D.
Publisher: Holt Paperbacks; 2007

Sexuality and Fertility After Cancer
Leslie R. Schover, Ph.D.
Publisher: Wiley; 1997

Timeless Healing
Herbert Benson, M.D., Marg Stark
Publisher: Scribner; 1997

COPING SKILLS

The Feeling Good Handbook
David D. Burns
Publisher: Plume; 1999

**The Human Side of Cancer: Living With
Hope, Coping With Uncertainty**
Jimmie C. Holland, M.D., Sheldon Lewis
Publisher: Harper Paperbacks; 2001

I Am Not My Breast Cancer
Ruth Peltason
Publisher: Harper Paperbacks; 2009

**Life Strategies: Doing What Works,
Doing What Matters**
Phillip C. McGraw, Ph.D.
Publisher: Hyperion; 2000

**The Courage to Grieve:
The Classic Guide to Creative Living,
Recovery, and Growth Through Grief**
Judy Tatelbaum
Publisher: William Morrow; 2008

**The Portable Therapist: Wise and
Inspiring Answers to the Questions
People in Therapy Ask the Most**
Susanna McMahon, Ph.D.
Publisher: Dell; 1994

**You Don't Have to Suffer: A Handbook
for Moving Beyond Life's Crises**
Judy Tatelbaum
Publisher: Skyhorse Publishing; 2012

DIET AND EXERCISE

**The Breast Cancer Survivor's Fitness
Plan (Harvard Medical School Guides)**
Carolyn M. Kaelin, M.D., M.P.H.,
Francesca Coltrera, Josie Gardiner, Joy Prouty
Publisher: McGraw-Hill; 2006

Complete Guide to Nutrition
for Cancer Survivors

Abby S. Bloch, PhD, RD and Barbara Grant, MS,
RD, CSO, LD

Publisher: American Cancer Society; 2010

Dr. Ann's 10-Step Diet:
A Simple Plan for Permanent Weight
Loss and Lifelong Vitality

Ann Kulze, M.D.

Publisher: Top Ten Wellness & Fitness; 2008

Eating Well Through Cancer

Holly Clegg, Gerald Miletello, M.D.

Publisher: Self-Published; 2006

INSPIRATIONAL

Cancer: 50 Essential Things to Do

Greg Anderson

Publisher: Plume; 2009

Chicken Soup for the
Breast Cancer Survivor's Soul:
Stories to Inspire, Support and Heal

Jack Canfield, Mark Victor Hansen, Mary Olsen
Kelly

Publisher: Health Communications; 2012

Finding the "CAN" in Cancer

Terri Schinazi, Nancy Emerson, Susan Moonan

Publisher: Lulu.com; 2007

The Triumphant Patient:
Become an Exceptional Patient in the
Face of Life-Threatening Illness

Greg Anderson

Publisher: iUniverse, Inc.; 2000

APPENDIX F

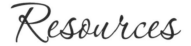

"Knowledge is of two kinds. We know a subject ourselves, or we know where we can find information on it."

—*Samuel Johnson*

One of the most important ways to gain control over your cancer and reduce anxiety is to get answers to your questions. Because you are an individual, your questions and needs may be different from other women, and may not be addressed by your healthcare team. When you are confused, reach out to support resources and find out what you need to know. The good news is that most resources are available online and are free of charge.

Tips for Organizing Resources:

■ Start a notebook for keeping information about your disease, treatment and recovery.

■ Remove the tear-out pages in the back of this book and place them in your notebook.

■ Write down your questions, and then read through the following list of resources for breast cancer patients.

■ Call or email the identified resource. In your notebook, record your questions, the telephone number, date you called and with whom you spoke.

■ Print out the information you want to keep.

■ Ask your healthcare team for the names of local sources of support.

Finding Information on the Internet

The Internet is a valuable resource, but be sure that the sites you visit are recognized as having sound clinical information. Most national cancer organizations, medical schools and universities have reputable websites. If you do not have a computer, Internet access is available at most public and hospital libraries.

Suggestions for Internet Use:

■ Always seek breast cancer information from reputable organizations only.

■ Make sure the information is current. Look for the last update of the information on the site.

■ Never substitute information found on the Internet for seeing or asking your healthcare provider about your concerns.

ADVOCACY GROUPS / ORGANIZATIONS

National Breast Cancer Coalition

www.breastcancerdeadline2020.org

Grassroots advocacy group of hundreds of member organizations and tens of thousands of individuals fighting breast cancer through action, advocacy and public education.

National Coalition for Cancer Survivorship

www.canceradvocacy.org

Advocates for quality cancer care for all Americans and the empowerment of cancer survivors through federal policy initiatives.

Patient Advocate Foundation

(Employment, Insurance and Debt Issues)

www.patientadvocate.org

A national non-profit organization that serves as an active liaison between the patient and her insurer, employer or debt holders in matters relating to a diagnosis through case managers, doctors and attorneys. Seeks to safeguard patients through effective mediation, ensuring access to care, maintenance of employment and preservation of financial stability.

Susan G. Komen for the Cure

www.komen.org

Provides information on all areas of breast cancer treatment and support.

BREAST RECONSTRUCTION

American Cancer Society

www.cancer.org
Search: breast reconstruction

Provides information about breast reconstruction after mastectomy.

BreastCancer.org

www.breastcancer.org/pictures/treatment/

Pictures of breast cancer patients with different types of breast reconstruction.

Breast Implants

www.fda.gov
Search: breast implants

Information on choosing an implant, the associated risks, FDA regulations and manufacturers of implants.

Microsurgical Breast Reconstruction

www.diepflap.com

Provides a description of DIEP and SGAP reconstruction; includes timelines and before and after photos.

Medline Plus

www.nlm.nih.gov
Search: breast reconstruction

Guide to different types of breast reconstruction.

Reconstruction Procedure Articles

www.mauricenahabedian.com

Clinical articles written by Dr. Nahabedian, Professor of Plastic Surgery at Georgetown University and an Associate Professor of Plastic Surgery at Johns Hopkins University.

CANCER TREATMENTS
CLINICAL ASPECTS

American Society of Clinical Oncology (ASCO)

www.asco.org

Provides educational resources and general standards of practice.

Cancer.gov: Breast Cancer Clinical Trials

www.cancer.gov/clinicaltrials

Information on choosing and participating in clinical trials, results of recent trials and resources for finding a trial.

Inflammatory Breast Cancer Research

www.ibcresearch.org

General information, research, articles, news articles, discussion and commentary on inflammatory breast cancer.

National Cancer Institute

www.cancer.gov

A cancer treatment database providing prognostic, stage and treatment information on more than 1,000 protocol (treatment) summaries.

National Comprehensive Cancer Network: Breast Cancer Treatment Guidelines for Patients

www.nccn.org

Provides decision trees to aid patients in choosing treatment and follow-up options. Also available in Spanish.

CHILDREN AND FAMILIES

Caring Bridge

www.caringbridge.org

Non-profit service that provides a free website to anyone going through a health crisis.

Kids Konnected

www.kidskonnected.org

A non-profit organization that provides for the needs of the children of cancer patients. Informative website, a 24-hour hotline, leadership training, support groups, online forums, a teddy bear outreach program and support tools for children and families.

COMPLEMENTARY AND ALTERNATIVE MEDICINE (CAM)

Office of Dietary Supplements, NIH

www.ods.od.nih.gov

Research resources, frequently asked questions and fact sheets about supplements to help the public make informed decisions.

CAM-CANCER

http://www.cam-cancer.org/
Select: CAM

Evidence-based summaries on different types of complementary care for cancer patients.

EMPLOYMENT CONCERNS

Americans With Disabilities Act

www.ada.gov

Provides basic information about the Americans with Disabilities Act.

Family and Medical Leave Act

www.dol.gov/whd/fmla

Provides a fact sheet about FMLA. The toll-free number reaches the Wage and Hour Division at the Department of Labor. They can provide the number of the office nearest to you.

National Coalition for Cancer Survivorship (NCCS) Employment

www.canceradvocacy.org

Provides information on your employment rights as a cancer survivor, including a free download of their publication, *Working It Out*.

The US Equal Employment Opportunity Commission

www.eeoc.gov

Includes frequently asked questions about cancer in the workplace and patients' and survivors' rights under the Americans with Disabilities Act.

GENERAL RESOURCES

Association of Cancer Online Resources

www.listserv.acor.org

Cancer information site that archives online support groups, information on treatments and clinical trials, links to other cancer education, advocacy groups on the Internet and much more.

BreastCancer.org

www.breastcancer.org

Breast cancer education site that includes articles, news, newsletters and chats. Archives the latest news about breast cancer and allows quick and specific searches.

CancerIndex.org

www.cancerindex.org

Index of cancer resources that provide information and support, along with a collection of media clips on the various breast cancers. To access media clips, choose "Breast Cancer" from the list on the main screen and then click on "Multimedia Breast Cancer Resources."

Chemocare.com

www.chemocare.com

Provides the latest information about chemotherapy side effects and self-care for patients, families and caregivers. Regularly updated by Cleveland Clinics.

Merck Manual Online Medical Library

www.merck.com/mmhe/index.html

Explains disorders, their symptoms, how they are diagnosed and how they can be treated.

National Cancer Institute (NCI)

www.cancer.gov

Provides comprehensive information on breast cancer diagnosis, treatment, statistics, research, clinical trials and breast cancer news.

HAIR CARE AND MAKEUP

Look Good … Feel Better

www.lookgoodfeelbetter.org

A comprehensive online guide about caring for your hair and skin during cancer treatment. Contact your local American Cancer Society for free classes and instructions on make-up application and hair care during treatment.

HEREDITARY BREAST CANCER

Facing Our Risk Empowered (FORCE)

www.facingourrisk.org

A national nonprofit organization devoted to hereditary breast and ovarian cancer. The mission includes support, education, advocacy, awareness and research specific to hereditary breast and ovarian cancer.

LYMPHEDEMA

National Lymphedema Network

www.lymphnet.org

Provides education and guidance to lymphedema patients and healthcare professionals.

MALE BREAST CANCER

American Cancer Society

www.cancer.org
Search: male breast cancer

Information and links to other websites focusing on male breast cancer.

PREGNANCY AND BREAST CANCER

Breast Cancer.org

www.breastcancer.org
Search: pregnant

Information about treatment during pregnancy.

Fertile Hope

www.fertilehope.org

A national, non-profit organization dedicated to providing reproductive information, support and hope to cancer patients whose medical treatments present the risk of infertility.

Pregnant With Cancer Network

www.pregnantwithcancer.org

Connects pregnant women with cancer to women who have lived through the experience.

PROSTHESIS, WIGS, CAMISOLES

American Cancer Society

www.tlcdirect.org

Boutique offering prostheses, bras, camisoles, wigs and other post-surgical products.

ReForma

www.myreforma.com

Offers reusable, hypoallergenic and self-adhering prosthetic nipples. Available in two sizes and three colors.

Softee

www.softeeusa.com

Offers a wide selection of post-surgical products for recovery, including camisoles.

Wigs.com

www.wigs.com

Offers a full selection of wigs, including baseball caps with attached bangs and ponytails.

SEXUALITY

International Academy of Compounding Pharmacies

www.iacprx.org

Allows patients to search for a local compounding pharmacist.

Pure Romance

www.pureromance.com

Offers a range of sexual products and in-home parties. The Sensuality, Sexuality, Survival (SSS) program serves as a resource for patients who have questions about restoring their intimacy.

SUPPORT GROUPS / ORGANIZATIONS

African-American Breast Cancer Alliance (AABCA)

www.aabcainc.org

Provides education to African-American women on breast health, early detection and breast cancer support groups.

Cancer Care, Inc.

www.cancercare.org

Offers free counseling, education, referral and direct financial assistance to cancer patients.

Living Beyond Breast Cancer

www.lbbc.org

Provides interactive conferences, toll-free information and support line, teleconferences, free newsletters and a networking program.

Local Support Groups

1-800-ACS-2345

Call the national American Cancer Society number and ask for local support group information. Call your cancer center and ask for local support group information.

National Coalition for Cancer Survivorship (NCCS)

www.canceradvocacy.org
Search: Cancer Survival Toolbox

Survivorship information and support. The Cancer Survival Toolbox, a CD of survival skills, is provided free (also available in Spanish).

Pink-Link

www.pink-link.org

A free online breast cancer support network with access to a member forum, online journals and breast cancer resources.

Sharsheret (Jewish Women)

www.sharsheret.org

Provides support for young Jewish women facing breast cancer. Offers a peer support network that connects young women with others who share similar diagnoses and experiences, as well as education and outreach programs.

Sisters Network Inc. (African-American Women)

www.sistersnetworkinc.org

An African-American breast cancer survivorship organization. Promotes the importance of breast health through support, breast education programs, resources, information and research.

The Young Survival Coalition

www.youngsurvival.org

Advocacy and awareness organization for young women who are diagnosed with breast cancer. Offers support, information and education.

SURGERY

Breast Cancer Network of Strength

1-800-221-2141 (24-Hour Hotline-English)

1-800-986-9505 (24-Hour Hotline-Spanish)

www.networkofstrength.org

Gives referral information to major cancer treatment centers for second opinions or treatments not offered in some localities.

Caring Connections

www.caringinfo.org/stateaddownload

Provides free advance directives and instructions for each state.

SURVIVORSHIP MAGAZINES

Breast Cancer Wellness

www.breastcancerwellness.org

The mission of the magazine is to empower the mind, body and spirit of women diagnosed with breast cancer. Offers a paid subscription.

Coping With Cancer

www.copingmag.com

Magazine for people whose lives have been touched by cancer. Offers a paid subscription.

CURE

www.curetoday.com

CURE provides information on recent advancements in diagnosis, treatment and prevention of cancer. Offers a free subscription.

SURVIVORSHIP RESOURCES

Imaginis

www.imaginis.com

Provides education and the latest news in breast cancer for professionals and patients. Sign up for the online newsletter to receive the latest news and breast cancer information.

Reach To Recovery

www.cancer.org
Search: Reach To Recovery

American Cancer Society program offers in-home visits from volunteers. Volunteers will share helpful information for recovery, including range of motion exercises for the surgical arm.

Survivorship A-Z: Practical Information for Living Successfully After a Diagnosis

www.survivorshipatoz.org

Provides practical information survivors need to thrive in the new normal that exists after a life-changing diagnosis.

References

American Cancer Society Consumer's Guide to Cancer Drugs
Wilkes, G., R.N., M.S., A.O.C.N., and Ades, T., R.N., M.S., A.O.C.N.,
Sudbury, Massachusetts: Jones and Bartlett Publishers, 2003.

American Joint Committee on Cancer (AJCC)
https://cancerstaging.org

American Society of Clinical Oncology
http://www.asco.org

Atlas of Breast Surgical Techniques
Kimberg, V. S., Townsend, C. M., Evers, B. M.
St. Louis: Saunders Company, 2010.

The Breast: Comprehensive Management of Benign and Malignant Disorders, Third Edition
Bland, K., M.D., and Copeland, E., III, M.D., St. Louis: Elsevier Science, 2009.

Clinical Practice Guidelines in Oncology: Breast Cancer
National Comprehensive Cancer Network, 2016.
http://www.nccn.org/professionals/physician

Core Curriculum for Oncology Nursing
Itano, J., and Taoka, K., St. Louis: Saunders Company, 2005.

Diseases of the Breast, Fifth Edition
Harris, J., Lippman, M., Morrow, M., and Osborne, C.K., Philadelphia: Wolters Kluwer, 2014.

Ferri's Clinical Advisor 2012: Instant Diagnosis and Treatment
Ferri, F., M.D., F.A.C.P., St. Louis: Mosby, 2012.

Guidelines for Detection, Prevention and Risk Reduction:
Breast Cancer Risk Reduction
National Comprehensive Cancer Network, 2016.
http://www.nccn.org/professionals/physician

Guidelines for Detection, Prevention, and Risk Reduction:
Genetic/Familial High Risk Assessment Breast and Ovarian Cancer
National Comprehensive Cancer Network, 2016.
http://www.nccn.org/professionals/physician

REFERENCES

Kuerer's Breast Surgical Oncology
Kuerer, Henry M., M.D., Ph.D., F.A.C.S., Houston: McGraw-Hill Companies, 2010.

Pocket Radiologist: Breast
Birdwell, R., M.D., Philadelphia: Saunders, 2003.

Psycho-oncology
Holland, J., M.D., New York: Oxford University Press, 2010.

Glossary

It is important to understand the medical terminology related to your diagnosis and treatments. The following is a list of the most common medical terms used in breast cancer. If you do not understand the technical language used by your doctors or nurses, ask them to explain what they mean. Understanding these terms will enable you to make more informed decisions.

A

ABSCESS — A collection of pus from an infection.

ABSOLUTE RISK REDUCTION — Absolute number of patients who will benefit from a treatment.

ACCELERATED BREAST RADIATION — External beam radiation delivered to the breast at a higher dose over a shorter period of time than traditional radiation. Reduces treatment time to three weeks.

ACELLULAR DERMAL MATRIX — Donated human skin processed to remove any cells that cause a rejection response when used as a skin graft. Eliminates need for skin graft and harvesting surgery for breast reconstruction procedures. Used in expander-implant reconstruction, direct-to-implant reconstruction and in breast reconstruction revision procedures when additional tissue is required.

ACINI — The parts of the breast gland where fluid or milk is produced (singular: acinus).

ACUTE — Occurring suddenly or over a short period of time.

ADENOCARCINOMA — A form of cancer that involves cells from the lining of the walls of many different organs of the body. Breast cancer is a type of adenocarcinoma.

ADJUVANT TREATMENT — Treatment that is added to increase the effectiveness of a primary treatment. In cancer, adjuvant treatment usually refers to chemotherapy, targeted therapy, hormonal therapy or radiation therapy after surgery to increase the likelihood of killing all cancer cells.

ALKYLATING AGENT — Type of chemotherapy drug used in cancer treatment.

ALLERGIC REACTION — Various physical symptoms that may include rash, hives, itching, nasal congestion, watery and red eyes, swelling of the throat or difficulty breathing that occur when the body reacts to a substance that it is exposed to or that is ingested.

ALOPECIA — Refers to hair loss as a result of chemotherapy or radiation therapy administered to the head. Hair loss from chemotherapy is temporary. Hair loss from radiation therapy may be permanent.

ALTERNATIVE MEDICINE — Treatment used instead of standard treatments. They generally are not recognized by the medical community as standard or conventional medical approaches.

AMENORRHEA — Absence or discontinuation of menstrual periods.

ANALGESIC — Medicine given to control pain; for example: Aspirin or Tylenol®.

ANEMIA — Condition marked by a decrease in the blood component hemoglobin; causes symptoms of fatigue, weakness, dizziness, inability to concentrate and shortness of breath. Many chemotherapy drugs cause a reduction in hemoglobin levels.

ANESTHESIA — Medication that causes entire or partial loss of feeling or sensation.

ANESTHESIOLOGIST — A doctor who specializes in giving drugs to prevent or relieve pain during surgery or other procedures.

ANDROGEN — A male sex hormone. Androgens may be used in patients with breast cancer to treat recurrence of the disease.

ANEUPLOID — The characteristic of having either fewer or more than the normal number of chromosomes in a cell. This is an abnormal cell.

ANGIOGENESIS — Development of new blood vessels (angio=vessel; genesis=new). Caused by secretion of an enzyme from a malignant tumor. Process called neovascularization (neo=new; vascularization=abnormal blood vessel formation).

ANOREXIA — Severe, uncontrolled loss of appetite.

ANTIEMETIC — A medicine that prevents or relieves nausea and vomiting; used during, and sometimes after, chemotherapy.

ANTIMETABOLITES — Anticancer drugs that interfere with the process of DNA production, thus preventing cell division.

AREOLA — The circular field of dark-colored skin surrounding the nipple.

AROMATASE INHIBITOR — Drugs that block production of estradiol, a female hormone. Given to women who have positive estrogen receptors to block production of estradiol and lower potential of recurrence.

ASPIRATION — Removal of fluid or cells from tissue by inserting a needle into an area and drawing the fluid into the syringe.

ASYMPTOMATIC — Without obvious signs or symptoms of disease. While cancer may cause symptoms and warning signs, it may develop and grow without producing any symptoms, especially in its early stages.

ATYPICAL CELLS — Not usual; abnormal. Cancer is the result of atypical cell division.

AUTOLOGOUS — Tissue from your own body.

AXILLA — The armpit.

AXILLARY DISSECTION — Surgical removal of lymph nodes from the armpit. The removed nodes are sent to a pathologist to determine if the breast cancer has spread outside of the breast.

AXILLARY NODES — Lymph nodes in the axilla. These nodes may be cut out and examined during surgery to see if the cancer has spread past the breast. The number of nodes in this area varies.

AXILLARY SAMPLING — Procedure that removes lymph nodes under the arm during breast cancer surgery to evaluate whether cancer is present.

B

BENIGN TUMOR — An abnormal growth that is not cancerous and does not spread to other parts of the body.

BILATERAL — Pertains to both sides of the body. For example, bilateral breast cancer would be on both sides of the body or in both breasts.

BIOLOGICAL RESPONSE MODIFIER — Treatment that alters the body's natural response to stimulate bone marrow to make specific blood cells. Referred to as a colony-stimulating factor.

BIOPSY — The surgical removal of a small piece of tissue or a small tumor for microscopic examination to determine whether cancer cells are present. A biopsy is the most important procedure in diagnosing cancer.

BIOTHERAPY — Treatments used to stimulate the body's immune system.

BLOOD COUNT — *See Complete Blood Count*

BONE MARROW — The soft, fatty substance filling the cavities of the bones. Blood cells are manufactured in the bone marrow. Chemotherapy affects the bone marrow, resulting in a temporary decrease in the number of cells in the blood.

BONE MARROW BIOPSY AND ASPIRATION — A procedure in which a needle is inserted into the center of a bone, usually the hip, to remove a small amount of bone marrow for microscopic examination.

BONE SCAN — A procedure in which a trace amount of radioactive substance is injected into the bloodstream to illuminate the bones. A special camera is used to see if the cancer has spread to the bones.

BRACHYTHERAPY — Radiation therapy administered by placement of radioactive seeds directly into the site of the removed tumor after breast cancer surgery. Also called interstitial radiation therapy.

BRCA 1 AND BRCA 2 — Genes identified to increase risk of hereditary breast cancer.

BREAST CANCER — A potentially fatal tumor, because of its ability to leave the breast and go to other vital organs. Will continue to grow if it is not removed from the body. These are breast cells that are abnormal with uncontrolled growth.

BREAST IMPLANT — A round or teardrop-shaped sac inserted into the body to restore the shape of the breast. May be filled with saline water or synthetic material.

BREAST-CONSERVING SURGERY — *See Lumpectomy*

BREAST MASTOPEXY — Surgery to lift the opposite breast to match contour of the reconstructed breast

BREAST SELF-EXAM (BSE) — A procedure to examine the breasts thoroughly once a month to detect any changes or suspicious lumps.

C

CALCIFICATIONS — Calcium deposits in breast tissue seen on mammography. Deposits are the result of cell death. Occurs with benign and malignant changes.

CANCER — A general term used to describe more than 100 different uncontrolled growths of abnormal cells in the body. Cancer cells have the ability to continue to grow, invade and destroy surrounding tissue, leave the original site and travel via lymph or blood systems to other parts of the body where they can set up new cancerous tumors.

CANCER CELL — A cell that divides and reproduces abnormally with uncontrolled growth. This cell can break away and travel to other parts of the body and set up another site; this is referred to as metastasis.

CAPSULAR CONTRACTURE — Fibrous tissues that form around an implant and cause changes in the shape of the implant and may cause pain.

CARDIOLOGIST — Physician specializing in heart disease.

CLAVICLE — The collarbone.

CARCINOEMBRYONIC ANTIGEN (CEA) — A blood test used to monitor women with metastatic breast cancer to help determine whether the treatment is working.

CARCINOGEN — Any substance that initiates or promotes the development of cancer. Example: Asbestos is a proven carcinogen.

CARCINOMA — A form of cancer that develops in tissues covering or lining organs of the body, such as the skin, uterus, lung or breast.

CARCINOMA IN SITU — An early stage of development, when the cancer is still confined to the tissues of origin and has not spread outside the area. In situ carcinomas are highly curable.

CELL — The basic structural unit of all life. All living matter is composed of cells.

CELLULITIS — Infection occurring in soft tissues. The surgical arm has an increased risk for cellulitis due to the removal of lymph nodes. Pain, swelling and warmth occur in the area.

CHEMOTHERAPY — Treatment of cancer by use of chemicals. Usually refers to drugs used to treat cancer.

CLINICAL TRIAL — A scientific study, generally involving a large number of test subjects (or patients), that is conducted to prove or determine the effectiveness of a drug or treatment program.

COBRA — Consolidated Omnibus Budget Reconciliation Act of 1985. A health insurance available if you are terminated or laid off from your job. Insurance remains in effect for a period of 18 months after the job is terminated.

COMBINATION CHEMOTHERAPY — Treatment consisting of two or more chemicals to achieve maximum kill of tumor cells.

COMBINED MODALITY THERAPY — Two or more types of treatments used to supplement each other. For instance, surgery, radiation, chemotherapy, targeted therapy, hormonal therapy or immunotherapy may be used separately or together for maximum effectiveness.

COMPLEMENTARY THERAPY — Treatment often used to enhance or complement standard treatments. Example: Massage therapy.

COMPLETE BLOOD COUNT (CBC) — A test to determine the number of red blood cells, white blood cells, platelets, hemoglobin and other components of a blood sample.

CONTRALATERAL BREAST — Opposite, nonsurgical breast.

CONTRAST AGENT — Compounds used to improve the visibility of internal bodily structures during an X-ray image or an MRI.

COOPER'S LIGAMENTS — Flexible fibrous elastic bands of tissue passing from the chest muscle into the breast tissues between the lobes of the breasts, providing shape and support for the breasts.

CORE BIOPSY — Removal (with a large needle) of a section (core) of a lump. The core is sent to a lab to see if the lump is benign or malignant.

COSMESIS — Final appearance of a breast.

CT SCAN OR CAT SCAN — An imaging exam that uses X-rays to create cross-sectional pictures of the body. These specialized X-ray studies detect cancer or metastasis.

CYST — An abnormal sac-like structure that contains liquid or semi-solid material; is usually benign. Lumps in the breast are often found to be harmless cysts.

CYTOLOGY — The study of cells that have been sloughed off, cut out or scraped off organs; cells are microscopically examined for signs of cancer.

CYTOTOXIC — Drugs that can cause the death of cancer cells. Usually refers to drugs used in chemotherapy treatments.

D

DELAYED RECONSTRUCTION — Reconstruction performed at any time after breast cancer surgery.

DEPRESSION — A mental condition marked by ongoing feelings of sadness, despair, loss of energy, difficulty dealing with normal daily life, feelings of worthlessness and hopelessness, loss of pleasure in activities, changes in eating or sleeping habits, and thoughts of death or suicide.

DETECTION — The discovery of an abnormality in an asymptomatic or symptomatic person.

DEXA SCAN — Dual Energy X-ray Absorptiometric scan. An imaging test that measures bone density to diagnose osteoporosis.

DIAGNOSIS — The process of identifying a disease by its characteristic signs, symptoms and laboratory findings. With cancer, the earlier the diagnosis is made, the better the chance for a cure.

DIAPHANOGRAPHY (DPG) — A non-invasive procedure (no cutting) that uses ordinary light as an investigative tool to detect breast masses. Also called transillumination.

DIEP RECONSTRUCTION — A type of breast reconstruction in which blood vessels called Deep Inferior Epigastric Perforators (DIEP) are removed with the skin and fat connected to them from the lower abdomen. Muscle is not used.

DIFFERENTIATED — The similarity between a normal cell and the cancer cell; defines what degree of change has occurred. Cancer cells that are well differentiated are close to the original cell and are usually less aggressive. Poorly differentiated cells have changed more and are more aggressive.

DIPLOID — The characteristic of having two sets of chromosomes in a cell. This is normal for a breast cell.

DISTANT RECURRENCE — When cancer recurs in a distant site, such as the bones, lungs, liver, brain or other sites in the body.

DNA — One of two nucleic acids (the other is RNA) found in the nucleus of all cells. DNA contains genetic information on cell growth, division and cell function.

DOSE-DENSE CHEMOTHERAPY — Same amount (dose) of chemotherapy drugs given in a shorter period of time. Usually every two weeks rather than every three weeks.

DOUBLING TIME — The time required for a cell to double in number. Breast cancer has been shown to double in size every 23 to 209 days. It would take one cell, doubling every 100 days, eight to ten years to reach one centimeter ($\frac{3}{8}$ inch, or the size of the tip of your small finger).

DUCTAL CARCINOMA IN SITU (DCIS) — A cancer inside the ducts of the breast that has not grown through the wall of the duct into the surrounding tissues. Sometimes referred to as a precancer. In situ cancers have a good prognosis.

DUCTAL PAPILLOMAS — Small, noncancerous, finger-like growths in the mammary ducts that may cause a bloody nipple discharge. Commonly found in women 45 to 50 years of age.

E

EDEMA — Excess fluid in the body or a body part that is described as swollen or puffy.

ENDOCRINE MANIPULATION — Treating breast cancer by changing the hormonal balance of the body to prevent hormone-dependent cancer cells from multiplying.

ESTROGEN — A female hormone, secreted by the ovaries; essential for menstruation, reproduction and the development of secondary sex characteristics, such as breasts.

ESTROGEN RECEPTOR ASSAY (ERA) — A test to reveal if your cancer is estrogen receptor positive or negative. ER positive cancer may be treated with hormonal therapy.

ESTROGEN RECEPTORS (ER) — Describes cells that have a protein to which the hormone estrogen will bind. Cancer cells that are estrogen receptor positive require estrogen to grow.

ESTROGEN REPLACEMENT THERAPY — Estrogen hormone derived from plant or animal sources that replaces estrogen in a woman's body after natural or chemical menopause.

EXCISIONAL BIOPSY — Surgical removal of a lump or suspicious tissue by cutting the skin and removing the tissue.

EXTERNAL BEAM RADIATION — High dose of X-ray beams delivered to the site of cancer by a machine called a linear accelerator.

F

FAMILIAL CANCER — Cancer occurring in families more frequently than would be expected by chance.

FAMILY AND MEDICAL LEAVE ACT (FMLA) — Law that allows eligible employees to take up to 12 work weeks in any 12-month period off from work for personal illness.

FATIGUE — A condition marked by extreme tiredness and inability to function due to lack of energy.

FAT NECROSIS TUMOR — A hard, noncancerous lump caused by the destruction of fat cells in the breast due to trauma or injury.

FERTILITY — The ability to have children.

FIBROADENOMA — A noncancerous, solid tumor most commonly found in younger women.

FIBROCYSTIC BREAST CHANGES OR CONDITION — A noncancerous breast condition in which multiple cysts or lumpy areas develop in one or both breasts. It can be accompanied by discomfort or pain that fluctuates with the menstrual cycle. Large cysts can be treated by aspiration.

FINE NEEDLE ASPIRATION (FNA) — A procedure to remove cells or fluid from tissues using a needle with an empty syringe. Cells or breast fluid, extracted by pulling back on the plunger, are analyzed by a physician.

FLAP NECROSIS — Cell death of flap tissues that have been transplanted from another area of the body during reconstruction; caused by lack of blood supply to the tissues.

FLOW CYTOMETRY — A test done on cancerous tissues to show the aggressiveness of the tumor. It shows how many cells are in the dividing stage at one time, commonly referred to as the "S" phase, and the DNA content of the cancer, referred to as the ploidy. This reveals how rapidly the tumor is growing.

FREE FLAP — Tissues (skin and fat with or without muscle) removed from an area of the body that are cut free from their original blood supply and reattached at the new reconstruction site.

FROZEN SECTION — A technique in which a part of the biopsy tissue is frozen immediately, and a thin slice of frozen tissue is mounted on a microscope slide for a diagnostic examination by a pathologist.

FROZEN SHOULDER — Surgical shoulder which is painful and has a severely restricted range of motion.

G

GALACTOCELE — A clogged milk duct; often associated with childbirth.

GAMMA-DETECTION PROBE — Instrument used during sentinel node biopsy to identify radiation uptake of first nodes that drain a tumor.

GENES — Segments of DNA that contain hereditary information transferred from cell to cell; genes are located in the nucleus of the cell.

GENETIC — Refers to the inherited pattern located in genes for certain characteristics.

GENETIC TESTING — Blood or saliva testing to determine the presence of a gene mutation that increases the risk of hereditary cancer. The most common breast cancer mutations are BRCA1 and BRCA2.

GLUTEAL (GLUTEUS) FLAP — Tissues composed of muscle, fat and blood vessels removed from the buttocks and used to reconstruct the breast.

GLYCEMIC INDEX — Measure of the increase in the level of blood glucose (a type of sugar), caused by eating a specific carbohydrate.

H

HEALTHCARE DIRECTIVES — A written document that instructs others about your healthcare wishes, appoints a healthcare agent and provides specific healthcare instructions, should you be unable to make decisions on your own.

HEMATOMA — A collection of blood that forms in a wound after surgery, aspiration or injury.

HEMOGLOBIN — A component inside red blood cells that binds to oxygen in the lungs and carries it to all of the tissues in the body.

HER2/NEU — Human epidermal growth factor receptor 2 is a protein identified in breast cancer which indicates increased aggressiveness.

HORMONAL THERAPY — Treatment of cancer by alteration of the hormonal balance. Some cancers will only grow in the presence of certain hormones.

HORMONES — Chemicals secreted by various organs in the body that help regulate growth, metabolism and reproduction. Some hormones are used as treatment following surgery for breast, ovarian and prostate cancers.

HORMONE RECEPTOR ASSAY — A diagnostic test to determine whether a breast cancer's growth is influenced by hormones or whether it can be treated with hormones.

HOT FLASHES — A sensation of heat and flushing that occurs suddenly. May be associated with menopause or with some chemotherapy medications.

HYPERPLASIA — An abnormal, excessive growth of cells that is benign.

I

IMMEDIATE RECONSTRUCTION — Breast reconstruction performed immediately after breast cancer surgery.

IMMUNE SYSTEM — A complex system by which the body protects itself from outside invaders that are harmful to the body.

IMMUNOLOGY — The study of the body's mechanisms of resistance against disease and invasion by foreign substances—the body's ability to fight a disease.

IMMUNOTHERAPY — A treatment that stimulates the body's own defense mechanisms to combat diseases, such as cancer.

IMMUNOSUPPRESSED — Condition of having a lowered resistance to disease. May be a temporary result of lowered white blood cell counts from chemotherapy administration.

INCISIONAL BIOPSY — A surgical incision made through the skin to remove a portion of a suspicious lump or tissue.

INFERTILITY — The inability to have children.

INFILTRATING CANCER — Cancer that has grown through the wall of the breast area in which it originated and into surrounding tissues.

INFILTRATING DUCTAL CARCINOMA — A cancer that begins in the mammary duct and has spread to areas outside the duct.

INFILTRATING LOBULAR CARCINOMA — A cancer that originated in a lobule (milk-producing unit of the breast), and has grown through the wall and is infiltrating surrounding tissues.

INFLAMMATION — Reaction of tissue to various conditions that may result in pain, redness or warmth of tissues in the area.

INFLAMMATORY CARCINOMA — Very aggressive cancer in the lymphatics of the breast; requires immediate treatment with chemotherapy for disease control.

INFORMED CONSENT — Process of explaining the risks and complications of a procedure or treatment to the patient before it is performed. Most written informed consents are signed by the patient or a legal representative.

IN SITU CANCER — Cancer that is found only in the duct or lobule where it starts. It has not grown through the duct or lobular wall into surrounding tissue.

INTEGRATIVE MEDICINE — Combination of evidence-based (mainstream) medicine and complementary therapies (massage, yoga, etc.).

INTERNAL BREAST RADIATION — Radiation therapy that places the radiation source inside of the breast for short periods of time; given after breast cancer surgery.

INTERNAL MAMMARY NODES — Lymph nodes located in the area near the breastbone.

INTRADUCTAL — Residing within the duct of the breast; may be benign or malignant.

INTRAMUSCULAR (I.M.) — To receive a medication by needle injection into a muscle.

INTRAVENOUS (I.V.) — To receive a medication by needle injection into a vein.

INVASIVE CANCER — Cancer that has spread outside its site of origin and is growing into the surrounding tissues.

INVERTED NIPPLE — The turning inward of the nipple. Usually a congenital condition; but, if it occurs where it had not previously existed, it can be a sign of breast cancer.

K

KI-67 — Cell protein that increases prior to cell division. Pathology study measures percentage of positive cells, indicating how quickly a tumor is dividing and forming new cells.

L

LACTATION — Process of being able to produce milk from the breasts.

LATISSIMUS DORSI — Muscle tissue from the back used for breast reconstruction.

LESION — An area of tissue that is diseased.

LEUKOCYTE — A white blood cell or corpuscle.

LEUKOPENIA — A decrease in white blood cells (where the count is less than 5000); increases a person's susceptibility to infection.

LINEAR ACCELERATOR — A machine that produces high-energy X-ray beams to destroy cancer cells.

LIVER SCAN — A small dose of a radioactive substance is injected into the bloodstream, which helps visualize the liver during X-ray.

LIVING WILL — Signed document stating wishes in medical care issues if one is unable to properly communicate or make decisions.

LOBULAR — Pertaining to the part of the breast that is furthest from the nipple, the lobes.

LOCALIZED CANCER — A cancer still confined to its site of origin.

LOCAL RECURRENCE — When cancer returns to the local area of removal. Occurs because surgery or radiation left behind microscopic cells.

LUMP — Any kind of abnormal mass in the breast or elsewhere in the body.

LUMPECTOMY — A surgical procedure in which only the cancerous tumor and an area of surrounding tissue is removed. Usually the surgeon will remove some of the underarm lymph nodes at the same time.

LYMPH — A clear fluid circulating throughout the body in the lymphatic system that contains white blood cells and antibodies.

LYMPH NODES (LYMPH GLANDS) — Rounded body tissues in the lymphatic system that vary in size from a pinhead to an olive. May appear in groups or one at a time. The principal lymph nodes are in the neck, underarm and groin. Lymph nodes are usually sampled during surgery to determine whether the cancer has spread outside of the breast area.

LYMPHATIC VESSELS — Vessels that remove cellular waste from the body by filtering through lymph nodes and eventually emptying into the vascular (blood) system.

LYMPHEDEMA — Swelling in the arm caused by excess fluid that collects after the lymph nodes have been removed by surgery or from fibrosis after radiation treatments.

M

MACROCYST — A cyst that is large enough to be felt with the fingers.

MAGNETIC RESONANCE IMAGING (MRI) — A magnetic scan using magnets instead of radiation. MRI gives a more clearly defined picture of fatty tissue than an X-ray.

MAGNIFICATION VIEW — Special, enlarged mammography views to magnify a specific area for greater detail of suspicious finding.

MALIGNANT TUMOR — A mass of cancer cells. These cells have uncontrolled growth and will invade surrounding tissues and spread to distant sites of the body, setting up new cancer sites; this process is called metastasis.

MAMMARY GLANDS — The breast glands that produce and carry milk, by way of the mammary ducts, to the nipples during breastfeeding.

MAMMOGRAM — An X-ray of the breast that can detect benign and cancerous changes.

MARGINS — The area of tissue surrounding a tumor when it is removed by surgery.

MASTALGIA — Pain occurring in the breast.

MASTECTOMY — Surgical removal of the entire breast, including nipple, areola, lymph nodes and some of the surrounding tissue.

MASTITIS — An infection occurring in the breast. Pain, tenderness, swelling, redness and warmth may be observed. Usually responds to antibiotic treatment.

MENOPAUSE — The time in a woman's life when the menstrual cycle ends and the ovaries produce lower levels of hormones; usually occurs between the ages of 45 and 55.

METASTASIS — The spread of cancer from one part of the body to another through the lymphatic system or the bloodstream. The cells in the new cancer location are the same type as those in the original site.

MICROCALCIFICATIONS — Particles appearing as small spots on a mammogram. Usually occur from calcium deposits caused by death of breast cells that may be benign or malignant. When clustered in one area, may need to be checked more closely for a malignant change in the breast.

MICROCYST — A cyst that is too small to be felt but may be observed on mammography or ultrasound screening.

MICROINVASION — Most often used to describe early infiltration of ductal carcinoma (DCIS) into surrounding tissue; measures 1.0 mm or less.

MICROMETASTASIS — Area of cancer that has spread from original tumor (metastasized); measures between 0.2 to 2.0 mm in size.

MITOTIC RATE — Rate of cell division and growth of a cancerous tumor.

MODIFIED RADICAL MASTECTOMY — The most common type of mastectomy. Breast skin, nipple, areola and underarm lymph nodes are removed. The chest muscles are saved.

MULTICENTRIC — Describes cancers or suspicious microcalcifications located in more than one quarter (quadrant) of the breast.

MULTIFOCAL — Describes cancers or suspicious microcalcifications located within one quarter (quadrant) of the breast.

MYELOSUPPRESSION — A decrease in the ability of the bone marrow cells to produce blood cells, including red blood cells, white blood cells and platelets. This condition increases susceptibility to infection, increases risk of bleeding and produces fatigue.

N

NADIR — The time after chemotherapy when blood cell counts reach their lowest levels. According to the type of blood cells affected by different drugs, an increase in infection, fatigue and bleeding occur.

NECROSIS — Death of a tissue.

NEEDLE BIOPSY — Removal of a sample of tissue from the breast using a large-core needle.

NEEDLE LOCALIZATION — *See Wire Localization*

NEGATIVE NODES — Lymph nodes that do not have evidence of cancer after surgical removal and pathological evaluation.

NEOADJUVANT CHEMOTHERAPY — Chemotherapy given before surgery to treat breast cancer.

NEOPLASM — Any abnormal growth. May be benign or malignant, but the term is usually used to describe a cancer.

NEUTROPENIA — Low blood count values of neutrophil cells (type of white blood cells that fight infection); increases potential for infections.

NIPPLE-SPARING MASTECTOMY — Surgery that removes all of the breast tissue without removing the nipple, areola or breast skin.

NODULARITY — Increased density of breast tissue, most often due to hormonal changes; causes the breast to feel lumpy in texture. This finding is called normal nodularity and usually occurs in both breasts.

NODULE — A small, solid mass.

NON-STEROIDAL ANTI-INFLAMMATORY (NSAID) — Drug that decreases fever, swelling, pain and redness. Ibuprofen (Advil®, Motrin®), naproxen sodium (Aleve®) or aspirin (Ascriptin®, Bayer®, Ecotrin®).

NUCLEAR GRADE — An evaluation of the size and shape of the nucleus in tumor cells and the percentage of tumor cells that are in the process of dividing or growing.

O

ONCOGENE — Certain stretches of cellular DNA. Genes that, when inappropriately activated, contribute to the malignant transformation of a cell.

ONCOLOGIST — A physician who specializes in cancer treatment.

ONCOLOGY — The science dealing with the physical, chemical and biological properties and features of cancer, including causes, the disease process and therapies.

ONCOTYPE DX® — Test performed by evaluating known genes in tumor cells of women with early stage breast cancer to assess the potential for breast cancer recurrence and the need for chemotherapy.

ONE-STEP PROCEDURE — A procedure in which a surgical biopsy is performed under general anesthesia. If cancer is found, a mastectomy or lumpectomy is done immediately as part of the same operation.

OOPHORECTOMY — The surgical removal of the ovaries, sometimes performed as a part of treatment for breast cancer to reduce hormonal stimulation.

ORGASM — A state of physical and emotional excitement that occurs at the climax of sexual intercourse.

OSTEOPOROSIS — Softening of bones that occurs with age, calcium loss and hormone depletion; increases risk of bone fractures.

P

PALLIATIVE TREATMENT — Therapy that relieves symptoms, such as pain or pressure, but does not alter the development of the disease. Its primary purpose is to improve the quality of life.

PALPATION — A procedure using the hands to examine organs such as the breast. A palpable mass is one that you can feel with your hands.

PATHOLOGIST — A physician with special training in diagnosing diseases from samples of tissue under a microscope.

PATHOLOGY — The study of disease through the microscopic examination of body tissues and organs. Any tumor suspected of being cancerous must be diagnosed by pathological examination.

PECTORALIS MUSCLES — Muscular tissues attached to the front of the chest wall and extending to the upper arms. These are under the breast and are divided into the pectoralis major and pectoralis minor muscles.

PEDICLE FLAP — Tissues to reconstruct the breast that are taken from another area of the body, such as the stomach, buttocks or back, and remain attached to their original blood supply.

PER ORALLY (P.O.) — To take a medication by mouth.

PERMANENT SECTION — A technique in which a thin slice of biopsy tissue is mounted on a slide to be examined under a microscope by a pathologist in order to establish a diagnosis.

PHLEBITIS — Inflammation in a vein or veins.

PHYTOCHEMICALS — Chemical components found in plants (vegetables, fruits and nuts) that have a beneficial effect on health.

PLATELET — A cell formed by the bone marrow and circulating in the blood that is necessary for blood clotting. Platelet transfusions are used in cancer patients to prevent or control bleeding when the number of platelets has decreased.

PLOIDY — The number of chromosome sets in a cell.

PORT, LIFE PORT, PORT-A-CATH — A device surgically implanted under the skin, usually on the chest, that enters a large blood vessel and is used to deliver medication, chemotherapy, blood products and is also used to obtain blood samples. A port is usually inserted if a person has veins in the arm that are difficult to use for treatment or if certain types of chemotherapy drugs are to be given.

POSITIVE NODES — Lymph nodes removed during surgery that have cancer cells present after being studied by a pathologist.

PRECANCEROUS — Abnormal cellular changes that are potentially capable of becoming cancer. These early lesions usually respond well to treatment and cure. Also called pre-malignant.

PRIMARY TUMOR — First or original site of a cancer.

PROGESTERONE — Female hormone produced by the ovaries during a specific time in the menstrual cycle. Causes the uterus to prepare for pregnancy and the breasts to get ready to produce milk.

PROGESTERONE RECEPTOR ASSAY (PRA) — A test that is performed on cancerous tissue to determine whether breast cancer is progesterone hormone dependent and can be treated by hormonal therapy.

PROGESTERONE RECEPTORS (PR) — A receptor protein in breast cells to which progesterone will attach. Breast cancer cells that are PR+ depend on the hormone progesterone to grow and usually respond well to hormonal therapy.

PROGNOSIS — A prediction of the course of the disease; the future prospect for the patient.

PROPHYLACTIC MASTECTOMY — A preventative procedure sometimes recommended for patients at a very high risk for developing cancer in one or both breasts.

PROSTHESIS — An artificial breast form that can be worn inside a bra.

PROTOCOL — A schedule of selected drugs and treatment time intervals known to be effective against a certain cancer.

PTOSIS — The natural drooping of an organ, such as the breast, caused by aging.

Q

QUACKERY — Treatments, drugs or devices that claim to prevent, diagnose or cure diseases (including cancer) that are known to be false or have no proven scientific evidence on which to base their claims.

R

RADICAL MASTECTOMY (HALSTED RADICAL) — The surgical removal of the breast, breast skin, nipple, areola, chest muscles and underarm lymph nodes.

RADIATION ONCOLOGIST — A physician specifically trained in the use of high energy X-rays to treat cancer.

RADIATION THERAPY (RADIOTHERAPY)— Treatment of cancer with high-energy X-ray radiation. Radiation therapy may be used to reduce the size of a cancer before surgery or to destroy any remaining cancer cells after surgery. Radiation therapy can be helpful in shrinking recurrent cancer to relieve symptoms such as pain and pressure.

RADIOLOGIST — A physician who specializes in diagnoses of diseases by the use of X-rays.

RANGE OF MOTION — The normal movement capability of a limb; measured in degrees of a circle.

RECONSTRUCTION — The rebuilding of the breast mound after surgical removal. Surgery is performed by a reconstructive surgeon using implants or body tissues.

RECURRENCE — Reappearance of cancer after a period of remission.

RED BLOOD CELLS — Portion of the blood that carries oxygen to cells in the body.

REGIONAL RECURRENCE — The spread of cancer outside the breast. This spread may be to the underarm lymph nodes, chest muscles, internal mammary nodes located under the breastbone or to the nodes above the collarbone.

REHABILITATION — Programs that help patients adjust and return to full, productive lives. May involve physical therapy, the use of a prosthesis, counseling and emotional support.

RELAPSE — The reappearance of cancer after a disease-free period.

RELATIVE RISK REDUCTION — Figures derived by taking the absolute number of women benefiting from a therapy and translating it into a percentage of increase or decrease.

REMISSION — Complete or partial disappearance of the signs and symptoms of disease in response to treatment. The period during which a disease is under control. Remission, however, is not necessarily a cure.

RETRACTION (DIMPLING) — The process of skin pulling in toward breast tissue.

RISK FACTORS — Anything that increases an individual's chance of getting a disease such as cancer. Example: Having a first-degree relative with breast cancer.

RISK REDUCTION — Techniques used to reduce your chances of getting a certain cancer.

S

S PHASE — A test that is performed to determine how many cells within the tumor are in a stage of division.

SALINE — Substance containing salt.

SARCOMA — A form of cancer that arises in the supportive tissues, such as bone, cartilage, fat or muscle.

SECONDARY SITE — A second site in which cancer is found. Example: Cancer in the lymph nodes near the breast is a secondary site.

SECONDARY TUMOR — A tumor that develops as a result of metastasis or spreads beyond the original cancer.

SENTINEL LYMPH NODE MAPPING — A procedure that uses radioactive contrast agent or blue dye to identify the first nodes draining a cancerous tumor.

SENTINEL LYMPH NODE(S) — First identified node or nodes that drain lymphatic fluid from a cancerous tumor.

SERMS (SELECTIVE ESTROGEN RECEPTOR MODULATORS) — Antihormonal drugs that can slow down or stop the growth of cancers that need estrogen to grow. Drugs in this group include tamoxifen, toremifene and raloxifene.

SEROMA — Collection of fluid (noncancerous) under the skin that feels soft and spongy.

SIDE EFFECTS — Usually describes situations that occur after treatments. Example: Hair loss may be a side effect of chemotherapy; fatigue may be a side effect of radiation therapy.

SKIN-SPARING MASTECTOMY — Mastectomy that spares the skin for reconstruction but removes the nipple and areola. Most commonly used for DCIS or prophylactic mastectomy.

SPICULATED — Describes the shape of a tumor margin that has long needle-like protrusions into surrounding tissues.

SSRIs (SELECTIVE SEROTONIN REUPTAKE INHIBITORS) — A class of drugs that increases serotonin in the brain. Used in the treatment of depression.

STAGING — An evaluation of the extent of a disease, such as breast cancer. A classification based on stage at diagnosis, which helps to determine the appropriate treatment and prognosis. In breast cancer, the classification is determined by whether the lymph nodes are involved; whether the cancer has spread to other parts of the body (through the lymphatic system or bloodstream) and set up distant metastasis; and the size of the tumor. Five different stages (0 – 4) are used in breast cancer with levels in each stage. Stage 4 is the most serious.

STELLATE — Appearing on mammography as a star-shape because of the irregular growth of cells into surrounding tissue. May be associated with a malignancy or some benign conditions.

STEREOTACTIC NEEDLE BIOPSY (STEREOTACTIC CORE BIOPSY) — A biopsy done while the breast is compressed under mammography. A series of pictures locate the lesion, and a radiologist enters information into a computer. The computer positions a needle to remove the finding. A needle is inserted into the lump, and a piece of tissue is removed and sent to a lab for analysis.

STOMATITIS — Inflammation of the gastrointestinal tract that causes discomfort and a potential for infection. May be caused by chemotherapy drugs or radiation.

SUBCUTANEOUS (S.Q. OR S.C.) — To receive a medication by needle injection into the fatty tissues of the body.

SUPRACLAVICULAR NODES — The nodes located above the collarbone in the area of the neck.

SYMPTOMS — Changes you can feel that may or may not be visible to others.

SYSTEMIC — Pertaining to the whole body.

T

TAMOXIFEN — Anti-estrogen drug given to women with estrogen-receptive tumors to block estrogen from entering the breast tissues. May produce menopause-like symptoms, including hot flashes and vaginal dryness. Currently being used with high-risk women in clinical trials to prevent breast cancer and with women who have had breast cancer to prevent recurrence.

TARGETED THERAPY — Treatment attacks only a specific cell characteristic. Example: Herceptin targets only HER2 cells on a HER2 positive cancer.

TESTOSTERONE — Major male hormone found in lower amounts in females. Testosterone in females increases the sex drive and impacts the ability to experience orgasm.

THROMBOCYTOPENIA — A decrease in the number of platelets in the blood, resulting in the potential for increased bleeding and decreased ability for clotting.

TISSUE — A collection of similar cells. There are four basic types of tissues in the body: epithelial, connective, muscle and nerve.

TISSUE EXPANDER — A balloon-like device placed under the chest muscle, gradually filled with saline water over several months to stretch the muscle. The expander is removed when the muscle is stretched to the size required for the permanent implant placement.

TRAM (TRANSVERSE RECTUS ABDOMINIS MUSCLE) — Tissue that is used to reconstruct a breast using the major stomach muscle attached to its original blood supply.

TREATMENT MODALITIES — Different types of treatment. Example: Surgery, chemotherapy, radiation therapy and hormonal therapy.

TRIPLE NEGATIVE BREAST CANCER — Breast tumor that tests negative for three receptors: estrogen, progesterone and HER2.

TUMOR — An abnormal tissue, swelling or mass; may be either benign or malignant.

TUMOR GROWTH RATE — Time required for a specific tumor to double in size. Same type of tumor varies in time from person to person.

TWO-STEP PROCEDURE — When surgical biopsy and breast surgery are performed in two separate surgeries.

U

ULTRASOUND EXAMINATION — The use of high frequency sound waves to locate a tumor inside the body. Helps determine if a breast lump is solid tissue or filled with fluids.

ULTRASOUND GUIDED BIOPSY — The use of ultrasound to guide a biopsy needle to obtain a sample of tissue for analysis by a pathologist.

V

VACUUM-ASSISTED BIOPSY — Biopsy procedure in which an instrument cuts tissues and uses a vacuum to withdraw them into a container.

W

WET/MOIST DESQUAMATION — Condition where the top layers of the skin peel or slough off, exposing red, tender skin that oozes fluid. May occur in late stages of radiation therapy.

WHITE BLOOD CELLS — Components of the blood, also known as leukocytes, that are able to kill bacteria and other invaders in the body. Low white blood cell count—identified after a complete blood count is performed—causes one to be more susceptible to infections.

WIRE LOCALIZATION — Placement of a fine wire(s) to mark the location of nonpalpable tumor or DCIS for surgical removal. The wire is placed by a radiologist under mammography or ultrasound guidance to locate the specific area. The wire is secured in place and later removed by the surgeon.

Index

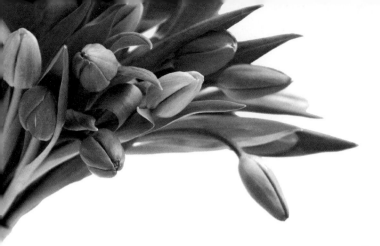

Tear-Out Worksheets

The following tear-out worksheets are designed to help you custom-manage your cancer experience. You may wish to tear the worksheets out and place them in a notebook to carry to physician appointments.

Cancer Can't Rob Me

Today is another new day, and I can choose to use it in many ways. I did not choose to have cancer, but I can choose how I am going to respond and what I plan to do with today. Today is mine to make choices. This day can be a new beginning for me, if I so choose.

Today can be the day that I decide to exchange those things which weigh my spirit down for a lighter load of faith and trust. I can change my perception of cancer as a robber of my health and my future and change it into a vehicle to transport me into a life rich in understanding. This understanding will strengthen me and make me valuable to others who will walk the same path after me.

I can choose:

◊ To see cancer as a challenge instead of as a defeat.
◊ To demystify cancer by learning about my disease, rather than cowering in fear of the unknown.
◊ To give up concentrating on the things I can't control and replace them with thoughts of what I can control.
◊ To respond with a spirit of "I can" instead of "I can't."
◊ To ask for help and not try to face the challenge alone.
◊ To face my fears with a plan for steps of action against them.
◊ To look for the blessings in the events of today, instead of focusing on losses.
◊ To add to my life the things I have always wanted to do but postponed until the right time.

Today is the time:

◊ To use my spiritual faith as a vehicle to understand why and to give me hope.
◊ To let go of anger, bitterness and resentments, which only slow down my recovery.
◊ To see my cancer experience as a new tool for personal growth.
◊ To offer my support and share what I'm learning with others who may need my help.

Therefore, I choose for today:

◊ Peace and not anxiety.
◊ Good and not evil.
◊ Love and not hate.
◊ Gain and not loss.

When today becomes tomorrow, this day will be gone forever, leaving in its place what I choose today. I, alone, can choose to use today wisely —

Cancer can't rob me of this day!

— Judy Kneece, RN, OCN

PATIENT TREATMENT BARRIERS ASSESSMENT   WORKSHEET

Patient Name:_____   **Date:** _____

Listed below are obstacles (barriers) that may prevent you from getting the healthcare you need during your cancer treatment. It is essential that your healthcare team understand your needs. This sheet is designed to help you identify your current situation. Please read the following list and mark the items that identify your present situation. Return this sheet to the physician.

Communication

☐ Primary language other than English   Language: _____

☐ Cannot read or write

☐ Hearing Obstacle: ○ Hard of Hearing   ○ Hearing Aid   ○ Deaf

☐ Vision Obstacle: ○ Vision Impairment   ○ Blind

☐ Problems understanding medical language

☐ Problems filling out medical forms

☐ No telephone

☐ No permanent address

☐ Other: _____

Financial

☐ Insurance: ○ No Insurance   ○ Underinsured

☐ Pre-existing financial debts or obligations impacting decisions

☐ No funds for food

☐ No paid leave from work for illness

☐ Prescription medication assistance needed

☐ Medical equipment or supplies assistance needed

☐ Other: _____

Transportation

☐ No transportation available

☐ Public transportation needed

☐ No funds for public transportation

☐ Other: _____

Family Care

☐ Child care during treatment needed

☐ Responsible for older adults living in my home

☐ Housing

☐ Other: _____

Patient Name: _____ Date: _____

Personal Care

☐ Need home care assistance for eating, bathing, dressing, toileting and/or walking

☐ Need prosthesis

☐ Need wig

☐ Need medical equipment

☐ Need help with nutrition

☐ Need help learning new job skills

☐ Other: _____

Coping

☐ I have a history of coping difficulties (depression or anxiety).

☐ I am presently under the care of a: ○ Counselor   ○ Psychologist   ○ Psychiatrist

☐ I have no personal support system at home.

☐ I would like to speak with a spiritual leader. My faith: _____

☐ I am concerned about the impact of my diagnosis on my present career or occupation.

☐ Other: _____

Treatment

☐ I would like a second opinion.

☐ I do not understand how treatment decisions will be made.

☐ I do not understand my treatment plan recommendation.

☐ I have religious beliefs that need to be considered by my healthcare team during treatment:
   ○ Blood transfusions   ○ Narcotics for pain control   ○ Medications containing alcohol   ○ Abortion

☐ I have questions that need to be answered by a: ○ Doctor   ○ Nurse

☐ Other: _____

Cultural

☐ I have citizenship problems.

☐ Other: _____

MANAGING MY FEARS

In the first column, list all of the fears and worries you are presently facing. In the second column, list the name of the most appropriate person with whom to verbalize these fears. In the third column, think about and list things you can do to change or reduce these fears.

Fears	Person(s) Involved	Things I Can Do

"You can gain strength, courage and confidence by every experience in which you really stop to look fear in the face. The danger lies in refusing to face the fear, in not daring to come to grips with it. You must do something you think you cannot do."

—Eleanor Roosevelt

"Nothing in life is to be feared; it is only to be understood. Now is the time to understand more, so that we may fear less."

—Marie Curie

MANAGING MY FEARS

Fears	Person(s) Involved	Things I Can Do

"Fear comes as a warning sign that we do not understand how to solve a problem we are facing. We confront fear when we acknowledge its presence and seek to understand what we need to do about the fear. We diminish a fear when we act."

—Judy C. Kneece

"I learned that courage was not the absence of fear, but the triumph over it. The brave man is not he who does not feel afraid, but he who conquers that fear."

—Nelson Mandela

"To fight fear—ACT. To increase fear—wait, put off, postpone."

—David Joseph Schwartz

Check the questions you would like to have answered.
Tear out this sheet and take it to your surgical consultation.

Surgeon's Name: _____ **Date:** _____

General Questions

☐ What is the name of the type of breast cancer I have?

☐ How large is the tumor?

☐ Is the tumor in situ (inside ducts or lobules) or invasive (has grown through walls of ducts or lobules)?

☐ Do you think cancer cells may be found in my lymph nodes?

☐ Do you think the cancer has invaded anything else (skin, muscle, bones, other organs)?

☐ Is there any evidence from my mammogram that there might be cancer anywhere else in this breast or in the opposite breast?

☐ Does my type of cancer have an increased risk of being found in the same breast or occurring, at a future time, in the opposite breast?

Additional Questions:

_____

_____

Lumpectomy Questions

☐ Am I a candidate for a lumpectomy?
If so, how do you expect my breast to appear after surgery, considering the size of the lump and tissue you need to remove compared to the size of my breast, or the position of the lump in the breast?

☐ Do you think the cosmetic results will be acceptable?

☐ Am I a candidate for sentinel lymph node biopsy?
If so, do you evaluate the removed sentinel lymph node(s) for cancer during surgery or after surgery?

☐ Will you remove lymph nodes by a separate incision under my arm?

☐ What do you consider the advantages and disadvantages of a lumpectomy for my case?

☐ Will a lumpectomy give me the same chance for control of my cancer as a mastectomy?

☐ Will I need to have radiation therapy after a lumpectomy?

☐ Will my surgery require hospitalization?

☐ Will I have drains in the incision after surgery? If so, will I go home with drains?

☐ When do you expect the drains to be removed?

☐ How long will I need to be away from my job?

Additional Questions:

_____

_____

Mastectomy Questions

- ☐ Which type of mastectomy do you plan to perform? (Refer to *Chapter 7: Surgical Treatment Decisions*)
- ☐ What do you think are the advantages and disadvantages of having a mastectomy?
- ☐ In my particular case, does mastectomy offer a better chance to control my cancer?
- ☐ Will my surgery require hospitalization? If so, how long?
- ☐ Am I a candidate for sentinel lymph node biopsy? If so, do you evaluate the removed sentinel lymph node(s) for cancer during surgery or after surgery? If not, how many lymph nodes do you plan to remove?
- ☐ Will I have drain bulbs in my incision after surgery? If so, how many?
- ☐ Will I go home with drains in place?
- ☐ When are drains usually removed?
- ☐ Will I need to have my surgical bandage changed?
- ☐ Will I need to have stitches/sutures removed? When and where will this be done?
- ☐ When should I be able to resume my normal activities?
- ☐ Are there any types of limitations that I should expect in my surgical arm in the future?
- ☐ When can I plan to return to work?

Additional Questions:

_____

_____

Reconstruction Questions

- ☐ Am I a candidate for immediate reconstruction?
- ☐ Can you provide me with information about immediate reconstruction?
- ☐ Can you explain the advantages and disadvantages of immediate reconstruction?
- ☐ Can you provide me with information on the use of implants and the potential use of my body tissues for reconstruction?
- ☐ Do you foresee anything in my present health status which could prevent me from having either type of reconstruction?

Additional Questions:

_____

_____

Final Questions

- ☐ Is there anything else you need to tell me about my cancer or surgery?
- ☐ Do you have any written information on my type of cancer or surgery?
- ☐ Will I be assigned a nurse navigator?
- ☐ Do you recommend a support group or a professional counselor?
- ☐ If I have additional questions, whom should I call and with whom should I speak (nurse/physician)?

Additional Questions:

_____

_____

Tumor Location

Ask your physician to draw where your tumor is located in your breast, and the estimated amount of tissue that will be removed during surgery.

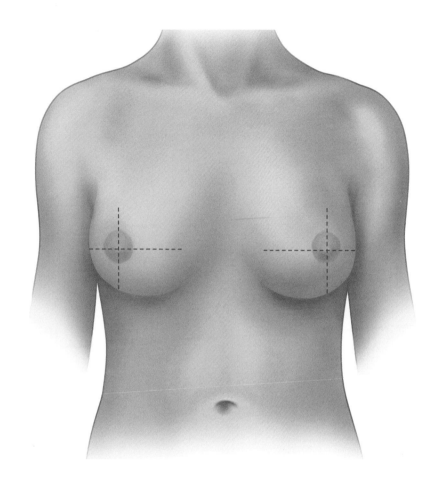

Tumor Size

Ask your physician to draw the estimated size of your tumor on this chart.

Tumor size is the largest dimension of the tumor.

Results are reported in centimeters (cm) or millimeters (mm).

- 10 mm equals 1 cm
- 1 cm equals ⅜ inch
- 1 inch equals 2.5 cm

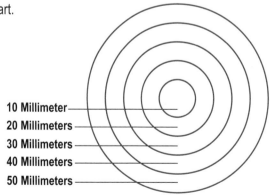

10 Millimeter
20 Millimeters
30 Millimeters
40 Millimeters
50 Millimeters

APPEARANCE AFTER SURGERY

Ask your surgeon to draw in the location of your planned incision(s).

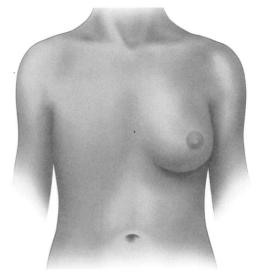

Lumpectomy Scar(s)

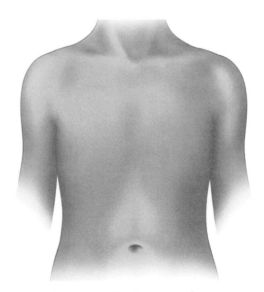

Right Mastectomy Scar

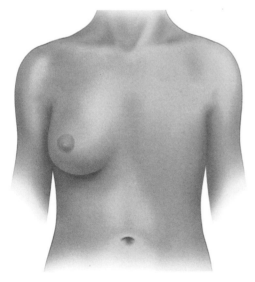

Left Mastectomy Scar

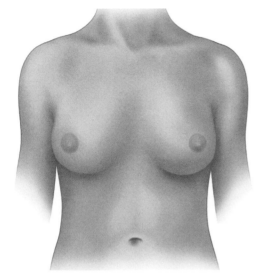

Bilateral Mastectomy Scars

264

If you have been told that you are a candidate for a lumpectomy or a mastectomy, making a decision between the two surgeries is often difficult. This self-questionnaire is designed to help you explore your innermost thoughts and desires about outcomes of the surgical options by choosing between sets of two probing questions that only you can answer. Take this short assessment to help make a decision that agrees with your desired outcomes.

Answer the following questions to help uncover your true feelings. The statements are in pairs. Read both statements before you answer. **Choose only one answer between the two statements that best states how you feel at this time.** You will circle either A or B in the column on the right for each section.

A. I would resent losing my breast. B. I would accept losing my breast.	A B
A. My breasts are very important to how I feel about my self-image. B. My breasts are not that important to how I feel about my self-image.	A B
A. My goal is to preserve my body image (breast), if possible. B. My goal is to reduce my chances of local recurrence (in breast) to the lowest level possible.	A B
A. I don't want to lose my breast and be required to wear a prosthesis or have reconstructive surgery. B. I would prefer to lose my breast to reduce the chance of recurrence to the lowest level.	A B
A. I would not worry about performing a breast self-exam or going for clinical exams on the lumpectomy breast. B. I would worry about recurrence in the remaining breast tissue after lumpectomy.	A B
A. I'm not a worrier; I would see my doctor as needed. B. I would worry about the cancer coming back in my remaining breast tissue.	A B
A. I would prefer to go to radiation therapy five days a week for up to six weeks to save my breast. B. I would rather not have to travel back to the hospital for up to six weeks for radiation therapy.	A B
A. I don't mind going to radiation for up to six weeks to keep my breast. B. I want to get this over. I don't have time to keep going back to the hospital.	A B
A. To keep my breast, I could accept changes after radiation therapy (increased lumpiness, decrease in size). B. I would be anxious about monitoring a breast that had lumpy changes after radiation.	A B
A. Breast changes (lumpiness, change in size) are minor compared to not having my breast. B. It would overwhelm me to feel my breast after having had cancer in it.	A B
A. I feel that my breast is important to my sexuality and self-esteem; without a breast I would feel less sexually attractive to my partner. B. My partner does not care if I have a breast or not; our relationship would not change if I lost my breast.	A B
A. I do not think I would ever feel sexy again without my breast. B. I do think I could feel sexy again without my breast.	A B

Add the number of A's and B's you selected: **Total A's _____   Total B's _____**

The highest number shows your **inclination** to prefer this type of surgical procedure: **A = Lumpectomy   B = Mastectomy**

This is a guide, not the answer, as to your inclination toward surgical options.

If your initial choice is mastectomy, continue with questions about reconstruction on the next page.

Reconstruction or Prosthesis

If your total for mastectomy had the higher number, or if you simply prefer mastectomy, you now need to consider your options for reconstructive surgery. Continue to choose between the two statements in the same manner as the previous page.

A. I would dislike wearing an external prosthesis (breast form) daily. B. I would rather wear an external prosthesis than to have additional surgery.	A B
A. I prefer not to wear a prosthesis because it would be a daily reminder of having lost my breast to cancer. I want my body image to be back to normal as soon as possible. B. I would prefer to avoid additional surgery.	A B
A. I do want to be able to wear low-cut clothing or go braless. B. I do not want to wear low-cut clothing or go braless.	A B
A. I do not want to have to wear a prosthesis to maintain my body image. B. I would rather wear a prosthesis than have more surgery.	A B

Add the number of A's and B's you selected: **Total A's** _____ **Total B's** _____

The highest number shows your **inclination** to prefer: **A = Reconstruction   B = Prosthesis**

Delayed Reconstruction or Immediate Reconstruction

If your total for reconstruction had the higher number, or if you simply prefer reconstruction, you now need to consider your options between immediate and delayed reconstruction. Continue to choose between the two statements in the same manner.

A. I would rather have time to recover from my mastectomy and treatments before I have reconstructive surgery. B. I would rather have all of my surgeries performed at the time of my breast cancer surgery than to have to return after chemotherapy or radiation therapy.	A B
A. Additional surgery is too much to undergo when my anxiety is so high. B. Let's do it all now and get it over with; I don't like putting things off.	A B
A. I want to take my time to find a reconstructive surgeon and study the different types of reconstructive surgery. B. I do not need more time to decide. I understand my reconstructive options and feel comfortable with the recommended reconstructive surgeon.	A B
A. I cannot make a fast decision about reconstructive surgery while I am feeling overwhelmed about my cancer. B. I do not want to wait to have my body image restored.	A B

Add the number of A's and B's you selected: **Total A's** _____ **Total B's** _____

The highest number shows your **inclination** to prefer: **A = Delayed Reconstruction   B = Immediate Reconstruction**

Remember, *your decisions need to be made according to how you feel about the changes your surgical choice would have on you. Each option has advantages and disadvantages to consider. Survival rates are equal. Talking to a variety of healthcare professionals (surgeon, medical oncologist, radiation oncologist, plastic surgeon, nurse) and other women about the surgeries available will help you to arrive at your final conclusion.*

RECONSTRUCTIVE SURGERY QUESTIONS

Check the questions you would like to have answered.
Tear out this sheet and take it to your reconstructive consultation.

Surgeon's Name: _____ **Date:** _____

Questions

☐ Which type of reconstructive surgery do you recommend for me (autologous or implant)?

☐ If autologous (my own body tissues), which type of surgery do you recommend?

☐ If an implant, what kind of implant do you recommend? Will the implant be placed under the muscle?

☐ Will this surgery cause me to have additional scars?

☐ Will my surgery cause any restrictions on future physical activities (employment, sports or ability to exercise)?

☐ How many surgical procedures will my reconstruction require?

☐ Will hospitalization be required for each procedure?

☐ How long will I be in surgery for each of these procedures?

☐ How often will I need a return appointment with you?

☐ How long will it take to complete the reconstruction process?

☐ How long will it be after each procedure before I can return to work or normal activities?

☐ How much will it cost, and how much should my insurance cover?

☐ What are the advantages and disadvantages of the recommended surgery?

☐ What can I expect to look like after surgery?

☐ May I see photographs or talk to some of your patients?

☐ Will you reconstruct my nipple and areola?

☐ How much feeling (sensation) will I have in my reconstructed breast?

☐ How will my breast feel when touched (soft, firm)?

☐ In the future, what problems could potentially occur after reconstructive surgery?

Additional Questions:

_____

_____

_____

_____

_____

_____

_____

_____

_____

Additional Questions / Notes:

Prior to leaving the hospital, your nurse will provide you with verbal and written instructions concerning your care. You will also receive a list of symptoms that might occur and need to be reported to the doctor. During your hospitalization, it may be helpful to write down any questions as they occur. When your doctor makes the final hospital visit, you may want to be prepared to clarify the following. Check the questions you wish to have answered.

Discharge Questions

☐ Ask any questions you have about your diagnosis or surgery that have not been answered yet.

☐ Which activities should I avoid until my next appointment?

☐ Are there any special exercises or recommendations regarding the use of my arm?

☐ Will the numbness, tingling or sensations experienced be temporary or permanent?

☐ What type of pain is normal after my type of surgery?

☐ Will medications be prescribed for pain?

☐ Do I resume previous medications (especially estrogen-type medications)?

☐ When can I shampoo my hair?

☐ When can I shower or take a tub bath?

☐ How do I care for my surgical dressing?

☐ When can I remove my surgical dressing?

☐ When can I drive?

☐ When will my drains (if present) be removed?

☐ When will I have sutures or stitches removed?

☐ Will I be referred to any other doctors or have any other treatments?

☐ If so, when will I see these doctors? Who will make the appointments?

☐ When will my final pathology report be available?

☐ When do I need to make my next appointment?

☐ Is there anything that I can do to ensure a speedy recovery?

Ask your nurse to write down any appointment dates or names of doctors that you will be referred to for further evaluation concerning treatment.

Additional Questions:

_____

_____

_____

_____

_____

_____

_____

_____

_____

SURGICAL DISCHARGE NOTES

Additional Questions / Notes:

DRAIN BULB RECORD

Measure and record drainage of bulb(s) each time you empty a drain.

Take this record to your physician.

Date	Time	Drain 1	Drain 2	Total

DRAIN BULB RECORD

Measure and record drainage of bulb(s) each time you empty a drain.

Take this record to your physician.

Date	Time	Drain 1	Drain 2	Total

MEDICAL ONCOLOGIST QUESTIONS

Your medical oncologist specializes in treatment of cancer using chemotherapy, hormonal therapy and immunotherapy.

Check the questions you would like to have answered. Tear out this sheet and take it to your appointment with the oncologist.

Oncologist's Name: _____ **Date:** _____

My Treatment:

☐ What kind of treatment will I receive (chemotherapy, hormonal, targeted therapy)?

☐ On what schedule will I receive these treatments?

☐ How long will I receive treatments?

☐ How long will each treatment take?

☐ Where will I receive my treatments (office, clinic, hospital)?

☐ Can someone stay with me while I receive my treatments?

☐ Will I feel like driving myself home after my treatment, or will I need a driver?

☐ Will any other tests be needed before or during my chemotherapy?

☐ Will I need radiation therapy?

☐ Do you have written information on my cancer or treatment plans?

My Medications:

☐ What are the names of the drugs?

☐ Are the drugs given by mouth or into a vein?

☐ Will I need a port (device implanted under the skin) to receive I.V. medications, or will you use a vein in my arm?

Preparing for My Treatments:

☐ Should I eat before I come for my treatments?

☐ Can I take vitamins or herbs if I so choose?

During My Treatments:

☐ What side effects will I experience from the treatments (nausea, hair loss, changes in blood cell counts, etc.)?

☐ Will I be given medications to treat the side effects?

☐ What protective skin precautions should I take during chemotherapy (exposure to sunlight)?

☐ After I complete my treatments, how often will I return for checkups?

☐ How will you evaluate the effectiveness of the treatments?

Changes in My Body and Life:

☐ Will I continue to have menstrual periods during treatment? If not, when will they return?

☐ Should I use birth control during treatment? What type do you recommend?

☐ Will I be able to conceive and bear a child after treatment?

☐ What physical changes should I report to you or to your nurse during treatment?

☐ Can I continue my usual work or exercise schedules, or will I need to modify them during treatments?

☐ Are there any precautions that my family should take to limit exposure to the chemotherapy during my treatments (shared eating utensils, bathroom facilities)?

Additional Questions / Notes:

RADIATION ONCOLOGIST QUESTIONS

Check the questions you would like to have answered.

Tear out this sheet and take it to your radiation consultation.

Physician's Name: _____ **Date:** _____

Questions

☐ Which type of radiation will I receive (external beam, accelerated, brachytherapy)?

☐ How many radiation treatments will I receive?

☐ On what schedule will my treatments be given (how many weeks, what days of the week)?

☐ How long will my first visit take to mark the area?

☐ How do you mark the area that will be radiated (permanent or temporary markings)?

☐ What kind of soap and bathing do you recommend during my treatments?

☐ Is there anything that I can not use during my treatment (deodorant, perfume, lotions to the chest or back, etc.)?

☐ Can I wear a bra or my prosthesis during radiation treatments?

☐ What side effects are considered normal during radiation therapy?

☐ Which side effects, if they occur, should I report immediately?

☐ In the future, what changes could potentially occur in the radiated breast?

☐ Do you have written information on breast radiation therapy?

Additional Questions:

_____

_____

_____

_____

_____

_____

_____

_____

_____

_____

_____

_____

_____

_____

_____

_____

Additional Questions / Notes:

_____
_____
_____
_____
_____
_____
_____
_____
_____
_____
_____
_____
_____
_____
_____
_____
_____
_____
_____
_____
_____
_____
_____
_____
_____
_____
_____
_____
_____
_____
_____
_____
_____

PATHOLOGY REPORT QUESTIONS   WORKSHEET

Your pathology report contains the unique characteristics of your breast cancer. Your surgeon or oncologist can answer your questions about your pathology report. Some patients request a copy of their pathology report for their own records.

Listed below are questions you may want to ask about your pathology report. Check the questions you would like to have answered. If you desire to know only the components that impact your treatment decisions, refer to the next page.

Tear out this sheet and take it to your next appointment.

Physician's Name: _____   **Date:** _____

Tumor

What is the name of the type of cancer I have? _____

Was my tumor ☐ In situ (inside ducts or lobules)
　　　　　　　☐ Invasive (growing through the duct or lobule walls into surrounding tissues)?

What size was my tumor? _____

Lymph Nodes

Sentinel lymph node biopsy: How many nodes were removed? _____

Axillary dissection: How many lymph nodes were sampled or removed? _____

Were any nodes positive for cancer cells?　☐ Yes　☐ No

Tumor Markers

Were my estrogen or progesterone receptors positive or negative?　☐ Positive　☐ Negative

Was my tumor positive for HER2?　☐ Yes　☐ No

How fast was my tumor growing (cell proliferation status)? _____

Stage

What stage is my cancer?　☐ Stage 0　☐ Stage 1　☐ Stage 2　☐ Stage 3　☐ Stage 4

Other Things I Need to Know About My Cancer:

_____

_____

_____

_____

_____

_____

_____

_____

_____

The major components that determine your treatment are listed below. Ask your physician to provide the answers to the following characteristics of your cancer.

Tear out this sheet and take it to your next appointment.

Physician's Name: _____ **Date:** _____

Hormone Receptor Status
☐ ER positive (+)   PR positive (+)   ☐ ER negative (-)   PR positive (+)

☐ ER positive (+)   PR negative (-)   ☐ ER negative (-)   PR negative (-)

HER2 Receptor Status
☐ HER2 positive (HER2+)

☐ HER2 negative (HER2-)

Lymph Node Status
☐ Lymph node positive

☐ Lymph node negative

Ask your surgeon to identify the following surgical information:

Stage of My Cancer
☐ Stage 0   ☐ Stage 2   ☐ Stage 4

☐ Stage 1   ☐ Stage 3

Has My Cancer Metastasized?
☐ Yes   ☐ No

If Yes, Where Has My Breast Cancer Metastasized?
☐ Bones   ☐ Liver   ☐ Other: _____

☐ Lungs   ☐ Brain

Additional Questions / Notes:

_____

_____

_____

_____

_____

_____

_____

_____

_____

_____

Surgical arm exercises should be performed on a regular basis—preferably two or more 10 to 15 minute sessions every day. Persistence is the key to regaining complete range of motion. Do the exercises slowly, and hold the position when you get to the end of the range. This helps to strengthen the muscles.

If you have difficulty performing these exercises or feel you are not making progress, tell your surgeon. You may need the assistance of a physical therapist to help you regain your complete range of motion.

*Note: The **surgical arm** is the arm on the side of your surgery. The **non-surgical arm** is the opposite arm.*

Surgical Arm Lifts

- Lift your surgical arm away from your side toward the ceiling with your palm turned forward.
- Raise your arm as high as possible, and hold it there for a few seconds.
- Repeat six times.

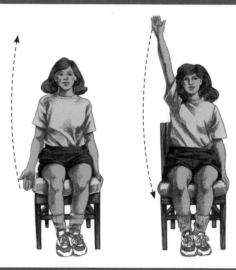

Surgical Arm Raises

- Clench a rubber ball in your surgical hand with your elbow bent.
- Slowly lift your arm toward your head, keeping your elbow away from your body.
- When you reach your head, hold this position for a few seconds.
- Repeat six times.

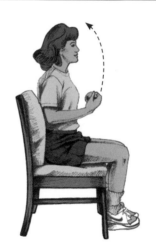
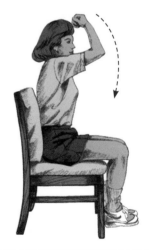

Surgical Arm Reach

- Hold your surgical arm straight beside your body.
- Slowly raise your arm as high as possible over your head while keeping your elbow straight.
- Hold the position for a few seconds.
- Repeat six times.

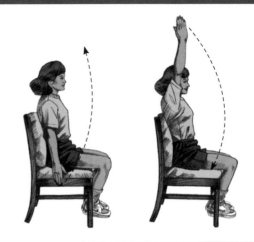

Surgical Arm Swing

- Place your non-surgical arm on a table to support your body.
- Put your surgical arm across your chest, placing your hand on the opposite shoulder.
- Move the surgical arm slowly away from your body until it is extended straight out.
- Keep your arm at shoulder level as you perform the exercise.
- Repeat six times.

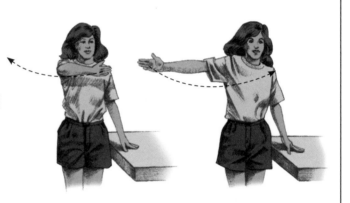

Lateral Range of Motion

- Hold a stick with your surgical hand palm up and your non-surgical arm palm down.
- Push your surgical arm directly out from your side toward the ceiling until you feel a stretch.
- Hold this position for several seconds.
- Repeat six times.

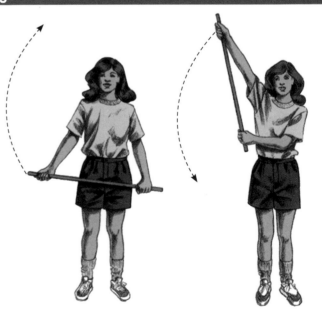

SURGICAL ARM EXERCISES

Surgical Arm Circles

- Lean on a table with your non-surgical arm.
- Move your surgical arm in a circle clockwise and then counter-clockwise.
- Repeat six times.

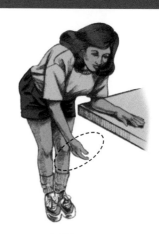

Surgical Arm Swings

- Lean on a table with your non-surgical arm.
- Swing your surgical arm up until you feel a stretch.
- When you feel the stretch, hold the position for a few seconds.
- Repeat six times.

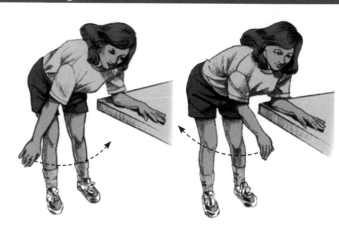

Overhead Range of Motion

- Hold a stick with both hands palm down.
- Without bending your elbows, bring the stick directly over your head, leading with the non-surgical arm.
- Reach back over your head until you feel a stretch.
- Hold the position for a few seconds.
- Repeat six times.

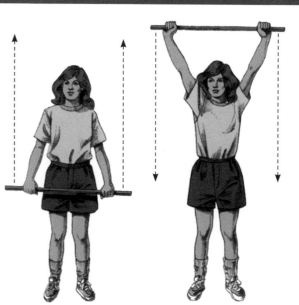

Full Range of Motion

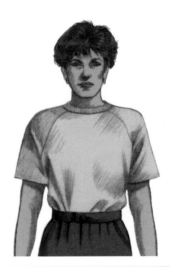
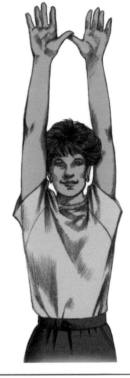

- With both of your arms straight by your side, raise both hands above your head and hold the position for several seconds.

- Repeat six times.

This exercise will be one of the last to be mastered and will be proof that your surgical arm has regained full range of motion.

Personal Healthcare Provider Record

Primary Physician

Name

Telephone

Address

Nurse

Surgeon

Name

Telephone

Address

Nurse

Reconstructive Surgeon

Name

Telephone

Address

Nurse

Oncologist

Name

Telephone

Address

Nurse

Radiation Oncologist

Name

Telephone

Address

Nurse

Breast Health Navigator / Nurse

Name

Telephone

Address

Notes

PERSONAL HEALTHCARE PROVIDER RECORD

Breast Health Center

Name

Telephone

Address

Notes

Hospital

Name

Telephone

Address

Notes

Pharmacy

Name

Telephone

Address

Notes

Social Worker

Name

Telephone

Address

Notes

Support Group

Name

Telephone

Address

Notes

Other

Name

Telephone

Address

Notes

Personal Treatment Record

Name _____ Diagnosis Date _____

Cancer Type _____ Tumor Size _____ Node Status _____

ER/PR Status _____ HER2_____ Oncotype DX® Score _____

Baseline Vital Signs: Blood Pressure _____ Pulse _____ Respirations _____ Weight _____

Allergies _____ Routine Medications _____

Surgery

Surgery Date: _____ Type: _____

Reconstructive Surgery Date: _____ Type: _____

Chemotherapy Treatments

Start Date: _____ End Date: _____

Name of Chemotherapy Drugs: Chemotherapy Treatment Dates:

_____   _____ _____ _____

_____   _____ _____ _____

_____   _____ _____ _____

_____   _____ _____ _____

_____   _____ _____ _____

_____   _____ _____ _____

_____   _____ _____ _____

_____   _____ _____ _____

Radiation Therapy

Start Date: _____ End Date: _____ Type: _____

Hormonal Therapy

Drug Name: _____ Start Date: _____ End Date: _____

Drug Name: _____ Start Date: _____ End Date: _____

Physical Therapy

Range of Motion: _____ Start Date: _____ End Date: _____

Lymphedema Treatment: _____ Start Date: _____ End Date: _____

Other Treatment: _____ Start Date: _____ End Date: _____

Treatment Notes:

_____

_____

_____

_____

_____

_____

_____

_____

_____

_____

_____

_____

_____

_____

_____

_____

_____

_____

_____

_____

_____

_____

_____

_____

_____

_____

_____

_____

_____

_____

_____

_____

_____

_____

_____

_____

_____

PATIENT APPOINTMENT REMINDER

Tear out this worksheet and place it where you can easily write down questions between visits.
Take this sheet with you to your next appointment to remind you of the questions you would like to have answered.

Next Scheduled Appointment

Physician's Name: _____ **Date:** _____

Questions To Ask Physician:

_____

_____

_____

_____

_____

_____

_____

_____

Questions To Ask Nurse:

_____

_____

_____

_____

_____

_____

_____

_____

Remember To Tell Physician/Nurse:

_____

_____

_____

_____

_____

Tear out this worksheet and place it where you can easily write down questions between visits.

Take this sheet with you to your next appointment to remind you of the questions you would like to have answered.

Next Scheduled Appointment

Physician's Name: _____ **Date:** _____

Questions To Ask Physician:

_____

_____

_____

_____

_____

_____

_____

_____

Questions To Ask Nurse:

_____

_____

_____

_____

_____

_____

_____

_____

Remember To Tell Physician/Nurse:

_____

_____

_____

_____

_____

Take the time to plan steps of action in every area of your life for maximum recovery.
Inventory your life and make the adjustments you feel will help you to restore a sense of control.

Support System

Personal:
Identify at least two people you can talk to openly.

_____ Phone: _____

_____ Phone: _____

Information:
Identify sources of correct information on breast cancer. Refer to the resource section of this book.

Physician: _____ Phone: _____

Physician: _____ Phone: _____

Physician: _____ Phone: _____

Nurse: _____ Phone: _____

Organization: _____ Phone: _____

Organization: _____ Phone: _____

Organization: _____ Phone: _____

Other: _____ Phone: _____

Other: _____ Phone: _____

Support:
Identify your local support groups by calling the American Cancer Society.

Breast Cancer Patients: _____ Phone: _____

Support Partner Groups: _____ Phone: _____

Children's Classes: _____ Phone: _____

Other: _____ Phone: _____

Spiritual:
Identify people who can help you deal with the spiritual aspects of your illness.

_____ Phone: _____

_____ Phone: _____

_____ Phone: _____

"Planning is like a road map.

It can show us the way and head us in the right direction and keep us on course.

Planning means mapping out how to get from here to where we want to be.

Planning is the power tool for achievement, the magic bridge to our goals and our success."

—Wynn Davis

☐ **Fears:** Name your fears, and plan steps of action to address them.
Complete the *Managing My Fears* worksheet on page 259.

Fears I need to address: _____

_____

☐ **Diet:** Evaluate your diet.

I plan to make the following changes: _____

_____

☐ **Exercise:** Plan a program of exercise to restore and maintain your physical condition.

I plan to: _____

I will check with my doctor about starting my exercise program on (date): _____

I am starting an exercise program on (date): _____

I am going to ask (person) to join me: _____

☐ **Personal Appearance:** Make plans to enhance your self-esteem and personal appearance during treatment.
If taking chemotherapy, check out a "Look Good...Feel Better" class, sponsored by the American Cancer Society.

I plan to: _____

_____

☐ **Time Management:** Plan to make lifestyle changes (employment, social, civic duties).

I plan to start: _____

I plan to stop: _____

☐ **Family Management:** Make changes in your household.

I need to delegate chores for: _____

I need to hire help for: _____

I need to stop doing: _____

☐ **Personal Fulfillment:** Think of things you want to do more of, or things you want to begin to do. Think selfishly. You deserve it!
Add goals, hobbies or pleasurable events to your life.

I plan to: _____

_____

☐ **Reaching Out:** A spirit of gratefulness and an effort on your part to help others is very rewarding. Plan to say "thank you" to those who play an important part in your life and recovery. Plan to give back to others who are in need.

People to write or to thank: _____

Things I would like to do to help others: _____

Congratulations!
You have just taken steps to plan your psychological and social recovery.
Refer to this sheet when in doubt of what you can do to speed your recovery.

HEALTH SYMPTOMS RECORD WORKSHEET

Your physician needs to know about changes in your health. Use this chart to record any symptoms you have experienced since your last visit. Take this chart with you to your next checkup and give it to your healthcare provider.

Pain Scale: 0=None; 10=Severe

General Symptoms	Frequency	Notes
Fever	□ Never □ Occasional □ Frequent □ Daily	Highest Temperature: _____ °
Fatigue	□ Never □ Occasional □ Frequent □ Daily	
Dizzy	□ Never □ Occasional □ Frequent □ Daily	
Headaches	□ Never □ Occasional □ Frequent □ Daily	Pain Scale (0-10): ____
Hot flashes	□ Never □ Occasional □ Frequent □ Daily	
Night sweats	□ Never □ Occasional □ Frequent □ Daily	
Nervous/Anxious	□ Never □ Occasional □ Frequent □ Daily	Scale (0-10): _____
Depressed	□ Never □ Occasional □ Frequent □ Daily	Scale (0-10): _____
Forgetful	□ Never □ Occasional □ Frequent □ Daily	Scale (0-10): _____
Problems sleeping	□ Never □ Occasional □ Frequent □ Daily	
Poor appetite	□ Never □ Occasional □ Frequent □ Daily	
Vaginal dryness	□ No □ Yes	
Painful intercourse	□ No □ Yes	
Loss of sexual desire	□ No □ Yes	
Vision change	□ No □ Yes	
Weight change	□ No □ Yes	_____ Pounds □ Lost □ Gained
Numbness in extremities	□ No □ Yes	□ Hands □ Feet
Pain	□ No □ Yes	Location: _____; Pain Scale (0-10): ___
Gastrointestinal		
Nausea	□ Never □ Occasional □ Frequent □ Daily	
Vomiting	□ Never □ Occasional □ Frequent □ Daily	
Indigestion	□ Never □ Occasional □ Frequent □ Daily	
Constipation	□ Never □ Occasional □ Frequent □ Daily	
Diarrhea	□ Never □ Occasional □ Frequent □ Daily	
Stomach pain	□ Never □ Occasional □ Frequent □ Daily	
Stomach swelling	□ Never □ Occasional □ Frequent □ Daily	
Blood in stool	□ Never □ Occasional □ Frequent □ Daily	
Problems swallowing	□ Never □ Occasional □ Frequent □ Daily	
Urinary		
Painful/frequent urination	□ Never □ Occasional □ Frequent □ Daily	
Inability to control urine	□ Never □ Occasional □ Frequent □ Daily	
Dark-colored urine	□ Never □ Occasional □ Frequent □ Daily	
Respiratory		
Shortness of breath	□ Never □ Occasional □ Frequent □ Daily	□ At rest □ After activity
Chest pain	□ Never □ Occasional □ Frequent □ Daily	□ At rest □ After activity
Cough	□ Never □ Occasional □ Frequent □ Daily	Phlegm □ No □ Yes
Breast/Chest Wall		
Breast changes	□ Lump □ Discharge □ Rash	
Breast pain	□ Never □ Occasional □ Frequent □ Daily	Location: _____
Overall Health		
Quality of Life	□ Poor □ Acceptable □ Good □ Great	

HEALTH SYMPTOMS RECORD

Your physician needs to know about changes in your health. Use this chart to record any symptoms you have experienced since your last visit. Take this chart with you to your next checkup and give it to your healthcare provider.

Pain Scale: 0=None; 10=Severe

General Symptoms	Frequency	Notes
Fever	□ Never □ Occasional □ Frequent □ Daily	Highest Temperature: _____°
Fatigue	□ Never □ Occasional □ Frequent □ Daily	
Dizzy	□ Never □ Occasional □ Frequent □ Daily	
Headaches	□ Never □ Occasional □ Frequent □ Daily	Pain Scale (0-10): ____
Hot flashes	□ Never □ Occasional □ Frequent □ Daily	
Night sweats	□ Never □ Occasional □ Frequent □ Daily	
Nervous/Anxious	□ Never □ Occasional □ Frequent □ Daily	Scale (0-10): _____
Depressed	□ Never □ Occasional □ Frequent □ Daily	Scale (0-10): _____
Forgetful	□ Never □ Occasional □ Frequent □ Daily	Scale (0-10): _____
Problems sleeping	□ Never □ Occasional □ Frequent □ Daily	
Poor appetite	□ Never □ Occasional □ Frequent □ Daily	
Vaginal dryness	□ No □ Yes	
Painful intercourse	□ No □ Yes	
Loss of sexual desire	□ No □ Yes	
Vision change	□ No □ Yes	
Weight change	□ No □ Yes	_____ Pounds □ Lost □ Gained
Numbness in extremities	□ No □ Yes	□ Hands □ Feet
Pain	□ No □ Yes	Location: _____; Pain Scale (0-10): ___
Gastrointestinal		
Nausea	□ Never □ Occasional □ Frequent □ Daily	
Vomiting	□ Never □ Occasional □ Frequent □ Daily	
Indigestion	□ Never □ Occasional □ Frequent □ Daily	
Constipation	□ Never □ Occasional □ Frequent □ Daily	
Diarrhea	□ Never □ Occasional □ Frequent □ Daily	
Stomach pain	□ Never □ Occasional □ Frequent □ Daily	
Stomach swelling	□ Never □ Occasional □ Frequent □ Daily	
Blood in stool	□ Never □ Occasional □ Frequent □ Daily	
Problems swallowing	□ Never □ Occasional □ Frequent □ Daily	
Urinary		
Painful/frequent urination	□ Never □ Occasional □ Frequent □ Daily	
Inability to control urine	□ Never □ Occasional □ Frequent □ Daily	
Dark-colored urine	□ Never □ Occasional □ Frequent □ Daily	
Respiratory		
Shortness of breath	□ Never □ Occasional □ Frequent □ Daily	□ At rest □ After activity
Chest pain	□ Never □ Occasional □ Frequent □ Daily	□ At rest □ After activity
Cough	□ Never □ Occasional □ Frequent □ Daily	Phlegm □ No □ Yes
Breast/Chest Wall		
Breast changes	□ Lump □ Discharge □ Rash	
Breast pain	□ Never □ Occasional □ Frequent □ Daily	Location: _____
Overall Health		
Quality of Life	□ Poor □ Acceptable □ Good □ Great	

HEALTH SYMPTOMS RECORD WORKSHEET

Your physician needs to know about changes in your health. Use this chart to record any symptoms you have experienced since your last visit. Take this chart with you to your next checkup and give it to your healthcare provider.

Pain Scale: 0=None; 10=Severe

General Symptoms	Frequency	Notes
Fever	□ Never □ Occasional □ Frequent □ Daily	Highest Temperature: _____°
Fatigue	□ Never □ Occasional □ Frequent □ Daily	
Dizzy	□ Never □ Occasional □ Frequent □ Daily	
Headaches	□ Never □ Occasional □ Frequent □ Daily	Pain Scale (0-10): ____
Hot flashes	□ Never □ Occasional □ Frequent □ Daily	
Night sweats	□ Never □ Occasional □ Frequent □ Daily	
Nervous/Anxious	□ Never □ Occasional □ Frequent □ Daily	Scale (0-10): _____
Depressed	□ Never □ Occasional □ Frequent □ Daily	Scale (0-10): _____
Forgetful	□ Never □ Occasional □ Frequent □ Daily	Scale (0-10): _____
Problems sleeping	□ Never □ Occasional □ Frequent □ Daily	
Poor appetite	□ Never □ Occasional □ Frequent □ Daily	
Vaginal dryness	□ No □ Yes	
Painful intercourse	□ No □ Yes	
Loss of sexual desire	□ No □ Yes	
Vision change	□ No □ Yes	
Weight change	□ No □ Yes	_____ Pounds □ Lost □ Gained
Numbness in extremities	□ No □ Yes	□ Hands □ Feet
Pain	□ No □ Yes	Location: _____; Pain Scale (0-10): ___
Gastrointestinal		
Nausea	□ Never □ Occasional □ Frequent □ Daily	
Vomiting	□ Never □ Occasional □ Frequent □ Daily	
Indigestion	□ Never □ Occasional □ Frequent □ Daily	
Constipation	□ Never □ Occasional □ Frequent □ Daily	
Diarrhea	□ Never □ Occasional □ Frequent □ Daily	
Stomach pain	□ Never □ Occasional □ Frequent □ Daily	
Stomach swelling	□ Never □ Occasional □ Frequent □ Daily	
Blood in stool	□ Never □ Occasional □ Frequent □ Daily	
Problems swallowing	□ Never □ Occasional □ Frequent □ Daily	
Urinary		
Painful/frequent urination	□ Never □ Occasional □ Frequent □ Daily	
Inability to control urine	□ Never □ Occasional □ Frequent □ Daily	
Dark-colored urine	□ Never □ Occasional □ Frequent □ Daily	
Respiratory		
Shortness of breath	□ Never □ Occasional □ Frequent □ Daily	□ At rest □ After activity
Chest pain	□ Never □ Occasional □ Frequent □ Daily	□ At rest □ After activity
Cough	□ Never □ Occasional □ Frequent □ Daily	Phlegm □ No □ Yes
Breast/Chest Wall		
Breast changes	□ Lump □ Discharge □ Rash	
Breast pain	□ Never □ Occasional □ Frequent □ Daily	Location: _____
Overall Health		
Quality of Life	□ Poor □ Acceptable □ Good □ Great	

HEALTH SYMPTOMS RECORD

Your physician needs to know about changes in your health. Use this chart to record any symptoms you have experienced since your last visit. Take this chart with you to your next checkup and give it to your healthcare provider.

Pain Scale: 0=None; 10=Severe

General Symptoms	Frequency	Notes
Fever	□ Never □ Occasional □ Frequent □ Daily	Highest Temperature: _____°
Fatigue	□ Never □ Occasional □ Frequent □ Daily	
Dizzy	□ Never □ Occasional □ Frequent □ Daily	
Headaches	□ Never □ Occasional □ Frequent □ Daily	Pain Scale (0-10): ____
Hot flashes	□ Never □ Occasional □ Frequent □ Daily	
Night sweats	□ Never □ Occasional □ Frequent □ Daily	
Nervous/Anxious	□ Never □ Occasional □ Frequent □ Daily	Scale (0-10): _____
Depressed	□ Never □ Occasional □ Frequent □ Daily	Scale (0-10): _____
Forgetful	□ Never □ Occasional □ Frequent □ Daily	Scale (0-10): _____
Problems sleeping	□ Never □ Occasional □ Frequent □ Daily	
Poor appetite	□ Never □ Occasional □ Frequent □ Daily	
Vaginal dryness	□ No □ Yes	
Painful intercourse	□ No □ Yes	
Loss of sexual desire	□ No □ Yes	
Vision change	□ No □ Yes	
Weight change	□ No □ Yes	_____ Pounds □ Lost □ Gained
Numbness in extremities	□ No □ Yes	□ Hands □ Feet
Pain	□ No □ Yes	Location: _____; Pain Scale (0-10): ___
Gastrointestinal		
Nausea	□ Never □ Occasional □ Frequent □ Daily	
Vomiting	□ Never □ Occasional □ Frequent □ Daily	
Indigestion	□ Never □ Occasional □ Frequent □ Daily	
Constipation	□ Never □ Occasional □ Frequent □ Daily	
Diarrhea	□ Never □ Occasional □ Frequent □ Daily	
Stomach pain	□ Never □ Occasional □ Frequent □ Daily	
Stomach swelling	□ Never □ Occasional □ Frequent □ Daily	
Blood in stool	□ Never □ Occasional □ Frequent □ Daily	
Problems swallowing	□ Never □ Occasional □ Frequent □ Daily	
Urinary		
Painful/frequent urination	□ Never □ Occasional □ Frequent □ Daily	
Inability to control urine	□ Never □ Occasional □ Frequent □ Daily	
Dark-colored urine	□ Never □ Occasional □ Frequent □ Daily	
Respiratory		
Shortness of breath	□ Never □ Occasional □ Frequent □ Daily	□ At rest □ After activity
Chest pain	□ Never □ Occasional □ Frequent □ Daily	□ At rest □ After activity
Cough	□ Never □ Occasional □ Frequent □ Daily	Phlegm □ No □ Yes
Breast/Chest Wall		
Breast changes	□ Lump □ Discharge □ Rash	
Breast pain	□ Never □ Occasional □ Frequent □ Daily	Location: _____
Overall Health		
Quality of Life	□ Poor □ Acceptable □ Good □ Great	

SURVIVORSHIP SURVEILLANCE GUIDELINES   WORKSHEET

You have completed your treatment for breast cancer. To monitor your future health, your healthcare team will recommend a follow-up schedule for physician visits and screening tests. It is important to understand when you are to return to your physician for your healthcare checkups. The American Society of Clinical Oncology (ASCO) recommends surveillance guidelines for breast cancer patients after completion of treatment. Your surveillance may be conducted by your oncologist or a primary care physician.

Physician Surveillance Visits

Physicians who will provide follow-up surveillance after cancer treatment:

Medical Oncologist   Name: _____   Phone: _____

Primary Care Physician   Name: _____   Phone: _____

Other: _____

Recommended Physician Visit Schedule:
(Ask a member of your healthcare team to mark the appropriate recommendations.)

1 – 3 years past treatment   ☐ Every 3 months   ☐ Every 4 months   ☐ Every 6 months   ☐ Other:_____

4 – 5 years past treatment   ☐ Every 3 months   ☐ Every 4 months   ☐ Every 6 months   ☐ Yearly

6 years or more past treatment   ☐ Every year   ☐ Other: _____

Returning to your physician for a physical exam and update of your history is the most important thing you can do to protect your future health. It has been proven that a physician's exam and review of your recent physical changes is the number one way that most recurrences are detected. Make the most of this opportunity by preparing to report any changes you have experienced since your last exam. Write down any changes you experience so that you don't forget. Report these changes early in the visit so that your physician will have time to further evaluate the change.

During your physical exam, your doctor will look for any physical changes that relate to your general health and/or any symptoms that may suggest that your cancer has recurred locally or spread to another part of your body (systemic disease). In addition to performing a careful breast exam, your doctor will closely examine your entire chest wall and check for lymph node enlargement in other areas of your body. Your physician will listen to your heart and lungs and check your abdomen, liver, spleen, neck and other areas will be checked for swelling or tenderness. The physician will also check your neurological (nerve) functioning for signs associated with recurrence.

Surveillance Recommendations

Breast Self-Exam   *Refer to Appendix D: Understanding Breast Self-Exam on page 215 for written instructions.*

Mammography   ☐ Every 6 months   ☐ Yearly   ☐ Not needed   ☐ Other: _____

Pelvic Examination   ☐ Yearly   ☐ Every 2 years   ☐ Every 3 - 5 years   ☐ Other: _____

Bone Density Scan   ☐ Yearly   ☐ Every 2 years   ☐ Every 3 - 5 years   ☐ Other: _____

Diagnostic Testing   Diagnostic tests are now recommended for surveillance testing only when you have symptoms that indicate a need. Your physician will order diagnostic tests (MRI, PET, CAT Scan, Chest X-ray, Bone Scan, Ultrasound, etc.) when needed.

Symptoms to Report to Physician: Breast or Chest Wall Changes

☐ Change in size, shape or contour of the lumpectomy breast or non-surgical breast

☐ Nipple discharge that is clear or bloody from the lumpectomy breast or non-surgical breast

☐ Nipple inversion from lumpectomy breast or non-surgical breast

☐ A new lump that may feel like a small pea in lumpectomy breast, non-surgical breast or on chest wall

☐ Thickening in breast tissues or on the chest wall after mastectomy

☐ Changes in the skin: dimpling (pulling in of skin), scaly appearance, orange peel appearance, rash, redness or discoloration on lumpectomy breast, non-surgical breast or chest wall

☐ A lump in the underarm area

Symptoms to Report to Physician: Body or General Health Changes

☐ New lump or thickening in the area above the collarbone

☐ Chronic bone pain or tenderness in an area

☐ Chest pain with shortness of breath

☐ Chronic cough

☐ Persistent abdominal pain or abdominal swelling

☐ Headaches, dizziness, fainting or rapid changes in vision

☐ Increasing fatigue unrelated to treatments

☐ Inability to control urine or bowels

☐ Persistent nausea or loss of appetite

☐ Changes in weight, especially weight loss

Do not hesitate to report any other changes you observe to your physician. The most common way recurrence is discovered is when a patient reports symptoms or changes she has experienced. Don't ignore any change as being unimportant. Instead, let your physician or nurse make the decision to determine if the symptom needs further evaluation. What may seem unimportant to you may be important to your healthcare team.

Thankfulness in My Circumstances

Today is another new day.

I can choose to reflect on the things that I have lost, or I can choose to reflect on the reasons I still have to be thankful.

I am thankful for:

◊ The diagnosis of cancer instead of a fatal heart attack, because I prefer to live.

◊ The alarm clock that jolts me awake in the morning, because it means that I am still alive.

◊ The cold floor under my feet, because I can still get out of bed on my own.

◊ The dirty dishes after breakfast, because my family and I have food to eat.

◊ The mounds of dirty laundry in the basket, because I am surrounded by people I love.

◊ The telephone that doesn't stop ringing, because I have friends who care about how I am doing.

◊ The covering of dust on my furniture, because I can still see.

◊ The lawn that needs mowing and the house that needs painting, because I have a home.

◊ The bills that I drop in the mailbox almost daily, because I still have an income.

◊ The doctor's appointment I have to make this afternoon, because I live in a country where I can receive medical care.

◊ The prosthesis that hugs my chest, because it reminds me that I am a survivor and not a statistic of breast cancer.

◊ The too-thin hair on my head, because there are treatments for my disease.

◊ The clothes that clinch my thighs and hug my waist after my weight gain, because I can still eat.

◊ The parking place I finally located at the top of the medical parking garage, because I can still walk.

◊ The shadow that trails behind me as I walk to the office, because I can be out in the sunshine.

◊ The long wait in the doctor's office, because I am not a hospitalized or homebound patient.

◊ The waiting room conversation complaining about high medical costs, because I live in a country with free speech.

◊ The repetitive blood draws I face, because I am still a candidate for treatment.

◊ The nurse's questions about my health over the past weeks, because I can still remember.

◊ The doctor's cold stethoscope on my chest, because I can still feel.

◊ The news about my blood work, because I can still experience hope.

◊ The insurance paperwork, because I have financial help with my medical bills.

◊ The overwhelming exhaustion I feel as I fall into bed at the end of the day, because it means I have been alive and productive for another day.

◊ The nighttime prayer I whisper, because I have a God who still cares about me.

My blessings may come in disguise, but I cherish every one of them.

— Judy Kneece, RN, OCN

Becoming a Cancer Survivalist

American Heritage Dictionary defines a **Survivalist** as: *"One who has personal survival as a primary goal in the face of difficulty, opposition and especially the threat of a natural catastrophe (death)."* Survivalists take a difficult situation and somehow manage to turn it into a challenge instead of a defeat. Survivalists learn to maximize the positives in their lives and deal with the negatives.

Survivalists are realistic. They accept their cancer diagnosis but refuse to accept it as an automatic death sentence. Rather, they view it as a caution light, warning them to take actions to better manage their health and build an even better quality of life.

Survivalists refuse to adopt the helpless, hopeless victim cliché. They are determined to influence their illness and, consequently, their future. They know that what they do can make a difference.

Survivalists know that coping and emerging from this disease means admitting their physical, mental and spiritual needs. Recovery means more than drugs and surgery. It also means facing the toughest demons—fear, anxiety and depression—and latching onto help when needed.

Survivalists feel responsible for their health. They depend on their physician, not as a dictator, but as a partner in recovery.

Survivalists reach out for valuable support—with partners, family, friends, support groups and healthcare professionals. They seek help without feelings of guilt, shame or inadequacy. They know that this is one of the most precious parts of being human—people helping people.

Survivalists take care of their bodies. They eat what is healthy, exercise regularly, get adequate rest, eliminate smoking, monitor alcohol intake and smile often.

Survivalists pay attention to the mental pollutants that seep into their lives. They identify their sources of stress. They learn how to modify the things they can and accept the things they cannot change.

Survivalists indulge themselves by saying "no" to those things that feel uncomfortable and "yes" to those things that feel good and right. They liberate themselves from stressful or unproductive situations and work to create pleasurable ones.

Survivalists apply their spiritual faith to make sense of suffering and find meaning and purpose in their situation.

Survivalists are grateful. They invest time in identifying their blessings. They share their love and appreciation generously and often with those who have blessed their lives.

Survivalists refuse to carry around the emotional baggage of resentment, anger, bitterness, envy or jealousy. They know that these things can only drag them down as they struggle to recover. Therefore, they abandon the things that make them powerless. They release others from the bondage of their expectations.

Survivalists know that life and death are inevitable and that both are business issues, so they take action. That includes preparing a will, a medical power of attorney, instructions for personal property, end of life directives (living will), and having frank discussions with family members about these decisions.

Survivalists give back to others who are struggling with the same challenges. They encourage, they teach, they support, they provide hope and they share what they have learned. They volunteer to make life better for others. They believe that a shared trial is half a trial and that a shared joy is a double joy.

Survivalists do not postpone happiness. They know that only this minute is guaranteed to anyone. They know that joy is not dependent on circumstances, but on how they view them. Joy is a product of the mind and not circumstances.

— Judy Kneece, RN, OCN